ELIZABETH MASON-WHITEHEAD
ANNETTE MCINTOSH
ANN BRYAN
TOM MASON

Key Concepts in
Nursing

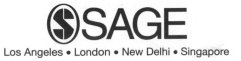

Los Angeles • London • New Delhi • Singapore

Editorial arrangement © Elizabeth Mason-Whitehead, Annette McIntosh, Ann
Bryan and Tom Mason 2008
© SAGE Publications Ltd 2008

First published 2008

SAGE Publications Ltd
1 Oliver's Yard
55 City Road
London EC1Y 1SP

SAGE Publications Inc.
2455 Teller Road
Thousand Oaks, California 91320

SAGE Publications India Pvt Ltd
B 1/I 1 Mohan Cooperative Industrial Area
Mathura Road, New Delhi 110 044

SAGE Publications Asia-Pacific Pte Ltd
33 Pekin Street #02-01
Far East Square
Singapore 048763

Library of Congress Control Number: 2007934799

British Library Cataloguing in Publication data

A catalogue record for this book is available from the
British Library

ISBN 978-1-4129-4614-8
ISBN 978-1-4129-4615-5 (pbk)

Typeset by C&M Digitals (P) Ltd, Chennai, India
Printed and bound in Great Britain by The Cromwell Press Ltd,
Trowbridge, Wiltshire
Printed on paper from sustainable resources

This book came into being with
Alice Poyner
and is dedicated to her.

contents

list of figures

list of tables

list of figures and tables

about the editors and contributors

EDITORS

Bryan, Ann, MSc, Cert.Ed., ADM, RGN, RM, HV, RMT is Head of Community and Child Health in the Faculty of Health and Social Care at the University of Chester.

Mason-Whitehead, Elizabeth, PhD, BA (Hons), HV, PGDE, ONC, SRN, SCM is Reader in Community Studies in the Faculty of Health and Social Care at the University of Chester.

Mason, Tom, PhD, BSc (Hons), RMN, RNMH, RGN is Professor of Mental Health and Learning Disabilities in the Faculty of Health and Social Care at the University of Chester.

McIntosh, Annette, PhD, BSc, Cert. Ed., Dip. CNE, SRN, SCM, RNT, RCNT is Associate Dean, Learning and Teaching, in the Faculty of Health and Social Care at the University of Chester.

CONTRIBUTORS

Astbury, Geoff, MA, Cert. Counselling, RNMH, RCNT is a Senior Lecturer, Learning Disabilities, in the Faculty of Health and Social Care at the University of Chester.

Bailey-McHale, Julie, MSc, BA (Hons), PGDE, PGCert., RMN is a Senior Lecturer, Mental Health, in the Faculty of Health and Social Care at the University of Chester.

Baldwin, Moyra, MMedSci., BSc (Hons), Dip.Adv.Nurs., Dip.Nurs., Cert.Ed., SRN, RCNT, RNT is a Senior Lecturer, Department of Professional Development in Health Care, in the Faculty of Health and Social Care at the University of Chester.

Barber, Paul, MSc, BSc (Hons), Cert. Ed., Dip. Nurs., RMN, SRN is a Senior Lecturer, Adult Nursing, in the Faculty of Health and Social Care at the University of Chester.

Barton, Janet, MA, PGCE, Dip. HE, RGN is a Senior Lecturer, Adult Nursing, in the Faculty of Health and Social Care at the University of Chester.

Bradshaw, Peter, MA, BNurs., RN, RMN, RHV, RNT is Professor of Health Care Policy at the University of Huddersfield.

Byatt, Kay, PhD, MN, Dip. N., RNT, RGN is Principal Lecturer and Divisional Leader of Complementary Medicine in the Department of Nursing at the University of Central Lancashire.

Capper, Carole, MSc, PGCE, RGN is a Senior Lecturer, Department of Professional Development in Health Care, in the Faculty of Health and Social Care at the University of Chester.

Carr, Helen, MEd, BSc (Hons), RN, Public Health Nurse is the Professional Development Lead for Wirral Primary Care Trust.

Cooke, Irene, MSc, BSc (Hons) PGCHE, RGN, RM, DN is a Senior Lecturer, Department of Community and Child Care, in the Faculty of Health and Social Care at the University of Chester.

Cooper, Heather, MSc, Cert Mgmt., RGN is Consultant Nurse, Critical Care, at East Cheshire Trust, Macclesfield District General Hospital.

Donovan, Tom, MPhil., BA(Hons), DN Cert., RN, RMN, RNT, PWT is a Lecturer in the Department of Health Sciences at the University of Liverpool.

Dulson, Julie, BSc (Hons), Dip. Nurs., RMN is a Senior Lecturer, Mental Health, in the Faculty of Health and Social Care at the University of Chester.

Edwards, Margaret, PhD, MSc, BA(Hons), PGCE, DN Cert., RN, RM, RHV is Head of Graduate Studies (taught programmes) at the Florence Nightingale School of Nursing and Midwifery, King's College London.

Flynn, Sandra, MSc, BA (Hons), RGN, ONC, DPSN is a Clinical Nurse Specialist in Orthopaedics at the Countess of Chester NHS Trust.

Gee, Alan, BA (Hons), PGCE, RGN is a Senior Lecturer, Adult Nursing, in the Faculty of Health and Social Care at the University of Chester.

Gidman, Jauice, MEd, BSc (Hons), PGCE, ONC, RN is Head of Department of Practice Learning, Development and Allied Health Care in the Faculty of Health and Social Care at the University of Chester.

Heyman, Bob, PhD, BA (Hons) is Professor of Health Research and Associate Dean for Research, St. Bartholomew School of Nursing & Midwifery at the City University, London.

Hinman, Peter, BSc (Hons), DipHE, RN is a Senior Lecturer, Adult Nursing, in the Faculty of Health and Social Care at the University of Chester.

Hobden, Alison, MSc, PGCAP, BN (Hons), RN, DN is a Lecturer in Nursing at the University of Liverpool.

Hosker, Neil, MSc, BA (Hons) RMN is a Senior Lecturer and e-learning co-ordinator in the Faculty of Health and Social Care at the University of Chester.

Keen, Adam, MSc, MEd, DipHE, RN is a Senior Lecturer, Adult Nursing, in the Faculty of Health and Social Care at the University of Chester.

Lovell, Andy, PhD, BA (Hons), Cert Ed., RNLD is a Reader in Learning Disabilities in the Faculty of Health and Social Care at the University of Chester.

Malone, Mary, MSc, BA (Hons), PGDip. (HV), PGDip. (teaching), RN, RM is the Programme Leader for Specialist Community Public Health Nursing in the Florence Nightingale School of Nursing and Midwifery at King's College London.

Mannix, Jean, BSc (Hons), SCPHN, RN, HV is Deputy Head of Community and Child Health in the Faculty of Health and Social Care at the University of Chester.

McAndrew, Sue, MSc, BSc (Hons), CPN, RMN is a Nurse Lecturer, Mental Health, in the School of Healthcare at the University of Leeds.

McCarthy, Jill, MSc, MA, BEd (Hons), RGN, DN, RNT is a Senior Lecturer, Department of Professional Development in Health Care, in the Faculty of Health and Social Care at the University of Chester.

McLaughlin, Andrea, MEd, Cert. Ed., RGN, RM, ADM is Head of Midwifery and Reproductive Health in the Faculty of Health and Social Care at the University of Chester.

Meredith, Linda, MSc, BSc, Dip. Counselling Skills, RGN, RNT is Associate Dean, Business Support, CIT and Learning Resources, in the Faculty of Health and Social Care at the University of Chester.

Phillips, Sue, MSc, BA (Hons), RGN, RHV is a Senior Lecturer and AP(E)L Co-ordinator in the Faculty of Health and Social Care at the University of Chester.

Phipps, Dianne, MA, PGCE, RNMH is Deputy Head, Department of Mental Health and Learning Disabilities, in the Faculty of Health and Social Care at the University of Chester.

Pierce-Hayes, Ian, BSc (Hons), Dip.HE, RGN is a Lecturer-Practitioner, Adult Nursing, in the Faculty of Health and Social Care at the University of Chester.

Quigley, Jane, MSc, PGDE, RGN, DN is a Senior Lecturer, Practice Learning, in the Faculty of Health and Social Care at the University of Chester.

Ridgway, Victoria, MA, BSc (Hons), PGDE, RN is a Senior Lecturer, Adult Nursing, in the Faculty of Health and Social Care at the University of Chester.

Rose, Pat, MSc, BSc, DipN., CertEd., RN, RHV is a Senior Lecturer, Practice Learning and Child Health, in the Faculty of Health and Social Care at the University of Chester.

Struthers, John, MN, BSc (Hons), DipN., Cert.Ed., RMN, RNT is Nurse Education Manager in the DHSS Education and Training Centre, Isle of Man.

Templeman, Jenni, BSc, Dip.ICN, RN, RM is Critical Care Practice Development Facilitator at East Cheshire Trust, Macclesfield District General Hospital.

Thomas, Mike, PhD, MA, BNurs., CertEd., RMN, RNT is Professor of Mental Health and Dean of the Faculty of Health and Social Care at the University of Chester.

Thompson, Cathy, MSc, ADM, PGCEA, DipNurs., SRN, SCM is Directorate Manager of Learning and Development at Wirral Hospital NHS Trust.

Warne, Tony, PhD, MA, MBA, BNurs., RN, RMN, RNT, JP is a Professor of Mental Health Care at the University of Salford.

Watts, Geoff, MEd, DipAd.Nurs., Dip.Nurs., CertEd, RCNT, RNT is a Senior Lecturer, Department of Professional Development in Health Care, in the Faculty of Health and Social Care at the University of Chester.

Waugh, Anne, MSc, BSc(Hons), CertEd., SRN, RNT is a Senior Lecturer in the School of Nursing, Midwifery and Social Care, Faculty of Health, Life and Social Sciences at Napier University.

While, Alison, PhD, MSc, BSc, CertEd., RGN, RHV is a Professor of Community Nursing at King's College London.

Wilkins, Maureen, MEd, RGN, RCNT, RNT is Head of Professional Development in Health Care in the Faculty of Health and Social Care at the University of Chester.

Wilson, Frances, MSc, PGDE, BSc, CPTC, RGN, RM, RHV is a Senior Lecturer, Department of Community and Child Health, in the Faculty of Health and Social Care at the University of Chester.

Woodhouse, Jan, MEd, BN(Hons) DipN., PGDE, RGN, OND, FETC is a Senior Lecturer, Department of Professional Development in Health Care, in the Faculty of Health and Social Care at the University of Chester.

preface

Nursing, like many other professions, has evolved at an alarming rate over the previous two decades. This is due to a number of factors including the move towards evidence-based practice, the advancements in technology, the growth in literature and the development of nursing as a profession. The move towards evidence-based practice has emerged from the advancements in technology and the growth in literature. There has been a focus on the need to provide evidence for the delivery of patient care rather than a traditional reliance on anecdotal, mythical or 'expert' opinion. We now face the future of delivering patient care that is underpinned by sound research and the logic of Western science. This has led to an expansion in nursing research, from both qualitative and quantitative paradigms, employing numerous methods, including multi-method approaches. This, in turn, has led to a different focus on nursing concepts and has changed, and continues to change, how we approach patient care. A glance at the key concepts list in the contents page of this book testifies to this changing focus, not only by clear key concepts relating to research and evidence-based practice but also in relation to how they affect other key concepts such as caring, nurturing and pain, for example. We can see no reason to anticipate a change in this focus in the foreseeable future.

Technological advances have paved the way for the expansion of computers in the field of healthcare and most students and qualified nurses will be familiar with the basics of information technology. The reliance on technology is apparent throughout nursing and is used to hold vast amounts of patient data and staff information as well as records relating to the general functioning of hospitals and wards. Related to this advancement in computers is the development in other equipment associated with patient care such as the systems of monitoring bodily functions, that is electrocardiography, temperature, pulse, respiration and so on. This technological advance has meant that nurses today must be able to use the basic systems related to data management and, again, a glance at the list of key concepts in this book will testify to this need.

With the advancements in technology there has also been a huge growth in the literature pertaining to nursing and its related disciplines. The number of journals now available on the market to hold relevant information for the nursing profession is expansive, and the number of databases used to hold these references are growing. Students, researchers and professionals keeping abreast of developments will be familiar with the amount of information that is available to us. Furthermore, this is growing weekly, with no sign of a slowing in the production of knowledge; in fact, if anything, it appears to continue to be a growth industry. Systems are constantly being developed to manage the amount of information, and databases grow in accordance with this. Literature reviews, systematic reviews and meta-analyses have been developed to manage this growth in the literature and also includes such approaches as taken in this book. Here fifty key concepts in nursing are concisely constructed and located within one volume to aid the reader to understand the basic constructs and indicate how they can be expanded upon.

The development of nursing as a profession is a global enterprise and one that is at differing stages around the world. In Western healthcare countries, nursing enjoys some degree of social status with varying levels of professional standing. Working with professional organisations and in tandem with national bodies, we note the increase in standards, benchmarks and service frameworks that govern nursing practice. These inevitably lead to pressures and practical conflicts with the demands on everyday working, and these can influence the key concepts within nursing. There can be little doubt that the National Health Service has come under intense scrutiny over recent decades, with intonations of funding restrictions, limited resources and increased working demands on staff. Key concepts emerge out of this tension and can be seen in such chapters as leadership, manager and managing change in this book. Thus, key concepts in nursing will evolve alongside the developments in healthcare professions.

This book will introduce the new student to the major key concepts in nursing and will also provide a linkage into other relevant key concepts as building blocks to a fuller understanding of the overall framework of nursing in contemporary times. It will also inform the reader where to look for exploration into a more detailed appreciation of the issues relating to the key concepts. We hope that this book will help the confused nurse who may be reeling with the abundance of issues surrounding modern-day healthcare delivery. Finally, we envisage that this book may also be of use to lecturers, mentors and clinical supervisors as an access point to the key concepts in nursing and the issues involved in employing them in practice.

Elizabeth Mason-Whitehead, Annette McIntosh, Ann Bryan and Tom Mason
Chester, UK
June 2007

acknowledgements

We have many to thank in the production of this book and none more important than all those who contributed as authors. However, we would also like to give special thanks to Olivia Guinan, who supported us with an outstanding administrative framework, and to Alison Poyner, Zoë Elliott-Fawcett, Anna Luker and all those at SAGE for their guidance, patience and encouragement.

acknowledgements

Introduction

Elizabeth Mason-Whitehead, Annette McIntosh, Ann Bryan and Tom Mason

The delivery of healthcare in modern settings relies upon a wide and diverse number of professionals who are required to work together in a unified team in order to function at the highest level resulting in the delivery of top quality patient care. This focus is dependent on many supporting personnel from diverse groups whose role in this healthcare may not be direct, but nonetheless is important. Whilst there will always be specific knowledge, terminology and areas of expertise within all groups there is also often a great deal of overlap which provides grounding for effective communication. Nursing, like the other professions, has developed considerably over the past two centuries but the speed of change over the previous two decades has far outpaced preceding periods of advancement. This has largely been due to technological advancements, an emphasis on the production of evidence and the prominence of managerialism (with all that it entails). Thus, nursing is a fast-changing and dynamic profession that deals with a wealth of theories, models, hypotheses, views and beliefs, not only from within its own branch of healthcare but also from many others with whom they closely work. Therefore, it is vitally important that modern-day nurses not only keep abreast of these numerous concepts but also further develop their knowledge in these areas. This book brings together the top fifty *Key Concepts in Nursing* in an attempt to outline their basic framework, for both newcomers to nursing and those who wish to keep abreast of the developments in our profession.

CONCEPTS

Human development involves the use of language, which is understood as a system of communication based on rules that allow for the use of various combinations of symbols. One of the most important symbols in language is the term 'concept'. Concepts can be understood as abstractions representing the reality of objects, properties of objects or particular phenomena. Thus, we can see that concepts become part of a particular group's framework of communication, known as their language, or sometimes as 'jargon'. They become known for their ability to formulate ideas within that group that employs a particular concept. For example, physicists use concepts such as 'black holes' and 'worm holes' in their language to produce known (to them) ideas about the universe. Thus, for physicists, these concepts are generalisable to other physicists. They are also not static but dynamic as the ideas involved in a concept grow, change, alter and develop in certain ways. Therefore, they may equally serve to create ambiguity and vagueness, and require constant refinement. This book attempts to dispel such uncertainty and bring, at least temporarily, a degree of clarity.

Concepts have a number of functions:

- Foundation stones of communication and thought – concepts transmit perceptions and information.
- Ways of perceiving empirical phenomena – concepts allow aspects of reality to have a common understanding.
- Means of classification and generalisation – concepts allow us to order, structure and categorise experiences and observations.
- Building blocks of theories, explanations and predictions – concepts are the critical components to larger-scale theories and need to be logically interrelated to be convincing.

This book is about nursing concepts as employed in modern-day health-care settings and which are part of our everyday professional language, much of which we share with our professional colleagues. They require careful consideration in order for them to produce the above functions, and will change over time as healthcare develops.

APPLICATION TO PRACTICE

An important element of the book is the grounding of the concepts within practice. It has to be stressed that key concepts are not purely theoretical constructs but are firmly embedded in, and driven by, practice. Nursing, as a practice-based profession, has long been required to demonstrate the application of theory to client care. Much has been written about the perceived theory-practice gap in nursing; this book aims to explicitly demonstrate this application of theory through the use of case studies. The book examines the application of evidence and theories at different levels: macro, meso and micro. The macro level incorporates aspects such as political and organisational agendas and imperatives, while the meso level involves communities, groups and unit level organisation. The micro level addresses patient and client care alongside personal and professional elements essential to the individual.

Throughout this book, due emphasis is placed on weaving together the theoretical and practical elements of each concept, thus demonstrating the evidence base, values and drivers underpinning the nursing profession of today.

Nursing is an expansive profession which draws upon a range of disciplines such as public health, sociology and pharmacology, to name but a few. For students who are new to nursing, this multitude of concepts can appear to be a complex web, which is difficult to navigate. Although these anxieties are understandable, students can take comfort in the knowledge that nursing, like nature, has its own order, patterns and logical connections (perhaps not always apparent). The chapters in this book provide the reader with sufficient connections to execute a number of tasks depending upon what the objectives are.

The levels at which you utilise this book are dependent upon your own stage of study and what your task will be, whether it be preparing for an exam, assignment or for your own professional interest. The fifty key concepts in nursing are arranged in alphabetical order. Each concept can be cross-referenced to others to provide further linkages in the conceptual framework of nursing. Thus, the book can be used in two inter-related ways: first, laterally across the key concepts as cross-references and, second, hierarchically to provide a leverage into establishing depth to a particular topic (see Figure 1).

Below are some practical examples of how you may use this book. We have used the key concept of inequalities in health to illustrate how you may achieve this:

Example A   You are required to write or discuss an overview of health inequalities. For this task the chapter on 'Inequalities in health' will be sufficient in providing you with a definition, key words and case history.

Example B   You are asked to discuss health inequalities within the broad context of nursing theory and practice. For this example we suggest you refer to the chapter on 'Inequalities in health' and also use the cross-reference concepts. This will give you a detailed framework of analysis for your discussion of health inequalities within the context of nursing.

Example C   Engaging with critical analysis of health inequalities. It is most likely you will not be expected to engage with critical analysis

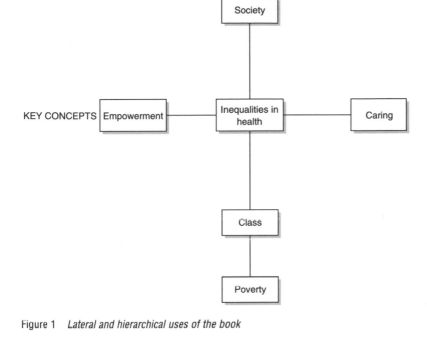

Figure 1 *Lateral and hierarchical uses of the book*

until you have progressed a considerable way into your nursing programme. However, when you arrive at this level of study, we suggest you incorporate the further reading sections of the chapters to examples A and B. Extending your reading and reviews of the related literature is an important component of any assignment requiring critical analysis.

Indeed, you may decide to read this book from beginning to end, and that will give you an overview of all the key concepts. You will also observe the varying perspectives, writing styles and interesting case studies from a wide range of academic and clinical nurses who are known for having made, and continue to make, an important contribution to the profession that they and you have chosen.

Key Concepts in Nursing

1 Accountability

Mike Thomas

DEFINITION

Accountability has two different areas of applicability and has two different definitions. In a narrow sense accountability is used in reference to financial and commercial transactions. It involves responsibility for recording and processing the balance of money so that the accounts can be scrutinised by others in authority (that is, auditing processes). A second wider definition has more relevance for healthcare workers. This describes accountability as that which is applied to a person having responsibility for certain activities and who has to provide rationales for these activities to those in authority so that both the actions and the reasons behind them can be judged. This concept of accountability is intrinsically related to responsibility and authority (the use of power). The application of authority and power can be seen in professional autonomy. This refers to the accountability and responsibility taken in certain situations where decisions for oneself or the actions of others are taken without direct supervision. The senior secular authority to which nurses are accountable is the law.

Accountability is a legal duty. This confers certain obligations and duties on the practitioner which empowers decision making and the improvement of care for patients. It also provides constraints on the abuse of power and authority through the process of legal proceedings. The system of healthcare law in the United Kingdom confers the responsibility and authority for ensuring nurses comply with law to the Nursing and Midwifery Council (NMC). The Council has responsibility to protect the public. It monitors the compliance with its *Code of Professional Conduct* which came into force on 1 June 2002 (NMC, 2002).

The NMC code stipulates that there is a public expectation of the level of conduct which is required to be demonstrated in the practice setting. This is viewed as 'professional' accountability. Of equal value is the expectation that nurses and midwives actively protect the interests

accountability

9

and dignity of their patients and clients. This is the practitioner's 'personal' accountability. The nurse is answerable to the NMC in these areas. In turn the NMC is accountable to Parliament and the public.

KEY POINTS

- Accountability for nurses means that one is responsible to others for one's own actions and decisions (and in certain situations the actions of others).
- Accountability is intrinsically linked to responsibility and authority.
- There are professional, statutory and regulatory guidance on accountability in professional nursing and midwifery.
- Accountability can have applicability in different environments and circumstances.
- Related concepts are responsibility, authority, power and trust.

DISCUSSION

Being accountable for professional conduct is a requirement for all NMC registered practitioners. But accountability covers a wide range of different situations and can answer to a number of different statutory requirements. Pragmatically and in general terms accountability can be more easily presented in three different sections: personal accountability, professional accountability and public accountability.

Personal accountability

Personal accountability is related to issues of care, ethics, conscience and trust. The NMC code specifies the need for nurses to respect the dignity and interests of patients and clients. Within this section the code already covers the legal requirements under the European Union Equal Treatment Framework Directive. This requires all member states to extend their current discriminatory laws to include sexual orientation, religion or beliefs (including political beliefs), disability and age. The United Kingdom has combined the work of its three equality commissions and operates under a diversification agenda to meet the Equal Treatment Framework Directive.

The NMC code also covers the caring relationship, the information and advice regarding access to healthcare resources and the support and guidance on action to be taken in response to any conscientious objections to practice held by the nurse. Personal issues of conscience cannot override the care of others. There is a clear responsibility on the nurse to report issues of conscience to a person of authority as soon as possible and to continue to provide care until alternative arrangements are in place.

As well as personal ethics, personal accountability centres on the degree of trust that can be achieved in the nurse–patient relationship. Robinson (2001) discussed the importance of these relations in a moral context by professing that the psychological relationship between the carer and cared for can empower the client to make positive changes. This does not only mean changes to personal lifestyles but also positive changes to the system of care itself.

The accountable nurse has a duty to come to terms with their own understanding of the moral complexities of practice and to place this understanding in context. Furthermore, the level of insight has to be demonstrated in favour of the client or patient. The use of interpersonal skills is paramount to an effective nurse–patient relationship. The nurse communicates in order that the level of understanding of given information can be assessed; to determine the medium for providing knowledge and to establish the parameters of confidence in the care given and the confidentiality of information revealed. In essence, in its totality, communication can build rapport and trust so that there is some equality in the caring relationship.

Professional accountability

Professional accountability does not operate separately to personal accountability and whilst inherently an aspect of the nurses' own understanding of their part in care, it can be presented as a different type of accountability. In this area there is a more explicit applicability to the demonstration of practice and competence which is clearer than that contained in the complexity of conscience. Caulfield (2002) suggested professional accountability consists of the contract of employment, clinical law and regulatory guidance (personal ethics is also included).

The contract of employment is a legal document and stipulates the nature of responsibility and accountability for each employee. It also includes the constraints and flexibility for the application of authority and control for the post. This allows the employer to exercise their own accountability for public liability, health and safety issues and issues such as wages, benefits and entitlements. Clinical law applies to certain practices which seek to protect the interest of the patient.

Both contractual and clinical law provide a framework for the implementation of relevant national laws such as the Human Rights Act (HMSO, 1988); Freedom of Information Act (The Stationery Office, 2005) and the Data Protection Act (HMSO, 1998). Supporting such legislation are guidance and codes related to protection for 'whistle blowing', the requirements for good record keeping, confidentiality and access to health data and information.

The nurse is always accountable for the currency of their practice and the NMC code urges the practitioner to be aware of the limits of their competence and not carry out any activities which could not be supported demonstrably by knowledge and expertise. The other side of the coin is that the nurse is also accountable if she/he does not do something which would benefit the patient when they could clearly do so (an act of omission).

Public accountability

Public accountability is related to the public perception of the profession's trustworthiness. The actions of the individual nurse, therefore, obviously play a part. For example, the NMC forbids nurses to use their registration status to promote commercial products or services, or to accept any inducements or gifts to promote commercial services. Furthermore, nurses should be wary of using their qualifications to support products or services if the patient or client perceives such support as endorsement. Nurses cannot accept any gifts or favours in any form which could be perceived as inducement for favouritism or preferential treatment and must not ask for, or accept, loans from clients, their relations or friends.

This preoccupation with public trust reached its peak in the early 1990s when the Cadbury Report (HMSO, 1992) provided recommendations for Public Institutions and the selection of Board members, their terms of office, the disclosure of remunerations and the separation of the roles of Chair and Chief Executives. This was followed in 1994 by the Codes of Conduct and Accountability for NHS staff (HMSO, 1994), which highlighted the need to uphold public service values and also implemented the Cadbury recommendations. The Nolan Report (HMSO, 1995) provided further impetus and suggested there should be even more transparency in appointments and for a declaration of interest to be recorded and made public and appointments to be made on merit. The NMC code incorporates these recommendations and they are now deeply embedded in the profession's maintenance of public accountability.

Public accountability also covers research. This is broadly applied in the beneficence ethics of research (do no harm) and in the methodological approach and dissemination of data. Nurses active in research are expected to adhere to research guidelines and are accountable for their activities within research policies and regulatory requirements. This area of accountability also covers registered nurse academics and the organisations in which they practice their research and scholarly activities.

CASE STUDY

Julie, a district nurse with 17 years' experience, found herself working in a new community team following a local reorganisation. Julie experienced a degree of anxiety about the regularity checks on the home visit records which were carried out by the team leader. Her anxiety was based on the fact that she was unsure about the new assessments to be carried out on initial visits (both in the format to be used and the clinical skills to be applied) and that her seniority based on experience would be undermined in public. This was made worse by a colleague, Cathy, who had recently completed her District Nurse programme and seemed to take every opportunity to demonstrate her knowledge of new policies and local initiatives. Their working relations became increasingly strained and culminated in the involvement of the team manager, who called Julie and Cathy to a meeting. Julie was dismayed to hear Cathy outline her lack of confidence in Julie's record keeping and her view that Julie was a high risk to become a future legal case by a patient. Cathy expressed her anger at the lack of continuity of care because other team members did not know which assessment Julie had carried out.

Julie retorted that Cathy was not in a position to question her practice, was too inexperienced to understand, and had been undermining her role with team members because she lacked interpersonal skills. Julie then broke down in tears and revealed her anxiety to her manager. The manager pointed out to both that they were personally accountable under the NMC Code of Practice to co-operate with others in the team, and that Julie was professionally accountable to maintain her professional knowledge and competence and to identify and minimise risk to patients and clients. Her manager identified a development need and provided funds for Julie to attend a local Trust update course.

Both Julie and Cathy were accountable under their contract of employment to maintain good records of care. Julie had failed in her

accountability

13

responsibility to inform her manager of her development needs and was therefore derelict in her professional duty. Cathy was correct in bringing this issue to the attention of her manager despite her apparent lack of good communication skills.

CONCLUSION

A professional nurse or midwife is accountable for their actions at all times. Accountability occurs in different situations and can have simultaneous responsibilities to different authorities. The nurse is accountable for her or his own decisions, often without direct supervision and so is answerable to the patient/client, employer, regulatory legal guidelines and statutory bodies. Accountability is therefore not confined to a line manager and there is no situation wherein the nurse can abdicate their professional or personal responsibilities.

FURTHER READING

Gomm, R. (2004) *Social Research Methodology – A Critical Introduction*. Hampshire: Palgrave Macmillan.

Tadd, W. (2004) *Ethical and Professional Issues in Nursing – Perspectives from Europe*. Hampshire: Palgrave Macmillan.

Taylor, S. and Astra, E. (2006) *Employment Law – An Introduction*. Oxford: Oxford University Press.

REFERENCES

Caulfield, H. (2002) 'Law: issues for nursing practice', in J. Daly, S. Speedy, D. Jackson and P. Derbyshire (eds), *Contexts of Nursing – An Introduction*. Oxford: Blackwell.

HMSO (1988) *Human Rights Act*. London: HMSO.

HMSO (1992) *The Committee on the Financial Aspects of Corporate Governance – The Cadbury Report*. London: HMSO.

HMSO (1994) *Codes of Conduct and Accountability for NHS Staff*. London: HMSO.

HMSO (1995) *The Committee on Standards in Public Life – The Nolan Report*. London: HMSO.

HMSO (1998) *Data Protection Act*. London: HMSO.

Nursing and Midwifery Council (2002) *Code of Professional Conduct*. London: NMC.

Robinson, S.J. (2001) *Agape – Moral Meaning and Pastoral Counselling*. Cardiff: Aureus.

The Stationery Office (2005) *Freedom of Information Act*. London: HMSO.

Cross-References *Autonomy, Clinical governance, Competence, Empowerment, Evidence-based practice, Manager, Professional development, Record keeping.*

2 Advocacy

Moyra A. Baldwin

DEFINITION

Advocacy is an umbrella term for acting on behalf of another (Kohnke, 1982; Tschudin, 2003) by supporting and pleading that person's cause. The numerous definitions and explanations of advocacy in the nursing literature range from counsellor, 'watchdog' and representative (Abrams, 1978) to potential whistle-blower (Andersen, 1990). Copp (1986) claimed that advocacy is more than speaking for another. Advocacy involves intervening for 'vulnerable' people who require it. In similar vein Teasdale (1998), explaining that advocacy in healthcare is about power, stated that it involves intervening on behalf of the powerless by manipulating those who have power. In these terms Donahue (1978) reminds us that advocacy has existed as long as there has been a need for the powerless to be championed.

Advocacy is about making it possible for patients to exercise their right to freedom and self-determination (Gadow, 1980; Baldwin, 1994; Baldwin, 2003). A dictionary definition claims advocacy involves expressing active support for another (http://dictionary.cambridge.org). This notion of offering support is also evident in the Nursing & Midwifery Council's (NMC) (2006) advice as it recognises that patients may not have support from family or friends. In providing support the advocate helps people to express what they want and helps to secure their rights. The role of the nurse therefore is to advocate and to represent patients' interests. In today's health service where there is a requirement to provide a patient-led service (DoH, 2006), advocacy may be considered a necessary way of ensuring people's voices are heard.

advocacy

15

KEY POINTS

- Advocacy is an aspect of a therapeutic nurse–patient relationship.
- Advocacy is about promoting and protecting patients' autonomy.
- Advocacy is acting as an intermediary.
- Advocacy has a role to play in a modern patient-led service.

DISCUSSION

Advocacy has a long history of being explored in nursing literature (Corcoran, 1988; Mallik, 1997a; Mallik and Rafferty, 2000; Hewitt, 2002). Much of this work is USA based, although the UK contribution to the literature is expanding (see Mallik and Rafferty's (2000), bibliometric analysis). Advocacy first appeared in the curriculum of UK nurse education with Project 2000 (UKCC, 1988) and was followed by the publication of the *Code of Professional Conduct* (UKCC, 1992), which encouraged nurses to accept responsibility for advocacy when exercising accountability. The body of literature relating to advocacy suggests that there are numerous interpretations of the concept, each having potential to influence the way in which advocacy is practised. Mallik and Rafferty (2000), examining how advocacy has been disseminated, concluded that patient advocacy remains a risky activity but continues to have potential as new roles develop in nursing. While recognising that advocacy is a component of nursing, the nurse who acts as the patient's advocate faces both risks and rewards (Kohnke, 1982). Some express reservations about whether advocacy and nursing are, indeed, compatible (Allmark and Klarzynski, 1992; Copp, 1986; Mitchell and Bournes, 2000). This chapter will examine (a) advocacy as essential nursing practice, and (b) its implications for practice.

Advocacy as essential nursing practice

Healthcare reforms (DoH, 2006) are about making services responsive to patients' needs and preferences. This means putting people in control, and will require professionals to be in a position to empower them so that their voices are heard. As members of the healthcare team, nurses have a role to play in advocating for patients. A model of advocacy will be explored to demonstrate advocacy as essential nursing practice.

Characteristics of advocacy From a concept analysis Baldwin (1994, 2003) revealed that advocacy has three essential characteristics, summarised as valuing, apprising and interceding:

- Valuing encompasses a therapeutic nurse–patient relationship in which patients' freedom and self-determination may be secured.
- Apprising promotes and protects patients' rights to be involved in decision making and informed consent.

- Interceding involves acting as an intermediary between patients and their family or significant others, also between them and healthcare providers.

Valuing   The advocate is one who maintains the person's sense of individuality and humanity. These qualities have been identified by Gadow (1980) and Curtin (1979). They express valuing as 'the nurse being ideally placed to experience the patient as a unique human being with individual strengths and complexities ...' (Gadow, 1980: 81), and the nurse and patient as human beings who share humanity (Curtin, 1979). Gadow contends that the nurse, acting as advocate, helps patients to 'authentically' exercise their freedom of self-determination. What Gadow means here is the way in which one reaches decisions that are absolutely one's own. This means that the nurse acting as advocate respects the patient as an individual, a real person who has individual needs and preferences and one who can make decisions. In valuing the patient as a holistic being, nurses promote dignity. Evidence of valuing will be those activities that show nurses enabling and supporting patients to make decisions, freely and without pressure. They include encouraging patients to make their decision and supporting patient-centred goals and priorities. This aspect is stated by Curtin, who claims that advocacy is 'not-so-simple good nursing practice'. She recognised that it involves creating 'an atmosphere in which something intangible such as human values, respect and compassion can be realised' (1983: 10). Valuing affirms patients' dignity, respect, integrity and self-determination.

Apprising   Apprising involves informing, advising and educating. For Kohnke (1982), informing and supporting are at the heart of the role of patient advocacy. The likelihood of patients obtaining the healthcare of their choice in line with current reforms (DoH, 2006) requires that they are knowledgeable. The nurse acting as advocate needs to engage in informing patients, in advance of patients making their decision about the implications, consequences and alternative options on offer. From this we can see that apprising involves making it possible for patients to make their own decisions regarding healthcare. It is, however, more than merely assisting patients with their decisions. Apprising involves helping them to reason and deliberate. To be fully informed, is not only disclosing the consequences of proposed treatment it is also the consequences of refusing treatment. Apprising therefore promotes and protects patients' rights to be involved in decision making and giving their informed consent.

Interceding   Interceding involves coming between parties and intervening or mediating, where necessary. The notion of mediating suggests that there is conflict and/or an imbalance of power, as noted above (Teasdale, 1998). Bureaucratic healthcare systems and the power ascribed to healthcare professionals render patients vulnerable and impotent, as indeed does the disease process. In the position of powerlessness, patients require someone to speak for them, and in some cases mediate on their behalf. This aspect was evident in Mallik's (1997b) focus group of experienced nurses. Of the five conditions prompting a nurse to advocate, one specifically relates to the imbalance of power in the patient–doctor relationship. Nurses reported incidents in which patients were afraid to question doctors or voice their concerns, in fear of medical authority.

Preconditions for advocacy

Patient:

- Vulnerability whereby patients, simply being in the position of a patient, are at risk.
- In a vulnerable state patients might be facing conflict or find themselves in a situation which requires a decision.

Nurse:

- Willingness to act as an advocate.
- Willingness to take on the responsibility of advocating.

Consequences of acting as advocate

Patient:

- Positive – autonomy is secured.
- Negative – potential discomfort, for example where the decision made turns out not to be the best one.

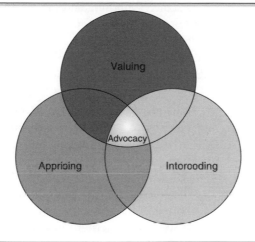

Figure 2   *Model of patient advocacy: characteristics, preconditions and consequences (Baldwin, 1994)*

Nurse:

- Positive – job satisfaction and self-actualisation.
- Negative – perceived and/or actual risks in terms of career.

Implications for practice

Advocacy was not a term explicitly used by Henderson. She stated that:

> The unique function of the nurse is to assist the individual, sick or well, in the performance of those activities contributing to health or its recovery (or to a peaceful death) that he would perform unaided if he had the necessary strength, will or knowledge. And to do so in such a way as to help him gain independence as rapidly as possible. (Henderson, 1961: 3)

This definition nevertheless encompasses the three characteristics of advocacy. The therapeutic nurse–patient relationship involves nurses assisting the individual with activities that in health could be performed without the need for assistance. Apprising and interceding are evident when individuals are no longer able to perform pertinent health-related activities themselves. Apprising is required when patients are not in possession of the 'necessary … knowledge'. Interceding involves nurses acting on behalf of patients when they are devoid of 'strength' or 'will'.

Assessment　Like the skills of problem solving, advocacy requires a deliberate, logical and systematic collection of information in order to determine whether advocacy is appropriate, or possible. Nurses are required to be vigilant to observe for opportunities other than vulnerability in which to advocate for patients. Additionally, they must be open to situations where there is potential to advocate. Assessment will also involve determining whether nurses have the necessary skills to advocate and whether they are willing to risk advocacy. Successful advocacy therefore rests on good assessment.

Planning　Planning for patient advocacy demands that nurses use the intellectual skills of decision making, observation, thinking and judgement as well as active patient involvement in all stages of care. This is important especially when patients may be experiencing conflict in making a decision. From the discussion above, advocating is a process of enabling patients to exercise autonomy. To be self-determining it is essential that patients are actively involved.

Implementing　Implementing advocacy involves the nurse engaging in those intellectual, interpersonal and technical skills associated with nursing. To engage in advocacy, there are the three essential characteristics that need to be present: valuing, apprising and interceding. Each characteristic on its own represents only one of a number of helping strategies. Only when all three are present is advocacy implemented.

Evaluating　Criteria to determine the effectiveness of advocacy will depend on patients' individual needs and subsequent consequences following advocating. A clearly written, unambiguous plan could be the instrument of evaluation.

CASE STUDY

James, a 78-year-old gentleman, was aware that he was losing his memory and confided this to the practice nurse, Mary, saying he was becoming forgetful and his loss of memory was causing friction between him and his wife. He was adamant that he did not want to go into a home. Mary detected that James was afraid that he may have dementia and thought he wanted more information about memory loss. She felt he was having difficulty deciding whether or not to mention his problem to his GP and family, fearing the consequences of the diagnosis and subsequent treatment options. She acknowledged that sharing his concern with her was probably difficult (valuing) and asked James whether he was asking her to speak with the GP so that tests could be arranged (apprising and interceding). She explained the nature of the tests and possible consequences depending on the outcome (apprising). Mary assured James that she would support his decision (valuing) to consent to, or refuse, for her to speak with the GP on his behalf.

The characteristics of valuing, apprising and interceding are necessary for advocacy. James, fearing dementia, was a vulnerable patient. Mary demonstrated valuing by respecting him as an individual. She recognised that he could make decisions about himself, and her actions were aimed at providing him with the necessary information to make an informed decision. Apprising and interceding were present. Mary acknowledged James's concern and gained his consent to speak with the GP. This she did having first provided him with information about the tests and the consequences of results. Mary was engaged in interceding when she took on the responsibility of speaking to the doctor – 'coming between' James and the GP.

CONCLUSION

In a contemporary patient-led healthcare service there are patients who, because of their illness, may be vulnerable. Nevertheless, in their capacity as patients they are required to make decisions, but they may not have the necessary knowledge, confidence or ability to communicate their wishes to healthcare professionals. In these circumstances patients require an advocate, someone who will promote and protect their autonomy, and act on their behalf.

advocacy

21

FURTHER READING

Gates, B. (1994) *Advocacy: Nurses' Guide*. London: Scutari Press.

Mitchell, G.J. and Bournes, D.A. (2000) 'Nurse as patient advocacy? In search of straight thinking'. *Nursing Science Quarterly*, 13(3): 204–9.

Vaartio, H., Leino-Kilpki, H., Salanterä, S. and Suominen, T. (2006) 'Nursing advocacy: how is it defined by patients and nurses, what does it involve and how is it experienced?' *Scandinavian Journal of Caring Science*, 20: 282–92.

REFERENCES

Abrams, N. (1978) 'A contrary view of the nurse as patient advocate'. *Nursing Forum*, xvii(3): 258–67.

Allmark, P. and Klarzynski, R. (1992) 'The case against nurse advocacy'. *British Journal of Nursing*, 2(1): 33–6.

Andersen, S. (1990) 'Patient advocacy and whistle-blowing in nursing: help for the helpers'. *Nursing Forum*, 25(3): 5–13.

Baldwin, M.A. (1994) *'Patient Advocacy: A Concept Analysis'* Unpublished M.Med.Sci. Dissertation, University of Sheffield.

Baldwin, M.A. (2003) 'Patient advocacy: a concept analysis'. *Nursing Standard*, 17(21): 33–9.

Cambridge Dictionary (2006) 'Advocacy'. Retrieved 27 November 2006 from http://dictionary.cambridge.org

Copp, L.A. (1986) 'The nurse as advocate for vulnerable persons'. *Journal of Advanced Nursing*, 11(3): 255–63.

Corcoran, S. (1988) 'Toward operationalizing an advocacy role'. *Journal of Professional Nursing*, 4(4): 242–8.

Curtin, L.L. (1979) 'The nurse as advocate: A philosophical foundation for nursing'. *Advances in Nursing Science*, 1(3): 1–10.

Curtin, L.L. (1983) 'The nurse as advocate: a cantankerous critique'. *Nursing Management*, 14(5): 9–10.

Department of Health (2006) *Our Health, Our Care, Our Say: A New Direction for Community Services*. Norwich: The Stationery Office.

Donahue, P. (1978) 'The nurse as patient advocate?' *Nursing Forum*, xvii(2): 143–51.

Gadow, S. (1980) 'Existential advocacy: philosophical foundations of nursing' in S.F. Spicker and S. Gadow (eds), *Nursing: Images and Ideals*. New York: Springer Publications.

Henderson, V. (1961) *Basic Principles of Nursing Care*. London: International Council of Nurses.

Hewitt, J. (2002) 'A critical review of the argument debating the role of the nurse advocate'. *Journal of Advanced Nursing*, 37(95): 399–404.

Kohnke, M.F. (1982) *Advocacy Risk and Reality*. St. Louis, MO: Mosby.

Mallik, M. (1997a) 'Advocacy in nursing – a review of the literature'. *Journal of Advanced Nursing*, 25: 130–38.

Mallik, M. (1997b) 'Advocacy in nursing – perceptions of practising nurses'. *Journal of Clinical Nursing*, 6: 303–13.

key concepts in nursing

Mallik, M. and Rafferty, A.M. (2000) 'Diffusion of the concept of patient advocacy'. *Journal of Nursing Scholarship*, 32(4): 339–404.

Mitchell, G.J. and Bournes, D.A. (2000) '"Nurse as patients' advocate"?, in search of straight thinking'. *Nursing Quarterly*, 31(93): 204–9.

Nursing & Midwifery Council (2006) 'Advocacy and autonomy'. Retrieved 27 November 2006 from the NMC website www.nmc.uk.org/nmc/main/advice/patientAndClientAdvocacyAndAutonomy.html

Teasdale, K. (1998) *Advocacy in Health Care*. Oxford: Blackwell Science.

Tschudin, V. (2003) *Ethics in Nursing: The Caring Relationship*, 3rd edn. London: Butterworth-Heinemann.

United Kingdom Central Council for Nursing, Midwifery and Health Visiting (1988) *Consultation Paper: UKCC's Proposed Rules for the Standard, Kind and Content of Future Pre-registration Nursing Education*. London: UKCC.

United Kingdom Central Council for Nursing, Midwifery and Health Visiting (1992) *The Code of Professional Conduct*, 3rd edn. London: UKCC.

Cross-References *Accountability, Autonomy, Caring, Compassion, Dignity, Problem solving, Respect.*

3 Assessment: physical

Victoria Ridgway

DEFINITION

Assessment is defined by the Oxford Dictionary (1983) as an estimation of value of a given subject; however, in nursing terms assessment is seen as the first stage of the nursing process in which data is obtained and collected and from which a nursing care plan can be devised. Assessment is a multi-stage cyclic process viewed as the essence of nursing and involves initial ideas which are formed about clients' existing health needs followed by confirmation of the data obtained, clarification and understanding, reassessment and evaluation (Aggleton and Chalmers, 2000). Assessment and the use of the nursing process are embedded within nursing and together they constitute a standard proficiency for pre-registration nursing programmes at the point of registration.

KEY POINTS

- Assessment is multifaceted.
- Assessment is not a one-off activity but a continuous process.

DISCUSSION

Nursing assessment is a multi-stage complex process in which the nurse, client and their family develop a tangible relationship built on trust, respect and understanding. Assessment can be at the point of admission, or part of ongoing nursing care, for example pain assessment. In all encounters a nurse through experience will be able to recognise, collect and process useful information. This in turn will inform the care needs of the patient (Daly et al., 2002).

Nursing frameworks and philosophies

To organise information and data, the use of a nursing framework is recommended. First, the nursing process forms the backbone of care delivery and management. Yura and Walsh (1967) proposed that nursing is likened to a problem-solving process in which a partnership between patient and nurse together identified actual and potential problems requiring intervention, made plans to resolve these, took steps to alleviate them and then evaluated the outcome. Therefore, the four stages of the nursing process are assessment, planning, implementation and evaluation. In more recent years a fifth stage has been established between assessment and planning, in line with the changing role of the nurse, that of nursing diagnosis (Aggleton and Chalmers, 2000).

The nursing process then links directly to assessment, as it encourages the nurse to recognise and identify actual and potential problems. These may be linked to specific medical conditions or will consider an individual's psychological, social, spiritual or cultural needs.

Underpinning the nursing process, nursing models establish a framework upon which the nurse collects and processes information. How the nurse approaches the assessment depends upon the ideologies of the model. Roper et al.'s (1996) model is popular, in which a nurse forms

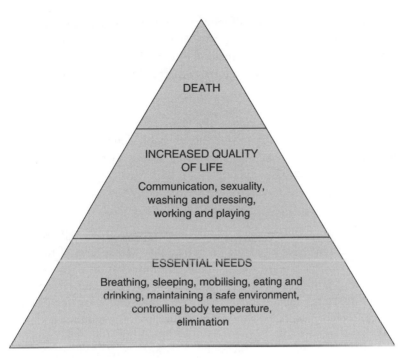

DEATH

INCREASED QUALITY
OF LIFE

Communication, sexuality,
washing and dressing,
working and playing

ESSENTIAL NEEDS

Breathing, sleeping, mobilising, eating and
drinking, maintaining a safe environment,
controlling body temperature,
elimination

Figure 3   *Hierarchy of needs (based on Maslow, 1954)*

the basis of assessment according to Maslow's hierarchy of needs (see Figure 3) in relation to activities of living. However, these models are tools and their application therefore depends upon the skills and knowledge of the nurse.

Sources of assessment

Assessment of a client is not an easy process and often complex skills and knowledge are required to complete the process. To gain a full assessment a variety of sources will be utilised. This will depend upon the age, physical status and mental capacity of the client. Sources of information may include the client, relatives, friends and significant others, multi-disciplinary documentation outlining previous and current history. Other sources may be police and ambulance records. Furthermore, the environment in which an assessment takes place will influence the quality of data obtained; for example, maintaining the dignity and privacy of a person in a busy surgical ward whilst asking personal questions is more difficult than asking the same questions in a private room. Continued along this theme is disclosure; asking clients information whilst a partner, relative or carer is present may inhibit the data collection or gain false information (Phillips et al., 2006; Hogston and Marjoram, 2007).

Other factors which are significant to the assessment process may also include the past experience of a client, the acute or chronic nature of an individual's health status, the probable length of time needed for health interventions, and a person's ability to participate in care (Hinchliff et al., 2003).

Assessment skills

In order to obtain the relevant data, there are several key skills required which if absent have a bearing on the quality and success of the intervention. These include listening skills, communication skills including verbal and non-verbal communication, use of open and closed questions, observing, taking and recording of measurements, for example weight, height, blood pressure, temperature, pulse, respiration and physical examinations. This is reinforced by Hinchliff et al., who maintain that the pre-requisites for effective assessment are reliant upon the skills of the nurse. Effective assessment depends upon:

- The nurse understanding and knowing the expected outcomes required and intervening to maintain life in an emergency.
- The nurse having appropriate social skills to establish a rapport and a relationship.
- The nurse having effective interviewing skills to gather data, including effective listening skills and summarising information obtained.
- The nurse observing verbal and non-verbal cues and attending to these.
- The nurse using appropriate language which the client understands.
- The nurse having the problem-solving and decision-making abilities to act on the information obtained.
- Recording the information obtained and establishing a baseline. (Hinchliff et al., 2003).

These elements are reinforced by Phillips et al. (2006), who add that healthcare professionals should also avoid making assumptions regarding the client or the purpose of the assessment.

Core elements of assessment

In order to plan care, nurses must be able to gather information. This is very much determined according to the individual; the nurse will collect both subjective and objective information. The nurse should begin by establishing the person's understanding and perceptions of their current health needs, their own priorities and goals regarding these and perceived areas of importance (Phillips et al., 2006). General biographical history should be obtained, such as name, age, address, GP, next of kin, marital status. Then the nurse should obtain information regarding a client using a bio-psychosocial approach. Typical health information would include:

- Current and past medical history; information on recent medical/nursing interventions and changes to health status, previous surgery, mental health problems, diagnosis of chronic conditions such as diabetes, heart disease, stroke, Parkinson's, allergies and adverse reactions.
- Information about coping strategies; ability to cope with transitions, changes in health and wellbeing.
- Self-perceived needs, current strengths and resources.
- Use of medicines; consideration of prescription drugs, over-the-counter medications, client's understanding and concordance.
- Knowledge and understanding of a patient's illness.
- Ability to self-care and functional ability; washing, dressing, shopping, cooking, mobility, continence.
- Mental health of the person.
- Nutrition and diet.
- Elimination; normal bowel and bladder function.
- The expression of sexuality and sexual activity.
- Vulnerability; possible abuse.
- Unhealthy behaviour; for example, excess alcohol, smoking, lack of exercise, poor diet.
- Physical measurement; body mass index (BMI), blood pressure (BP), temperature, pulse and respiration (TPR).
- Risk assessments; skin integrity, falls, mini-mental test, epilepsy, psychotic episodes.
- Observation of the individual and environment; pallor, physical appearance, such as is the client unkempt, malnourished, do they avoid eye contact, do they have food in the fridge, is the house/garden well maintained? Furthermore, assessing an individual in their own environment may mask problems (Phillips et al., 2006).

Psychological information would include coping ability, values, beliefs and communication, whereas assessment of a client's social history would examine a person's employment status, their personal history, the environment of care and living, key people in their network leisure and lifestyle including culture and religion, input from the inter-professional team and use of formal and informal carers (Hogston and Simpson, 2002; Hinchliff et al., 2003; Phillips et al., 2006; Hogston and Marjoram, 2007).

CASE STUDY

Robert Jones is an 84-year-old gentleman admitted with a general deterioration in his condition and severe pain in his right shoulder, radiating down his chest and arm. He has been bed-bound at home for the last few days and his wife Lillian has been taking care of him.

On admission, during data collection his wife informs the nurse that he has been unwell for a couple of months, has consulted his GP with this shoulder pain and been given an analgesic block one month ago to no effect. He has also been taking co-codamol and brufen, but again this has been ineffective. Two weeks ago the pain became so severe that the on-call GP prescribed oramorph. This controlled the pain to some degree, however, according to Lillian it made Robert drowsy and unsafe on his feet. Again the GP was called, the oramorph discontinued and he was prescribed co-proximal. This gave Robert some relief, but he has not eaten and in the last few days he has not managed to get out of bed. He has been incontinent of urine on occasions and has required all care from his wife Lillian, who is 81-years-old herself.

Following the assessment process Robert's functional ability was highlighted and although he has arthritic knees he was mobile, managing the stairs, was self-caring, could maintain his continence and was driving his car a month ago. Lillian informs the nurse that Robert's colostomy has not functioned for several days, but they both put this down to Robert eating and drinking a minimal amount.

His previous medical history includes a Myocardial Infarction five years ago, angina, and formation of a colostomy for bowel cancer 15 years ago.

The nurse having obtained relevant information can now identify actual and potential problems; priority should be given to pain management as it appears from the assessment process that Robert's functional and psychological wellbeing stems from poor pain management.

CONCLUSION

Effective assessment is a skill that a nurse learns and develops over a period of time. Assessment is not a one-off activity but rather a continuous process, which identifies actual and potential problems, prioritises need and balances this against resources and demands (Blackie, 1998). Furthermore, it is not solely problem centred. The underpinning philosophy allows the process to be holistic, interprofessional, needs led, reflect the individual's attitudes, beliefs and culture, giving empowerment to the client, thus allowing them to articulate their needs and concerns and finally be reliable and valid (Blackie, 1998; Phillips et al., 2006).

FURTHER READING

Aggleton, P. and Chalmers, H. (2000) *Nursing Models and Nursing Practice*, 2nd edn. Basingstoke: Palgrave.
Hinchliff, S., Norman, S. and Schober, J. (2003) *Nursing Practice and Health Care*. London: Arnold.

REFERENCES

Aggleton, P. and Chalmers, H. (2000) *Nursing Models and Nursing Practice*, 2nd edn. Basingstoke: Palgrave.
Blackie, C. (1998) *Community Health Care Nursing*. Edinburgh: Churchill Livingstone.
Daly, J., Speedy, S., Jackson, D. and Darbyshire, P. (2002) *Context of Nursing: An Introduction*. Oxford: Blackwell.
Hinchliff, S., Norman, S. and Schober, J. (2003) *Nursing Practice and Health Care*. London: Arnold.
Hogston, R. and Marjoram, B.A. (2007) *Foundations of Nursing Practice: Leading the Way*, 3rd edn. London: Palgrave Macmillian.
Hogston, R. and Simpson, P.M. (2002) *Foundations of Nursing Practice: Making a Difference*, 2nd edn. London: Palgrave.
Maslow, A.H. (1954) *Motivation and Personality*. New York: Harper and Row.
Oxford Paperback Dictionary (1983) Oxford University Press, 2nd edn. Oxford: Oxford University Press.
Phillips, J., Ray, M. and Marshall, M. (2006) *Social Work With Older People*, 4th edn. London: Palgrave.
Roper, N., Logan, W. and Tierney, A. (1996) *The Elements of Nursing*, 4th edn. Churchill, IL: Livingstone.
Yura, H. and Walsh, M. (1967) *The Nursing Process*. Norwalk, CT: Appleton-Century-Crofts.

Cross-References *Communication, Data, information, knowledge, Dignity, Problem solving.*

assessment: physical

4 Autonomy

Jill McCarthy

DEFINITION

Autonomy is regarded as the ability to make independent decisions; to be self-directing and self-determining. However, personal autonomy can never be viewed as pure and without restrictions because society places rules, regulations and restraints on its citizens through both legislation and cultural mores. Moreover, people are subject to direct and indirect influences from the media, workplace, family and acquaintances. So although autonomy is seen as self-determination, it is accepted that it will be operating within certain limits. Berofsky (1996) discussed three central concepts of personal autonomy, namely independence, rationality and personal integrity, believing that autonomous behaviour involves being true to oneself. This implies that choices are made independently and free from overt coercion by others, although, in order to reach an informed decision, it may be necessary to consult a range of outside opinions. Gillon described autonomy as 'the capacity to think, decide, and act on the basis of such thought and decision freely and independently' (1990: 60). Therefore, in order to function autonomously a person needs to be conscious and aware of their surroundings, and, in addition, for optimum autonomy a certain level of intelligence and physical ability is required.

KEY POINTS

- Autonomy is self-determination.
- Autonomy operates within society's guidelines.
- A person needs to be aware of their situation to be fully autonomous.
- Optimum autonomy requires optimum operational capacity.

DISCUSSION

The concept of autonomy was originally conceived by the philosopher Immanuel Kant, 1724–1804 (Guyer, 2004) and introduced into healthcare ethics as a result of The Belmont Report (National Commission, 1979), which examined research on human subjects. In healthcare, patient autonomy is closely linked to informed consent and implies that patients should make the final decisions in regard to their healthcare and treatments after being given the facts by the practitioners concerned. Respect for patient autonomy is regarded as one of the four ethical principles of healthcare alongside beneficence (seeking to do good), non-maleficence (avoidance of harm), and justice (Beauchamp and Childress, 2001). Of these four, autonomy is often cited as the most important principle in respect that it should be the one which takes precedent over the others (for example, Agich, 2003; Beauchamp and Childress, 2001; Gillon, 2003; O'Neill, 2002). Autonomy places emphasis on people being responsible for their own lives including decisions in regard to medical treatments, which might mean that a person chooses a path which could prove detrimental to health and wellbeing, and although this may oppose practitioner advice it must be respected. However, it can prove difficult for some practitioners to acknowledge and accept that patients may ignore their professional guidance and make decisions which are harmful to their health. Often cited in these cases are Jehovah's Witnesses who refuse lifesaving blood transfusions against medical opinion; however, there are many other examples of patients exercising their autonomy in opposition to the recommendations of practitioners.

It can be reasoned that healthcare professionals find it difficult to deal with patient autonomy when it contradicts their opinions, because the nature of their work is based upon obtaining optimum health for their clients. This is in keeping with two of the four ethical principles which are embedded in healthcare ethics, namely beneficence and non-maleficence (Beauchamp and Childress, 2001). Respect for patient autonomy in cases which go against clinical recommendations may be regarded as practitioners not seeking to do good and actually allowing harm to take place. Moreover, the ethical codes of practice belonging to the various healthcare professions provide guidance in terms of professional conduct in respect of ensuring and promoting patient health. For example, the Nursing and Midwifery Council (NMC) Code of Professional Conduct (2004) states that a nurse should 'protect and support the health of individual patients and clients' (Section 1.2). This guidance, at first glance, appears to contradict patient autonomy in certain cases. However, if the issues are examined in more detail it can be reasoned that supporting patient autonomy, even when it conflicts with medical advice, is to some degree both beneficent and non-maleficent to patients, as it supports both morale and emotional wellbeing. John Stuart Mill, 1806–1873, one of the early moral philosophers believed that 'the only purpose for which power can be rightfully exercised over any member of a civilised community, against his will, is to prevent harm to others' (Mill, 1985: 68). Moreover, the NMC Code of Professional Conduct states that as a nurse 'you must respect patients' and clients' autonomy – their right to decide whether or not to undergo any healthcare intervention' (Section 3.2), thus placing respect for autonomy at the forefront of the four ethical principles. Singleton and McLaren (1995) considered that respect for autonomy should occur in all situations, even when patient decisions are harmful to their health, because it is essential that relationships of trust are maintained between patients and healthcare workers.

It seems clear and unequivocal that respect for autonomy is regarded as an essential requisite of patient care. However, problems may arise when a person's ability to make informed choices and decisions is compromised, examples being in the cases of children, people who are unconscious or semi-conscious, people with learning disabilities or mental health problems, and older people with senility. As individual people within these client groups have different levels of cognitive ability, and as healthcare treatments have different levels of complexity, blanket policies about patient autonomy cannot be produced (DoH, 2001). Each person is individual, just as every healthcare scenario is different, and decisions need to be made independently on the merits of each case. When examining autonomy in regard to consent to treatment it is clear that if an adult does not have the capacity to understand the facts of the situation, then the healthcare professional should act in their best interests. However, the professional should first try to ascertain what the person's decision might have been or if an advance directive has been made in order to maximise patient autonomy (Hope et al., 2003). In the case of children under 16 years of age, the child's comprehension of the situation should be gauged in order to ascertain if they are capable of understanding the implications of the treatment in order to give informed consent. Failing this, parents, guardians or the court can consent on a child's behalf, but only if treatment is deemed in their best interests (Dimond, 2001). In some circumstances, people with profound senility or learning disabilities have flashes of clarity or insight. Should this occur and they are able to gain an understanding of the situation and, therefore, capable of giving or refusing consent, it is imperative that this autonomy be respected (Hart, 1999). In cases of people with mental health problems, including psychosis, the person's understanding of the individual treatment should be ascertained and, if comprehension is complete, consent or refusal should be respected. Delusions may not encompass every aspect of daily living and respect for autonomy is paramount (Parsons, 2003).

CASE STUDY

James Green is a 24-year-old student nurse studying on the second year of the Mental Health Branch of the BSc (Hons) Nursing programme. He is attending a clinical placement in a psychiatric admissions unit and on the second day of his placement he is approached by Peter, a 28-year-old patient with a diagnosis of depression and a history of attempted suicide, who asks him for razor blades as he wants to 'cut'. Confused, James discusses this with his mentor, Lucy, who tells him that after a risk assessment has been conducted, and after ascertaining the degree of intent, clean razor blades are sometimes issued to patients who self-harm in an attempt to reduce wound infections and minimise the severity of incisions. She explains that patients who self-harm may use other objects if refused blades, resulting in severe lacerations which can become infected. Lucy further explains that although treatment focuses on reducing self-harm this will not have immediate results and, meantime, the aim is to minimise harm. She instructs James to accompany her whilst she discusses with Peter his urge to cut himself, with the intention of persuading Peter to refrain from, or delay, the desire.

Following the discussion with Peter, in which he is still adamant that he wishes to self-harm, Lucy instructs James to issue Peter with a clean blade and to collect it from him after use and dispose of it in the sharps box. James is shocked by this instruction as he feels that Peter is mentally unstable and he regards this action as encouraging him to mutilate himself. James has had lectures at university on compulsory admission and treatment of patients with mental health problems under the Mental Health Act (1983), and he cannot reason why some patients can have their autonomy taken away from them and yet Peter's autonomous decision making is being encouraged. He also feels that he will not be adhering to the ethical principles of beneficence and non-maleficence should he follow his mentor's instructions, and, moreover, he intuitively feels uncomfortable with this action.

James is at a loss, and after briefly considering the issue he returns to his mentor and explains his dilemma. Lucy is understanding and advises

James to consider the situation from Peter's viewpoint; she also directs James to further reading on the topics of self-harm and patient autonomy and suggests that he discusses the incident and its implications with his tutor at university. Lucy explains the importance of building therapeutic relationships with patients/clients and how this hinges on trust and openness. She proposes that James concentrates on building such a relationship with Peter and further suggests that he broaches the topic of self-harm with him in order to understand the rationale for his actions. She discusses the necessity of understanding Peter's behaviour, and the triggers that precede it, before therapeutic behaviour changes can be introduced, and how all of these measures take place over time. Lucy timetables a meeting for herself and James in two week's time, when they can sit down and discuss the matter further, after he has had time to read around and consider the issues involved. Lucy reassures James that he will not be expected to conform to the directive of distributing blades to patients in order for them to self-harm until he has come to terms with this particular philosophy of care. She then leaves to go and give Peter a fresh razor blade.

CONCLUSION

Respect for autonomy is regarded as an ethical principle of healthcare and, as such, it involves consideration of the moral and legal implications. Patient autonomy is concerned with ensuring that people reach informed decisions and choices with regard to their healthcare, including consent to examinations and treatments. Autonomy should be respected and upheld wherever possible, but it is not an absolute principle. Optimally, every patient should control their own healthcare, but in circumstances where this is not practical, because of an inability to act independently, the healthcare practitioner should intervene with the best interests of the patient in mind. In many aspects of care whereby people are unable to arrive at independent decisions, or decisions are made in opposition to professional advice, much more is demanded from the practitioner involved, including their relationship with the patient and carers, in order that best interests are served.

FURTHER READING

Gillon, R. (1994) 'Medical ethics: four principles plus attention to scope'. *British Medical Journal*, 309: 184.

Hewitt-Taylor, J. (2003) 'Issues involved in promoting patient autonomy in health-care'. *British Journal of Nursing*, 12(22): 1323–30.

Parker, M. and Dickenson, D. (2001) *The Cambridge Medical Ethics Workbook. Case Studies, Commentaries and Activities*. Cambridge: University Press.

REFERENCES

Agich, G. (2003) *Dependence and Autonomy in Old Age: An Ethical Framework for Long-term Care*. Cambridge: Cambridge University Press.

Beauchamp, T.L. and Childress, J.F. (2001) *Principles of Biomedical Ethics*, 5th edn. New York: Oxford University Press.

Berofsky, B. (1996) *Liberation From Self: A Theory of Personal Autonomy*. New York: Routledge and Kegan Paul.

Department of Health (2001) *Reference Guide for Consent to Examination or Treatment*. London: Department of Health.

Dimond, B. (2001) 'Legal aspects of consent 8: children under the age of 16 years'. *British Journal of Nursing*, 10(12): 797–9.

Gillon, R. (1990) *Philosophical Medical Ethics*. Chichester: John Wiley.

Gillon, R. (2003) 'Ethics needs principles – four can encompass the rest – and respect for autonomy should be 'first among equals'. *Journal of Medical Ethics*, 29: 307–12.

Guyer, P. (2004) 'Kant, Immanuel', in E. Craig (ed.), *Routledge Encyclopedia of Philosophy*. London: Routledge.

Hart, S.L. (1999) 'Meaningful choices: consent to treatment in general healthcare settings for people with learning disabilities'. *Journal of Intellectual Disabilities*, 3(1): 20–6.

Hope, T., Savulescu, J. and Hendrick, J. (2003) *Medical Ethics and Law, the Core Curriculum*. Edinburgh: Churchill Livingstone.

Mental Health Act (1983) London: HMSO.

Mill, J.S. (1985) *On Liberty*. London: Penguin.

National Commission for the Protection of Human Subjects of Biomedical and Behavioural Research (1979) *The Belmont Report: Ethical Principles and Guidelines for the Protection of Human Subjects of Research*. 18 April 1979.

Nursing and Midwifery Council (2004) *The NMC Code of Professional Conduct: Standards for Conduct, Performance and Ethics*. London: NMC Publications.

O'Neill, O. (2002) *Autonomy and Trust in Bioethics*. Cambridge: University Press.

Parsons, A. (2003) 'Consent to treatment and mental health'. *Journal of the Royal Society of Medicine*, 96(6): 315–6.

Singleton, J. and McLaren, S. (1995) *Ethical Foundations of Health Care*. London: Mosby.

autonomy

Cross-References *Accountability, Advocacy, Empowerment, Equality, Ethics, Realism.*

5 Biological determinants of need

Jan Woodhouse

DEFINITION

What exactly are biological determinants of need? Why are they relevant in this book of concepts? It is hoped that these questions will be explored and briefly answered within the course of this chapter, because as a topic biological determinants is a vast subject and one that will merit further reading. Abraham Maslow, the influential psychologist of the 1970s and beyond, formulated a Hierarchy of Needs motivation model (Maslow, 1987). In it he suggested that the most important aspect of human need, that is, that which becomes the motivators for our actions, is the fundamental, homeostatic feature that protects us as individuals. Consequently, we address our thirst, our hunger, our breathing, sleeping, elimination, homeostatic and sexual needs before all other aspects of our self. These needs are biologically-driven, that is, they come from within us, and we have, one could argue, little control over them.

Therefore, if we give attention to our biologically-driven needs it should result in homeostasis and health. However, that is often not the case, and consequently environmental and lifestyle factors are frequently cited as being the causes of illness and disease (Brunner, 1997; Kue Young, 2003; Sharpe and Irvine, 2004). Locating such causes is important for healthcare professionals, not only in relation to the immediate treatment of the problem, but also in terms of prevention, policy making and healthcare provision.

Bortz (2005) suggests that there are four aspects of biological determinants. These are knowledge in respect to genes, 'external agency', 'internal agency' and the process of ageing. These aspects attempt to separate the demands of the body, that is, what nature gave us, from the external factors, which reflect how nurture might affect us. They prove to be useful pointers in the discussion of examining what biological determinants are, and how understanding of them helps the education of healthcare professionals.

KEY POINTS

Biological determinants of need are:

- Our genes.
- The number of external factors (such as disease and injury) that we meet.
- Our internal responses to stressors.
- The process of ageing.

DISCUSSION

Considering each of the above aspects helps us to explore how biological determinants impact upon us.

Genetics

The first aspect is that of genetics. Since the mapping of the human genome occurred, genetics has become a growing area of inquiry and knowledge (Porter, 2000). The history of genetics has, in some shape or form, been around for some time and it is noted that Darwinism considers how species adapt to their environment, with the possibility that biology plays its part in human behaviours (Porter, 2000). The concept of race acknowledges the existence of inherited genes (Chandrasoma and Taylor, 1995; Porter, 2000) in that body shape, body hair, facial features, height and skin colouring are determined in a fairly predictable way. Racial inheritance genes can also bring a tendency to particular diseases, such as the type of anaemia known as thalassemia, which is more prevalent in Mediterranean, African and Asian populations. McDowell et al. (2006) have also noted that some adverse reactions to drugs are linked to an individual's ethnicity.

Biological information, such as the race gene, is passed down, or inherited, through the deoxyribonucleic acid (DNA) in the chromosomes. Having the right amount and type of chromosomes helps us define whether we are male or female. So our gender, and all the resultant aspects of being that gender, impacts on our health needs. Females, by virtue of their reproductive role, may have diseases related to hormonal change and childbirth. Men, in their 'hunter-gatherer' role, may be more prone to accidents and injury. However, these aspects are, perhaps, logical and so the interest for many researchers are those ailments common to both sexes. Wilkinson et al. (2004) have noted, for example, that elderly women are slightly more at risk to succumbing to winter mortality than their male counterparts. However, problems can occur if the DNA is damaged by such agents as drugs, infections, radiation or chemicals. Damage to the DNA could result in an acquired genetic abnormality occurring, such as changes to the pairing and number of chromosomes, and giving rise to conditions such as Kline-Felter's syndrome, Turner's syndrome and Down's syndrome (Chandrasoma and Taylor, 1995). Hence, science has sought to overcome these problems with eradication of such genetic defects. The search for cures through gene manipulation is now the 21st-century's quest.

External agency

The external agency that Bortz describes is that of a 'by-product of an adverse encounter with a hostile threat' (2005: 390). Here, he is talking about the possibility of injury, acquiring an infection and the susceptibility to malignant change, and notes that threats to the person are usually confined to a part, rather than the whole of the body. These threats may emanate from sources that are in the individual's physical environment, such as sources of infection, chemical contaminants, housing, climate change and geography (Kue Young, 2003). All of these factors are noted as health determinants and may impact on the individual. Consequently, the role of the healthcare professional is to seek ways of preventing the sources from damaging the person. Part of this, for example, may be the monitoring of exposure to potentially harmful chemicals and matching this against individual susceptibility (Sharpe and Irvine, 2004). Some toxic substances, such as pesticides used in food production, can build up in the body, causing damage. This is a process known as bioaccumulation (Sharpe and Irvine, 2004), and it is thought to result in disrupting the endocrine system, causing illness and disease. Similarly, the healthcare professional will be trying to reduce the number of pathogens (that is, disease causing micro-organisms) (Marieb, 2004) that individuals are exposed to by attention to control of infection measures.

Internal agency

We are all individual, and our internal agency governs aspects such as digestion, metabolism, performance, sleep and so on, meaning we are going to differ from person to person. In addition, rather than affect a single part of the body, the internal agency tends to affect the whole body (Bortz, 2005). Bortz goes on to suggest that the 'healthy body has two primary expressions: fuel and energy' (2005: 390). Hence, the health professional needs to consider the role of nutrition, as a provider of fuel and energy, in maintaining a healthy status. Too little and you are faced with malnutrition, too much and you are meeting the problem of obesity.

The nutritional status of an individual can affect the hormone production in subtle ways, which in turn can have a knock-on effect on the level of spontaneous physical activity undertaken (Thorburn and Proietto, 2000). Hence, a vicious cycle may be entered into with an inadequate diet resulting in lack of exercise, which then causes additional problems such as a slow metabolism and disuse of muscles (Bortz, 2005). This is further compounded by the resulting weight gain and a loss of oxygen metabolism. Thus promoting exercise helps to break this downward spiral to ill-health. Exercise is also useful in the stabilisation of hormone secretion and is known to help in reducing stress (Brunner, 1997).

Reactions to stress are also very individual (Brunner, 1997; Bortz, 2005). Consequently, what causes distress to one person may not affect another. Brunner comments that humans have successfully adapted to 'the challenge of external, potentially lethal, but short term threats' (1997: 3, online version). However, we are less able to deal with sustained stressors and the 'fight or flight' response becomes maladaptive, forgetting to switch itself off. Therefore, healthcare professionals have an important role in identifying stress and coping mechanisms in their clients and patients, remembering that they may also be a cause of stress.

Ageing

Bortz (2005), when discussing this final aspect of biological determinants, gives a succinct definition of ageing: 'ageing is wear and tear minus repair'. He further comments that organs start to fall into disrepair from the age of 30 onwards. Chandrasoma and Taylor (1995) comment that although life expectancy varies between countries, there is a finite biological lifespan of 90–110 years, irrespective of diseases such as cancer and cardio-vascular problems. There are several theories of how we age, and it may be that it is not a single one that is responsible for the process but a combination of several.

The first theory is that of 'programmed ageing theory' (Chandrasoma and Taylor, 1995), where the notion is that cells are programmed to stop miotic division at a certain time. The second theory considers the DNA of the cells and suggests that ageing occurs as a consequence of 'DNA damage'. The third theory proposes that the ageing process is programmed into the brain cells, rather than other cells, which then have a direct influence over the hormones and neural connections. This is known as the 'neuroendocrine theory'. A fourth theory suggests that as we get older our immune system becomes overwhelmed by the number and frequency of responses it has had to make in a lifetime. Consequently, this is known as the 'immune theory'. On the other hand, the fifth 'free radical theory' proposes that there is a build-up of a substance known as lipofusin within the cells. Whilst the lipofusin is not harmful, it is an indication of free radical damage to cells and that the amount of circulating enzymes that normally inactivate free radicals are not sufficient. The sixth theory is the 'cumulative injury theory', where ageing is the result of repeated 'pathological insults' (Chandrasoma and Taylor, 1995: 242) on the body. This final theory suggests that if we could eradicate all diseases, then we might live forever.

For the healthcare professional an understanding of ageing helps in the promotion of a healthy lifestyle, as well as accepting that ageing and death are inevitable factors as we have not eradicated all diseases and removed external threats from our lives.

CASE STUDY

A useful case study to examine the biological determinants of need is the population of Australia. Here we can understand that genetics play their part in, say, protection from the harmful rays of the sun, where native Australians, the Aborigines, have more melanin in their skin than the settled white Europeans – hence the Europeans are more at risk of getting skin melanomas (The Melanoma Foundation, 2006). Similarly, the Europeans may have more resistance to an external agency, such as a childhood disease like measles, because previous generations have built up a level of immunity, unlike the Aboriginals who have only encountered the disease since arrival of the settlers (UNPO, 1991). If the two groups were given the same diet, as found in the bush, the Aborigine may thrive (being adapted to the diet), whilst the European might suffer from vitamin deficiency and malnourishment. However, both groups, Aborigines and Europeans, would undergo the same developmental and ageing process and, therefore, it is the differences in their lifestyles that ultimately decides the health of these two groups.

CONCLUSION

An understanding of the biological determinants of need helps us to consider the many factors that impact on the human. It demonstrates that we cannot give simple solutions to complex problems. A scientist may take a reductionist view of the human body in order to expand knowledge about one part of it, but will recognise that it is only a small part of the jigsaw. Considering the human being holistically, that is, thinking about all of the different factors that affect an individual, is the way forward in understanding disease, its treatments and its prevention.

FURTHER READING

Kelher, H. and Murphy, B. (2004) *Understanding Health: A Determinants Approach.* Melbourne: Oxford University Press.

Marieb, E.N. (2004) *Human Anatomy and Physiology,* 6th edn. (International Edition). San Franscisco, CA: Pearson Benjamin Cummings.

REFERENCES

Bortz, W.M. (2005) 'Biological basis of determinants of health'. *American Journal of Public Health,* 95(3): 389–92.

Brunner, E. (1997) 'Socio-economic determinants of health: stress and the biology of inequality'. *British Medical Journal,* 314: 1472 [online version accessed 25 Oct. 2006].

Chandrasoma, P. and Taylor, C.R. (1995) *Concise Pathology,* 2nd edn. Norwalk, CT: Appleton & Lange.

Kue Young, T. (2003) 'Review of research on aboriginal populations in Canada: relevance to their health needs'. *British Medical Journal,* 327: 419–22.

Marieb, E.N. (2004) *Human Anatomy and Physiology,* 6th edn. (International Edition). San Franscisco, CA: Pearson Benjamin Cummings.

Maslow, A. (1987) *Motivation and Personality,* 3rd edn. New York: Harper and Row.

McDowell, S.E., Coleman, J.J. and Ferner, R.E. (2006) 'Systematic review and meta-analysis of ethnic differences in risks of adverse reactions to drugs used in cardio-vascular medicine'. *British Medical Journal,* 332: 1177–81.

The Melanoma Foundation (2006) *2006 Melanoma Campaign,* at www.melanoma foundation.com.au/MACb.html (accessed 8 Jan. 2007).

Porter, D. (2000) 'Biological determinism, evolutionary fundamentalism and the rise of the genoist society'. *Critical Quarterly,* 42(3): 67–84.

Sharpe, R.M. and Irvine, D.S. (2004) 'How strong is the evidence of a link between environmental chemicals and adverse effects on human reproductive health?'. *British Medical Journal,* 328: 447–51.

Thorburn, A.W, and Proietto, J. (2000) 'Biological determinants of spontaneous physical activity. The International Association for the Study of Obesity'. *Obesity Reviews,* 1: 87–94.

Unrepresented Nations and Peoples Organisation (1991) *Aboriginals of Australia*, at www.unpo.org/member_profile.php?id=4 (accessed 8 Jan. 2007).

Wilkinson, P., Pattenden, S., Armstrong, B., Fletcher, A., Sari Kovats, R., Mangtani, P. and McMichael, A.J. (2004) 'Vulnerability to winter mortality in elderly people in Britain: population based study'. *British Medical Journal*, 329(7467): 647 online version (accessed 25 Oct. 2006).

Cross-References *Coping, Holistic care, Nurturing.*

6 Caring

Pat Rose

DEFINITION

A large volume of work has been published related to caring. A title search results in over 6000 hits in the Cumulative Index of Nursing and Allied Health Literature (CINAHL) alone. There have been a number of attempts by philosophers, nurses and others to define caring (see Table 1), although as Brilowski and Wendler (2005) noted, caring may be dependant on the circumstances, environment and people involved; an attribute of the concept that they describe as 'variability'. This suggests that there cannot be a single statement that accurately defines caring.

Caring is a particular emotional and behavioural response that draws on technical and interpersonal knowledge and skills. Roach (1987) identified 'compassion', 'conscience' and 'commitment' as the emotional element, whilst 'competence' and 'confidence' relate to the behavioural response. In Swanson's (1991) five categories of caring, 'doing for' is clearly a behavioural response and 'being with' is the emotional response. It is the integration of the emotional element within the behaviour that defines an action as caring. This discussion explores the concept in relation to two key themes in nursing: evidence-based practice and interpersonal relationships.

Table 1 *Defining attributes of caring*

Mayeroff (1971)	Roach (1987)	Swanson (1991)	Brilowski and Wendler (2005)	Morse et al. (1990)	Wolf et al. (1994)
Knowing	Compassion	Knowing	Relationship	Human trait	Respectful deference to others
Alternating rhythms	Competence	Being with	Action	Moral imperative	Assurance of human presence
Patience	Confidence	Doing for	Attitude	Affect	Positive connectedness
Honesty	Conscience	Enabling	Acceptance	Interpersonal relationship	Professional knowledge and skill
Trust	Commitment	Maintaining belief	Variability	Therapeutic intervention	Attentive to other's experience
Humility					
Hope					
Courage					

- Caring may be directed towards patients, artefacts or ideas.
- Caring is a moral obligation and a legal duty.
- A caring nurse will be a reflective practitioner who bases practice on evidence.
- Caring involves a relationship in which the carer is committed to the needs of the cared-for.

DISCUSSION

Caring is a normal human trait (Morse et al., 1990) and as such is the emotion that drives the nurse to act in the same way as it drives a mother to nurture a child, or a teacher to support a student (Noddings, 2003). To differentiate between caring in society and in nursing, one must establish what the object of caring in nursing is. The answer could, for example, be the patient, or keeping the patient alive or comfortable. The philosopher Mayeroff (1971) described the purpose of caring as helping another to grow and self-actualise. Perhaps, then, the object of caring in nursing is to enable the patient to self-actualise and become self-caring. However, Mayeroff (1971) and others (Kuhse, 1997; Noddings, 2003) identified that caring is not only directed towards people. It may also be directed towards artefacts or ideas. In nursing, the artefact might be an expensive piece of equipment, and the idea might be a research hypothesis.

Morse et al. (1990) noted that caring is not merely a moral ideal, but also a duty. Indeed, the duty of care is a legal obligation of all healthcare professionals. It is this moral and legal obligation that makes caring a key concept in nursing.

Caring and evidence-based practice

The study of caring has been undertaken within both the rationalistic and naturalistic paradigms. Kyle (1995) examined the findings of a range of studies from both paradigms. Although both had limitations, she identified that both had similar findings. Nurses tend to value the affective elements of caring, driven by emotions, such as providing comfort through listening. However, patients tend to value behaviours requiring knowledge and skill, such as knowing how to give injections and when to call a doctor. Thus, it is important for nurses to note that patients perceive the caring nurse as competent, skilled and knowledgeable.

In examining what caring actually is, Mayeroff listed eight major ingredients (see Table 1). Interestingly, his first ingredient is 'knowing'. He says that 'in order to care I must understand the other's needs and must be able to respond properly' (1971: 19). As an evidence-based profession, the importance of knowledge in nursing is paramount and is acknowledged in the profession's own analysis of caring. Roach (1987) equated competence with an appropriate level of knowledge and skill. Swanson (1991) expanded on this to suggest that a caring nurse will avoid assumptions and seek to understand the meaning of a situation in the life of the patient. To do this effectively the nurse must undertake a thorough assessment. This presupposes that the nurse has a detailed knowledge of the range of normal human experience and is able to identify any health-related deviations. The focus of assessment is to understand the needs of others, but responding to those needs requires a knowledge of nursing interventions and how to implement them. Thus, the caring nurse will be an educated nurse who keeps up to date with changes and developments in practice.

'Alternating rhythms' is Mayeroff's (1971) second major ingredient of caring. He suggests that the carer alternates between 'doing' and 'doing nothing'. Sometimes caring involves taking some form of action, and at other times standing back and allowing the person cared-for to take responsibility for her/himself. For Swanson (1991) this is characterised as enabling the patient to move towards self-care.

Because exactly the same circumstances are never presented twice to the nurse, reflection is a crucial element in evidence-based practice. Through reflection-in-action the expert nurse develops the skill of applying knowledge to the specific situation as it is unfolding, and after the event reflection-on-action enables the nurse to identify new knowledge gained and internalise it (Schön, 1983; Benner, 1984). In discussing the notion of caring for an idea, Mayeroff talks about 'the need to reflect on it again and again from similar and dissimilar points of view' (1971: 11). The same could be said of caring for a person.

Caring and interpersonal relationships

If the goal of caring is to help another to achieve self-actualisation, there must be a relationship between the carer and the cared-for. Roach (1987) suggested that 'compassion' within caring involves sharing in the world of the patient, and 'commitment' includes devotion to the needs of others. Swanson (1991) describes 'being with' as being emotionally

caring

there with the patient, whether physically there or not. Watson, who equated caring with 'the heart and soul of nursing' (1997: 54), adds another dimension, spirituality, when she describes the art of caring as 'soul to soul connecting' (1997: 60).

For Noddings (2003) the relationship between the carer and the cared-for is fundamental to the analysis of what caring is. She argued that whilst the relationship is not equal, and there is no agreement that it will be reciprocal, it is nevertheless the response of the cared-for that enhances or diminishes the caring relationship. For example, she suggested that the cared-for may respond in a positive way or the carer may be 'held off or ignored' (2003: 61). If the cared-for refuses to take on that role then, it is argued, caring cannot happen.

Mayeroff (1971), however, presented a different perspective. He suggested that there are one-sided caring relationships. The example he uses is that of a therapist caring for a patient. He argues that when the patient becomes able to care for himself, and could, therefore, care for others, the therapeutic relationship ends. The boundaries to professional relationships (Nursing and Midwifery Council, 2002) ensure that a reciprocal caring relationship cannot develop between the nurse and the patient. Whether care is received positively or not, Mayeroff (1971) suggested that patience is an essential ingredient. By patience he does not mean simply waiting passively, but rather creating time and space for the carer and cared-for to work their way through whatever situation they are dealing with. Swanson (1991) describes this as 'conveying ongoing availability' and Wolf et al. (1994) as 'assurance of human presence'.

To Mayeroff (1971) honesty as an ingredient of caring involves being able to look at oneself and the cared-for and seeing both as they are. Honesty is therefore about self-awareness and about not pretending to be what one is not. An example of this in practice might involve the ability to acknowledge to patients the limitations of one's knowledge and skill. It also involves a realistic understanding of the impact one has on the cared-for. For example, however much time a nurse may take explaining an aspect of treatment to a patient, or teaching an aspect of care, the patient may choose a different understanding of their situation. In this respect, honesty in caring is not only the ability to acknowledge the positive impact of the interaction with the patient, but also to acknowledge the patient's responsibility for, and choices regarding, her or his own health.

Another aspect of caring is its focus on the future. Mayeroff suggested that hope does not derive from dissatisfaction with the present compared to future possibility, but rather a belief that the 'plenitude of the present' (1971: 32) makes future growth a possibility. Swanson (1991) described this as 'maintaining belief' and discusses the hope-filled attitude of the nurse who offers realistic optimism and belief in the patient's capacity to face whatever the future holds. In doing this, the caring relationship is one of trust (Mayeroff, 1971). Not the trust the cared-for has in the carer, but the trust the carer must have in the cared-for to make autonomous choices.

CASE STUDY

Children's nurse Ann is caring for David, aged six months, and his mother. David was admitted to hospital following a febrile convulsion. He has been fretful all day and has finally settled to sleep. His mother is exhausted. Ann enters the room and the mother's look makes a silent appeal: 'Please don't wake my baby.' Ann knows that it is in David's best interests to have his temperature checked as, albeit rarely, a febrile convulsion can become prolonged and lead to brain damage or death so must be prevented. But she also knows that both mother and baby need rest. Quietly Ann approaches the cot. Very slowly she releases the catch and silently lowers the cot side. David barely stirs. Ann then very gently pats the sleeping baby with one hand while gesturing to the mother to indicate that she should take over patting him. Ann draws down the baby's ear lobe and positions the aural thermometer. It beeps as it takes the reading. David stirs and whimpers. Ann covers the mother's hand with her own and both briefly rock the baby who settles immediately. Ann raises the cot side as silently as she lowered it and with a nod leaves the room. David's mother, understanding the gesture, follows her. Ann reassures the now tearful mother that her baby's temperature is normal and gives her a quick hug. The encounter is over. Ann continues with her duties and the mother returns to watch over her baby.

CONCLUSION

This discussion, and the illustrative case study, has demonstrated that knowledge and competence are essential elements of caring. Caring also involves a relationship between the carer and the cared-for. Practice can be evidence-based and efficient, but it becomes true nursing when the caring element is introduced and the nurse engages emotionally with individuals and their needs.

FURTHER READING

Styles, M.M. and Moccia, P. (1993) *On Nursing: A Literary Celebration.* New York: National League for Nursing.

REFERENCES

Benner, P. (1984) *From Novice to Expert: Excellence and Power in Clinical Nursing Practice.* Menlo Park, CA: Addison-Welsley.

Brilowski, G.A. and Wendler, M.C. (2005) 'An evolutionary concept analysis of caring'. *Journal of Advanced Nursing,* 50(6): 641–50.

Kuhse, H. (1997) *Caring: Nurses, Women and Ethics.* Oxford: Blackwell.

Kyle, T.V. (1995) 'The concept of caring: a review of the literature'. *Journal of Advanced Nursing,* 21(3): 506–14.

Mayeroff, M. (1971) *On Caring.* New York: Harper Perennial.

Morse, J.M., Solberg, S.M., Neander, W.L., Bottorff, J.L. and Johnson, J.L. (1990) 'Concepts of caring and caring as a concept'. *Advancing Nursing Science,* 13(1): 1–14.

Noddings, N. (2003) *Caring,* 2nd edn. Berkley, CA: University of California Press.

Nursing and Midwifery Council (2002) *Practitioner–Client Relationships and the Prevention of Abuse.* London: NMC.

Roach, S. (1987) *The Human Act of Caring: A Blueprint for the Health Professions.* Ottawa: Canadian Hospital Association.

Schön, D.A. (1983) *The Reflective Practitioner.* San Francisco, CA: Harper Collins.

Swanson, K.M. (1991) 'Empirical development of a middle-range theory of caring'. Nursing Research, 40(3): 161–6.

Watson, J. (1997) 'Artistry of caring: heart and soul of nursing', in D. Marks-Maran and P. Rose (eds), *Reconstructing Nursing: Beyond Art and Science.* London: Baillière Tindall.

Wolf, Z.R., Giardino, E.R., Osborne, P.A. and Ambrose, M.S. (1994) 'Dimensions of nurse caring'. *Journal of Nursing Scholarship,* 26(2): 107–11.

Cross-References *Autonomy, Evidence-based practice, Reflection.*

7 Clinical governance

Linda Meredith and Ian Pierce-Hayes

DEFINITION

At the heart of clinical governance lie both the concept of quality in relation to patient care and accountability for the level of performance in its implementation. Attempts to improve the quality of clinical practice by nurses, doctors and indeed all healthcare professionals are not new. There have been a series of initiatives such as clinical audit, benchmarking and risk management strategies that have involved clinical staff in attempts to improve patient care. The central aim of clinical governance is to integrate all of these positive practices into a framework and create an environment where all levels of clinical and non-clinical staff are involved in improving patient care.

There have been several definitions of clinical governance but the one that is most widely quoted is in the consultation document *A First Class Service* (Department of Health) as 'a framework through which NHS organisations are accountable for continuously improving the quality of their services and safeguarding high standards of care by creating an environment in which excellence in clinical care will flourish' (1998: 33). Common to the majority of these definitions is the concept of clinical governance as a framework that leads to an integrated approach to care across the organisation (Som, 2004). This is achieved through co-ordination, co-operation and communication across departments and disciplines through a model of participation and shared decision-making at all levels (Garland, 1998). The legislation, *The Health Act* (DoH, 1999a), was warmly greeted by some healthcare professionals as putting clinical performance on a par with financial performance (Miles et al., 2001).

KEY POINTS

- Clinical governance is a framework for embedding quality improvement into service delivery.

- Both organisational and individual accountability for healthcare are central to clinical governance.
- Reducing risk and ensuring safe practices are an essential part of any quality assurance programme.
- Creating an environment and culture based on openness and mutual respect facilitates quality assured healthcare.
- Patient and user involvement is crucial at all levels of healthcare.

DISCUSSION

The election of a new Labour government in 1997 heralded a series of reforms. Referring to the NHS, the government's agenda explicitly highlighted quality as the key to development:

> The new NHS will have quality at its heart. Without it there is unfairness. Every patient who is treated in the NHS wants to know that they can rely on receiving high-quality care when they need it. Every part of the NHS and everyone who works in it should take responsibility for working to improve quality. (DoH, 1997: 18)

The background to the government's reforms within the NHS can be seen from political, economic and financial perspectives. The election of the Labour government came on the back of a series of unpopular financial changes within the NHS, revolving around the internal market implemented by the then Tory government which had been in office for nearly 20 years.

There had also been a growing public disquiet and concerns about the standards of the NHS following a series of high-profile cases during the 1990s, including the Bristol inquiry into the deaths of children following cardiac surgery (Bristol Royal Infirmary Inquiry, 2001) and the Alder Hey investigation into the lack of consent over organ/tissue donation. Public confidence in the NHS was further reduced following the Harold Shipman and Beverley Allitt inquiries, which investigated the harrowing cases where patients had been murdered by healthcare professionals. Thus, the government's initiatives could be seen as a response to public concern and, therefore, they emphasised in the 1999 Health Act that accountability for quality services was a statutory duty of all healthcare organisations and in particular the chief executives who lead them (Walshe, 2000).

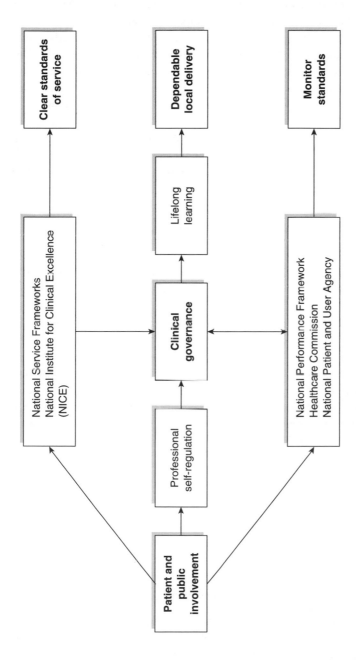

Figure 4 *Clinical governance: a model of improvement (adapted from Clinical Governance in the New NHS, Department of Health, 1999)*

The consultation document *A First Class Service* (DoH, 1998) identified three main components of quality assurance that are integral to clinical governance. These are the setting of quality standards both at a national and local level, and the delivery and monitoring of these benchmarks with subsequent actions to ensure the maintenance of standards. Clinical governance can be characterised as a control assurance framework embracing a whole-systems approach, to continuous quality improvement and a bridge between managerial and clinical approaches to quality (Freeman and Walshe, 2004). Figure 4 summarises the relationship between clinical governance and the drive for continuous quality improvement in healthcare and will form the basis for the discussion in this chapter.

Setting of quality standards

The setting of quality standards both at a national and local level are key components of the quality assurance process, which is pivotal to good clinical governance. This included the establishment of the National Institute for Clinical Excellence (NICE) with responsibility for developing, disseminating and monitoring clinical guidelines for treatment and care of patients, as well as reviewing the effectiveness of new technologies and drug therapies. The development of National Service Frameworks, for specific patient groups such as mental health, set out national standards for the treatment of particular conditions that are based on best-practice evidence. The *Essence of Care* (DoH), launched in February 2001, provided a tool to help practitioners to take a patient-focused and structured approach to sharing and comparing best practice. Patients, carers and professionals worked together to agree and describe good quality care. This resulted in benchmarks covering areas of care such as continence, bladder and bowel care, personal and oral hygiene and food and nutrition. *Essence of Care* has been described as the bedrock of clinical governance, with clinical practice benchmarking connecting the concepts of quality, clinical effectiveness and evidence-based practice (Badham et al., 2006).

Delivering quality standards

Quality assured healthcare delivery encompasses not only the achievement of national and local standards, but is also moving towards being underpinned by evidence and clinical effectiveness, supported by systems within a clinical governance framework across all NHS organisations. Clinical effectiveness can be applied to all professional practice and can be defined as the 'application of the best available knowledge, derived from research, clinical expertise and patient preferences, in order to achieve optimum processes and outcomes of care for patients' (Royal College of Nursing, 1996: 22). Clinical effectiveness has been promoted through the development of guidelines and protocols for particular diseases. These are based on evidence of effectiveness following randomised controlled trials, meta-analyses and systematic reviews (Starey, 2003). The main tenets of clinical governance are clear lines of responsibility, accountability for the overall quality of care, which is the responsibility of the Chief Executive and Board, with clear policies and processes for managing risk.

Minimising and managing risk is an essential part of any quality assurance process. Providing healthcare may inadvertently cause risks to patients, practitioners and the provider organisation. All NHS trusts are required to have clear policies and processes for managing such risks (Starey, 2003). Examples of these include a documented risk register which is regularly reviewed, incident reporting policy which is audited to assess compliance and schedules for risk assessment.

A real partnership between patients, carers, service users and professionals is at the centre of clinical governance (Nicholls et al., 2000). Service users can offer valuable insights into their experiences and perspectives on access to services, delivery of treatment and care, accessibility, efficiency and effectiveness of care delivery across different sectors; for example, between primary and secondary care or between health and social services (Stevenson, 2000). A variety of initiatives have been implemented across the NHS, including the development of questionnaires to assess patient satisfaction. The development of an expert patients' programme is a further example. Expert patients 'are those with experience of self-management of long-term conditions and the programme centres on developing a model of peer support for patients with similar conditions' (Squire, 2006: 17).

Monitoring quality standards

Monitoring is one of the key components of the quality assurance of healthcare. This is carried out at a national level through the Healthcare Commission, which replaced the Commission for Health Improvement in 2004. The Commission is a health watchdog whose slogan is 'inspecting, informing, improving'. These three main agendas are achieved through varying initiatives, including an annual review of the performance of every NHS trust with an award for performance rating, which is scored on the quality of the services they provide to patients and public. It also includes how well they manage their finances and other resources, such as their property and staff. These annual health check ratings are available on the Healthcare Commission's website.

CASE STUDY

Anna is a cardiac specialist nurse based in the A&E department of a district general hospital. Her role has developed and evolved from clinical audit data which showed that there were delays in patients with heart attacks receiving 'clot busting' treatment (thrombolysis). The time it takes from a patient having a heart attack being admitted to hospital and receiving thrombolysis (known as the door-to-needle time) has become a national target set by the government to measure the quality of patient care and the performance of hospital trusts. Anna sees her role as co-ordinating the evidence base supporting treatment with a partnership between different healthcare professionals to make a real difference to patient care. Clinical governance was used to establish new ways of working to enhance the quality of a service. Anna continues to collect audit data on all patients diagnosed with acute myocardial infarction and the data is presented on a monthly basis to the Trust's chief executive, senior managers and clinicians to ensure that the national target is being met, and any issues of quality are monitored and maintained. This approach to continuous quality improvement is essential for the success or failure of any changes in practice.

In tandem with patients' organisations she has been involved in producing publicity materials to highlight the need for members of the public not to delay treatment and to seek medical help early when experiencing chest pain. Part of her role is in educating staff in the benefits of prompt treatment as well as working alongside paramedics, nursing and medical staff to facilitate effective interventions. She has developed with nursing, medical and pharmacy professionals an integrated care pathway for patients presenting with chest pain, incorporating clear clinical guidelines to ensure that patients receive efficient, evidence-based treatment.

This case study demonstrates that through the implementation of clinical governance, new ways of working can bring improvements in the quality of patient care. By utilising collaboration within the multi-disciplinary team, partnerships are formed to create an environment and culture where all staff are not only involved in from the outset, but are also essential to its continuing success (McSherry and Pearce, 2002).

CONCLUSION

Clinical governance is the framework that builds on quality assurance mechanisms in order to facilitate continuous quality improvement in the delivery of healthcare. Clinical governance is the process that embeds quality improvement into service delivery. Quality assured healthcare is that in which national standards and guidance are reflected in the delivery of local services. Clinical governance involves the processes that support and enhance the provision of quality assured healthcare.

FURTHER READING

Healthcare commission www.healthcarecommission.org.uk/homepage.cfm
McSherry, R. and Pearce, P. (2002) *Clinical Governance: A Guide to Implementation for Healthcare Professionals*. Oxford: Blackwell.
Sale, D. (2005) *Understanding Clinical Governance and Quality Assurance: Making it Happen*. Basingstoke: Palgrave Macmillan.

REFERENCES

Badham, J., Wall, D., Sinfield, M. and Lancaster, J. (2006) 'The essence of care in clinical governance'. *Clinical Governance: An International Journal*, 11(1): 22–9.
Bristol Royal Infirmary Inquiry (2001) *Learning from Bristol: The Report of the Public Inquiry into Childrens' Heart Surgery at the Bristol Royal Infirmary 1984–1995*. London: HMSO.
Department of Health (1997) *The New NHS Modern and Dependable*. London: HMSO.
Department of Health (1998) *A First Class Service*. London: HMSO.
Department of Health (1999a) *The Health Act*. London: HMSO.
Department of Health (1999b) *Clinical Governance in the New NHS*. London: HMSO.
Department of Health (2001) *The Essence of Care: Patient-Focused Benchmarking for Healthcare Practitioners*. London: HMSO.
Freeman, T. and Walshe, K. (2004). 'Achieving progress through clinical governance? A national study of healthcare managers' perceptions in the NHS in England'. *Quality and Safety in Healthcare*, 13(5): 335–43.
Garland, G. (1998) 'Taking the first step'. *Nursing Management*, 5(6): 28–31.
McSherry, R.and Pearce, P. (2002) *Clinical Governance: A Guide to Implementation for Healthcare Professionals*. Oxford: Blackwell.

Miles, A., Hampton, J., and Hurwitz, B. (2001) *NICE, CHI and the NHS Reforms: Enabling Excellence or Imposing Control?* London: Aesculapius Press.

Nicholls, S., Cullen, R., O'Neill, S. and Halligan, A. (2000) 'Clinical governance: its origins and foundations'. *Clinical Performance and Quality Healthcare*, 8(3): 172–8.

Royal College of Nursing (1996) *The Royal College of Nursing Clinical Effectiveness Initiative- A Strategic Framework*. London: Royal College of Nursing.

Som, C.V. (2004) 'Clinical governance: a fresh look at its definition'. *Clinical Governance: An International Journal*, 9(3): 87–90.

Squire, P.H. (2006) 'The expert patient programme'. *Clinical Governance: An International Journal*, 11(1): 17–21.

Starey, N. (2003) 'What is clinical governance?'. *Haywood Medical Communications*, 1(12): 1–7.

Stevenson, K. (2000) 'Clinical governance'. *Health Services Management*, 3(1): 20–2.

Walshe, K. (2000) *Clinical Governance: A Review of the Evidence*. Birmingham: Health Services Management Centre, University of Birmingham.

Cross-References *Accountability, Communication, Data, information, knowledge, Equality, Evidence-based practice, Leadership, Managing change, Professional development, Researcher, Risk management, Teamwork.*

8 Common sense

Sue Phillips

'All truth, in the long run, is only common sense clarified'.

Thomas Huxley (www. famousquotes.com)

DEFINITION

'Common sense' is defined by the dictionary as 'practical good sense' (Chambers, 1997), by Wikipedia as 'beliefs or propositions that seem, to most people, to be prudent and of sound judgment, without dependence upon esoteric knowledge' and by Liu and Singh (2004) as the knowledge that is shared by the vast majority of people who live in a particular culture. However, Liu and Singh point out that when a statement is common sense in one culture, it does not mean that it is scientifically true, or even that it is common sense in other cultures. For example, wearing a seat belt in a car may be common sense in one culture, but may be seen as an imposition or irrelevant in another.

KEY POINTS

Three stances on common sense are:

- Common sense may be lost in the current healthcare climate of cost-effectiveness.
- Common sense may have a real place in clinical decision making in healthcare practice.
- The widespread views or common knowledge held by the population in general need to be taken into account when addressing health promotion or education.

DISCUSSION

Common sense and healthcare

Whether health professionals use common sense, or indeed are allowed to use common sense, depends largely on its definition and interpretation. Some argue that healthcare is so bound up in protocols, audits and so on that common sense is no longer a feature of healthcare, and this is to the detriment of patient care. But what does this mean?

McKeown suggests that 'healthcare has become so organised, codified, outcome analysed and protocol bound that it has lost sight of the rich common knowledge of its early teachers' (2000, www.cancerlynx. com/nurse). He argues that Florence Nightingale would put much of the current nursing practice into the 'Nursing . . . What it is not' category (Nightingale, 1860, cited by McKeown, 2000), and that the rush to codify and quantify everything in order to cost-account has tended to lose the caring needed in the profession. Nightingale's common-sense approach to the disposal of 'everything the patient passes', the need for public health principles of clean air and water, efficient drainage, cleanliness and light, and the value of observation and evaluation of the whole patient, is equally relevant today. McKeown (2000) suggests that in many instances, nursing care has become a financial risk analysis that is far from Nightingale's principles of what nursing care is, and approaching her principles of what it is not. Examples abound of patients who are unable to feed themselves being left unfed (Morrison, 2006) when staff are perhaps too busy, understaffed or uncaring to do so. As McKeown says, the concepts of patient nutrition are common sense, and a good indicator of whether a patient is 'getting better' is when they are hungry.

Common sense and critical decision making

How does common sense affect nursing and healthcare? Evidence-based decision making involves *combining* the knowledge arising from one's clinical expertise, patient preferences and research evidence within the context of available resources (Di Censo et al., 1998). Professional knowledge in nursing is gained from a variety of sources, based on experience as well as research (Thompson et al., 2004). Common sense should be integrated into this, not seen as separate from nursing knowledge.

Common sense can give weight to prioritising care; for example, looking after basic physical needs of the patient before filling in forms. Another example may be knowing when to report abnormalities; for example, finding a patient with a pulse of 40/min cannot wait to be reported until the end of a shift. It may be about weighing up options; for example, the questions arising may be 'has this been noticed before', 'is it something new', 'is it something the patient is having treatment for'?

Some critics of evidence-based medicine believe that evidence from experience is just as valid as traditional and established research methods, such as randomised controlled trials. For example, hitting a thumb with a hammer will cause pain – it doesn't need a randomised controlled trial to prove or disprove it (Michelson, 2004). Talking about clinical decision making, Michelson (2004) points out that the simplest explanations should be considered before going on to the more complicated possibilities (as he says, 'when you hear hoof beats, think horses, not zebras'), and suggests that one component of common sense is to 'intuitively' discard the avenues of inquiry that are unlikely to be fruitful. Similarly, the initial clinical problem has to be framed in an intuitive 'common-sense' way that correctly represents the actual clinical scenario. If this is incorrectly presented, the subsequent steps of accumulating evidence to support clinical decision making are likely to be flawed. Michelson (2004) and others (for example, Porta, 2003) feel that although 'pure' evidence-based medicine (that is, underpinned by randomised controlled trials (RCTs) or other good quality research) is laudable, it does not encourage the use of common sense, which may be a disadvantage in the realistic practice of medicine and healthcare. Indeed, Clinicians for the Restoration of Autonomous Practice (2002) suggest that practitioners who idealistically continue to apply available evidence to medicine will increasingly have to fear the wrath of the zealots when they 'resort to that most lay of clinical approaches: common sense' (Porta, 2003: 602). On a more serious note, it is suggested that funding may be withheld from some treatments that are tried and tested, simply because they are not based on RCTs or meta-analysis of RCTs (Porta, 2003).

Common sense and health promotion

Patients may hold 'common sense' or 'common knowledge' views about their illness, which may or may not be substantiated by medical or professional knowledge. These views stem from a variety of sources, for example, parents, upbringing, culture and own experiences, and are not lightly dismissed or overcome. This is particularly relevant to the health-care practitioner when planning health education and health promotion interventions. For example, Davison et al. (1989), in a study in South Wales, found a widespread belief that heredity plays a major part in the development of heart trouble in individuals, and that it is likely that these 'common sense' ideas have an important influence on personal decisions to adopt, or not to adopt, lifestyle behaviours currently promoted by health educators and primary care professionals. In other words, people may decide that there is no point in changing their risky behaviour, since their genetic make-up may be more likely to influence their health than, for instance, whether they smoke or not. For health promotion initiatives to be successful, health educators need to be aware of the cultural norms, values and beliefs – that is, the common sense – prevalent in the area. The beliefs that form an individual's understanding of an illness have been recognised as fundamental to how people react to new information and how they cope with illness (Donovan and Ward, 2001). Leventhal et al.'s (1992) common sense model is based on the idea that people have common sense beliefs, or representations, that guide how they cope with health problems. Donovan and Ward (2001) suggested that traditional educational interventions may try to teach new coping skills without first addressing the well-established beliefs that drive the selection of current coping strategies. Individuals are unlikely to accept new strategies that are inconsistent with long-held beliefs, and therefore are unlikely to change behaviour in line with health education advice.

CASE STUDY

Eileen is a patient with cancer who has been prescribed narcotics to control her pain. She is careful not to mix alcohol with her painkillers and so didn't take the narcotic on the morning of her birthday, as she thought she might be able to enjoy a glass of wine with her family that evening. By evening, she was feeling quite ill, and decided she was becoming addicted to the drugs, and so stopped them altogether. This stemmed from her reading and experience that people can become addicted to opiates. Within a few days, when seen by the nurse, she was in severe pain and distress. By talking with Eileen, the nurse was able to ascertain Eileen's concerns about addiction, discuss where these beliefs came from and reassure Eileen about the safe way to continue her medication and control her pain. Eileen was soon feeling much more comfortable and able to function more normally once her pain was under control.

(Adapted from Donovan and Ward, 2001.)

CONCLUSION

Common sense is acquired through life experiences, which are then applied to a particular problem that we are facing. It involves an assessment of a situation, having a set of 'tools' to do something about the problem, and being able to evaluate whether we have been successful or not. A certain degree of confidence is required to apply common sense to a situation, but it does allow for creativity in problem solving.

FURTHER READING

Backlar, P. (1996) 'Ethics in community mental healthcare: confidentiality and common sense'. *Community Mental Health Journal*, 32(6): 515–9.

Fowler, C. and Baas, L.S. (2006) 'Illness representations in patients with chronic kidney disease on maintenance hemodialysis'. *Nephrology Nursing Journal*, 33(2): 173–84.

Tilley, S. (1999) 'Altschul's legacy in mediating British and American psychiatric nursing discourses: common sense and the "absence" of the accountable practitioner'. *Journal of Psychiatric and Mental Heath Nursing*, 6: 283–95.

REFERENCES

Chambers (1997) *Chambers Super Mini Dictionary*. Edinburgh: Chambers.

Clinicians for the Restoration of Autonomous Practice (CRAP) Writing Group (2002) 'EBM: unmasking the ugly truth'. *British Medical Journal*, 325: 1496–8.

Davison, C., Frankel, S. and Davey Smith, G. (1989) 'Inheriting heart trouble: the relevance of common-sense ideas to preventive measures'. *Health Education Research*, 4(3): 329–40.

DiCenso, A., Cullum, N. and Ciliska, D. (1998) 'Implementing evidence-based nursing: some misconceptions'. *Evidence Based Nursing* 1: 38–40.

Donovan, H.S. and Ward, S. (2001) 'A representational approach to patient education'. *Journal of Nursing Scholarship*, 33(3): 211–6.

Leventhal, H., Diefenbach, M. and Leventhal, E.A. (1992) 'Illness cognition: using common sense to understand treatment adherence and affect cognition treatment'. *Cognitive Therapy and Research*, 16(2): 143–63.

Liu, H. and Singh, P. (2004) 'ConceptNet: a practical commonsense reasoning toolkit'. *BT Technology Journal*, 22(4): 211–26.

McKeown, M.J. (2000) 'What Ever Happened to Common Sense?' at www.cancerlynx.com/nurse_sense.html (accessed 5 Nov. 2006).

Michelson, J. (2004) 'Critique of (im)pure reason: evidence-based medicine and common sense'. *Journal of Evaluation in Clinical Practice*, 10(2): 157–61.

Morrison, B. (2006) 'I said to the nurse, please feed her', *Guardian*, Saturday, 7 January 2006.

Nightingale, F. (1860) *Notes on Nursing: What it is and What it is Not*. New York, Appleton.

Porta, M. (2003) 'Evidence b(i)ased medicine'. *British Medical Journal*, 326: 602.

Thompson, C., Cullum, M., McCaughan, M., Sheldon, T. and Raynor, P. (2004) 'Nurses, information use, and clinical decision making – the real world potential for evidence-based decisions in nursing'. *Evidence Based Nursing*, 68–72.

Wikipedia (2006) at www.wikipedia.org (accessed 5 Nov. 2006).

Cross-References *Accountability, Autonomy, Confidence, Dignity, Evidence-based practice, Problem solving, Sense of humour.*

common sense

9 Communication

Geoff Astbury

DEFINITION

Communication involves the encoding of thoughts and feelings, within the initiator of a message, into patterns of behaviour leading to the transmission of that message, via one or more of a range of potential communication channels, to one or more recipients. Decoding of this transmission exerts influence over the thoughts and feelings of the recipient(s), leading to an encoded feedback response to the transmission source. Communication is therefore a circular process occuring within influential social and physical contexts. Competence in communication results from the use of a range of learned cognitive, affective and behavioural skills which are open to enhancement through personal reflexivity and instruction.

KEY POINTS

- Communication skills influence the quality of nursing care.
- Nurse communications with patients should be directed at meeting functional and affective needs.
- Nursing communication can elicit patient emotional comfort or discomfort.
- Nursing communication must take account of patients' cultural background.
- The effective functioning of the multi-disciplinary/multi-agency team is influenced by the patterns of communication.
- Accurate and sufficient written communication is necessary for patient wellbeing and nurse protection.

DISCUSSION

Within interactions with patients and service users, peers, nursing and multi-professional teams, and the public, it is the effectiveness of communication that has salience. Effective communication has been identified by patients and carers as one facet of being a 'good nurse' (Rush and Cook, 2006), as leading to improved patient responses to healthcare, enhanced patient satisfaction (Johansson et al., 2002), team performance (Newson, 2006) and interagency communication (Day, 2006). Frequently expressed concern about nurses' communication (for example, Bowles et al., 2001), however, makes attention to ways of improving the communication skills of nurses critical.

Patient–nurse communication

Appropriate and therapeutically effective interactions between patient and nurse demand effective communication. Even the most 'basic' of nursing activities, such as the measurement of temperature, pulse and respiration, can be rendered accurate by appropriate communication and inaccurate by verbal and non-verbal behaviours which can provoke, for example, anxiety in the patient.

Kruijver et al. (2001) identify two forms of nurse communication behaviours directed at meeting the cognitive and the emotional needs of patients. Instrumental communication is described as that related to the provision of practical nursing care and the giving of information concerning the patient's illness and treatment, while affective communication behaviours are directed at 'giving comfort' and 'showing respect' towards the development of the nurse–patient relationship (2001: 773). The influence of both forms of communication in the development of emotional comfort in patients is articulated by Williams and Irurita (2004). Here, emotional comfort is described as being characterised by '... pleasant positive feelings, a state of relaxation that affected the physical status of the body' and contrasted with 'emotional discomfort' said to be experienced as '... unpleasant negative feelings, a state of tension' in patients (2004: 810). The development of emotional comfort is partly the product of information provision; nurses need to transmit '... with openness and honesty ...' (2004: 810) information concerning, for example, the patient's condition, the treatment and care which will be required and what the patient can expect to occur. Emotional comfort is said to be also associated with the demonstration of competence, the indication of availability and the characteristics of healthcare professionals' use of verbal and non-verbal communication skills. A suggested emphasis on the functional aspects of communication (McCabe, 2004) and on technical skills (Mok and Chiu, 2004) points to

communication

63

a need for nurses to seek balance in the features of their interactions with patients.

The patient–nurse relationship

The communication behaviours of nurses must be set within the context of the relationships that they form with patients. Patients must be seen as active in the process of relationship development, calling for the nurse to engage in ways which accommodate individual patient differences. A patient-centred approach to communication, defined by Langewitz et al. (cited by McCabe 2004) as 'communication that invites and encourages the patient to participate and negotiate in decision making regarding their own care' (2004: 42) is advocated.

Empathy is fundamental to relationship development; without seeking this, nurses cannot begin to develop an intellectual and emotional appreciation of the patient's predicament and the needs stemming from this. Empathic understanding of the patient is of little value unless it is communicated to the patient via a range of communication skills. The use of verbal skills, including questioning, explaining, reflecting and paraphrasing and the non-verbal skills of, for example, touch and body language along with the preparation of a conducive physical environment contribute to a process of active listening, which is generally held to be necessary for the generation of an appropriate, patient-centred approach to relationship development (e.g. Sully and Dallas, 2005). Within particular episodes of patient–nurse interaction, the nurse will additionally need skill in opening, closing and managing the duration of exchanges. For effectiveness such approaches must be conducted by nurses who are in possession of certain 'relational capacities' (Hartrick, cited by Mok and Chiu, 2004). The person-centred ideas of Carl Rogers (1957) involving 'genuineness', 'unconditional positive regard' and 'empathy' are often held up as qualities necessary to ensure that sincerity in the use of communication skills will be perceived by their recipients. Emphasis on the use of such 'helping skillls' does not negate the significance of less structured communications with patients. Burnard (2003) argues for the value of phatic communication; refering to the work of Malinowski, Burnard tells us that this form of communication is notable for its role in establishing and maintaining human contact rather than for the transmission of information or any explicit therapeutic intent. 'Hello, how are you?' as one illustration of this, acknowledges the presence of another person and opens up the possibility of further social exchanges. Phatic communication may not require the high levels of expertise and proficiency of those behaviours usually seen as required for relationship development, but it is socially skilled behaviour and therefore plays its part in the essentially human relatedness that effective nursing requires.

Culture and communication

The above approaches to communication must be seen as existing within a cultural frame which might not be appropriate in exchanges with patients whose culturally normative ways of thinking and behaving are drawn from contexts that lack congruence with values and forms of conduct which are essentially Western in origin. For example, Liu et al. (2005) describe the 'experiences and perceptions' of 'supportive communication' in Chinese patients who have cancer. Here, we are informed that 'The specific functions of Chinese communication dictate a set of communication behaviours that are unique to Chinese culture and might affect the communication processes between nurses and patients' (2005: 263). In illustration, we are told of differences in patterns of communication used in interactions with 'insiders' (including family members) and 'outsiders' (including health professionals); 'implicit' or communications characterised by superficiality are reserved for outsiders. Centrally, the study conducted by Liu et al. (2005) suggests that Chinese patients see the meeting of their psychological needs as being the preserve of family members and not that of nurses.

The multi-agency team

As Barrett et al. suggest, 'inter-professional working involves complex interactions between two or more members of different disciplines' (2005: 18) when approaches to meeting the holistic needs of patients extend beyond the expertise and responsibilities of any one professional group or agency. In a review of the literature, West (1999) has pointed to the outcomes of effective inter-agency working as being beneficial for both patients and members of the healthcare team. The need for collaboration and the imperative for effective communication between participants are obvious, but failures and their consequences have also been noted. Achieving effective multi-agency teamworking calls, according to Barrett et al. for knowledge of the roles and functions of other agencies and disciplines, willingness and motivation to engage in

communication

collaboration, the 'confidence and competence' of participants, 'trust and mutual respect' and 'open and honest communication' (2005: 20–21). Here, communication is viewed as necessary for 'joint decision making based upon shared professional perspective' which 'enables those involved to articulate their own perspectives, listen to the views of others and negotiate outcomes' (2005: 21).

Written communication

Attention to communication in nursing must extend to the documentation of nursing assessment, planning, implementation and evaluation processes. Patient wellbeing and personal and professional standing of nurses can be compromised by insufficient and/or inaccurate recording. The Nursing and Midwifery Council (NMC) state, for example, that:

> records should be factual, consistent and accurate, written as soon as possible after the event has occurred, providing current information on the care and condition of the patient or client, be written clearly, in such a manner that the text cannot be erased (and) should not include abbreviations, jargon, meaningless phrases, irrelevant speculation and offensive subjective statements. (NMC, 2002: 8)

An increase in the use of electronic recording and communication media is apparent, but a reluctance to its adoption has been suggested by Strople and Ottani (2006) in their report on the potential use of computer technology as an aid to nurses 'intershift report'. The use of a 'personal digital assistant' is advocated as a replacement for paper as a means of recording ongoing nursing actions 'at the point of care' and with the contents subsequently transmitted to a 'centralised patient database'. Strople and Ottani suggest that the use of such technology would potentially negate suggested deficits in traditional paper recording and oral reporting methods.

CASE STUDY

Mr and Mrs Cross had a son, Simon, who was 15 years old. During a hospital stay for unrelated treatment, examinations had raised the possibility that Mrs Cross had breast cancer. Confirmation of this was given to Mrs Cross prior to Mr Cross and Simon visiting her. On their arrival at the ward, it became immediately apparent to Mr Cross and Simon that

Mrs Cross was extremely distressed; she was running about the ward, talking loudly and shunned attempts made by Mr Cross to calm her; she ignored Simon. Nurses suggested that Mr Cross and Simon should leave while they attempted to calm Mrs Cross. Some fifteen minutes later, Mr Cross was called back to the ward; informed that his wife had calmed and that it would be possible for him to see her. It was suggested that it would be too distressing for Simon to see his mother. Mrs Cross was in bed and drowsy; Mr Cross's attempts to speak to his wife achieved only incoherent and slurred responses. Mr Cross stayed with his wife for thirty minutes before informing a nurse that he needed to leave to attend to Simon and to inform his daughter and other son of the events. On telephoning the ward later, Mr Cross was told that his wife had moved to an adjacent unit and he was informed of the times when visiting his wife would be possible. Following this call, he received a telephone call from a nurse who introduced herself as Mrs Cross's new key nurse; she summarised the care that Mrs Cross had received, asked how the family was coping and when they would like to visit. On arrival at the ward, Mr Cross, his daughter and sons were greeted warmly by the key nurse and offered the opportunity to meet with members of the multi-disciplinary team who had been involved in providing care for Mrs Cross. The family was provided with the details of the team members and with advice on how each could be contacted.

CONCLUSION

Nursing communication is inevitable and its effectiveness an imperative for the development of appropriate nurse–patient relationships and for collaboration between members of the multi-disciplinary and multi-agency team. Written communication, increasingly in electronic forms, is an important component of the nursing process. Concerns in relation to the communication skills of nurses are apparent, indicating the need for their emphasis in the preparation and in the personal and professional development of nurses.

FURTHER READING

Hargie, O.D.W. (ed.) (2003) *The Handbook of Communication Skills*, 2nd edn. London: Routledge.

Sully, P. and Dallas, J. (2005) *Essential Communication Skills for Nursing*. London: Elsevier Mosby.

communication

REFERENCES

Barrett, G., Selman, D. and Thomas, J. (eds) (2005) *Interprofessional Working in Health and Social Care*. London: Palgrave Macmillan.

Bowles, N., McKintosh, C. and Torn, A. (2001) 'Nurses' communication skills: an evaluation of the impact of solution-focussed communication training'. *Journal of Advanced Nursing*, 36(3): 347–54.

Burnard, P. (2003) 'Ordinary chat and therapeutic conversation: phatic communication and mental health nursing'. *Journal of Psychiatric and Mental Health Nursing*, 10: 678–82.

Day, J. (2006) *Interprofessional Working*. Cheltenham: Nelson Thornes.

Johansson, P., Oleni, M. and Fridlund, B. (2002) 'Patient satisfaction with nursing care in the context of healthcare: a literature study'. *Scandinavian Journal of Caring Sciences*, 16: 337–44.

Kruijver, I.P.M., Kerkstra, A., Bensing, J.M. and van de Wiel, H.B.M. (2001) 'Communication skills of nurses during interactions with simulated cancer patients'. *Journal of Advanced Nursing*, 34(6): 772–9.

Liu, J., Mok, E. and Wong, T. (2005) 'Perceptions of supportive communication in Chinese patients with cancer'. *Journal of Advanced Nursing*, 52(3): 262–70.

McCabe, C. (2004) 'Nurse–patient communication: an exploration of patients' experiences'. *Journal of Clinical Nursing*, 13: 41–9.

Mok, E. and Chiu, P.C. (2004) 'Nurse–patient relationships in palliative care'. *Journal of Advanced Nursing*, 48(5): 475–83.

Newson, P. (2006) 'Participate effectively as a team member'. *Nursing and Residential Care*, 8(12): 541–4.

Nursing and Midwifery Council (2002) *Guidelines for Records and Record-Keeping*. London: NMC.

Rogers, C. (1957) 'The necessary and sufficient conditions of therapeutic personality change'. *Journal of Consulting Psychology*, 21: 95–103.

Rush, B. and Cook, J. (2006) 'What makes a good nurse? Views of patients and carers'. *British Journal of Nursing*, 15(7): 382–5.

Strople, B. and Ottani, P. (2006) 'Can technology improve intershift report? What the research reveals'. *Journal of Professional Nursing*, 22(3): 197–204.

Sully, P. and Dallas, J. (2005) *Essential Communication Skills for Nursing*. London: Elsevier Mosby.

West, M. (1999) 'Communication and teamworking in healthcare'. *Ntresearch*, 4(1): 8–17.

Williams, A.M. and Irurita, V.F. (2004) 'Therapeutic and non-therapeutic interpersonal interactions: the patient's perspective'. *Journal of Clinical Nursing*, 13: 806–15.

Cross-References Confidence, Data, information, knowledge, Educator, Empowerment, Feedback, Nurturing, Problem solving, Record keeping, Teamwork.

key concepts in nursing

10 Compassion

Carole Capper

DEFINITION

Compassion is not easy to define, particularly in the context of nursing, but is often considered to be an essential component of nursing care. It is a concept thought to be synonymous with empathy and sympathy and is often used interchangeably with these terms. The English word compassion has been in use since the 14th century and is derived from the Latin *com* (together with) and *pati* (to suffer), literally to 'suffer with'. Compassion can be seen as a sense of shared suffering, most often combined with a desire to alleviate or reduce such suffering; to show special kindness to those who suffer. Blum (1980: 512) describes it as involving feeling with another person while recognizing that one's feelings are not the same as that other person's.

KEY POINTS

- Compassion requires action and is more than empathy or sympathy.
- Compassion is not just about an individual but about the community and has a sense of social justice.
- Compassionate care can be delivered at the cost of nurses' health.

DISCUSSION

Health is a precursor, as well as a consequence, of wellness and encompasses values of self-determination, caring and compassion, personal growth, democracy, equality and justice (Prilleltensky and Prilleltensky, 2003). A human orientated focus is considered a basic value for nurses (Bjorkstrom et al., 2006), and it is essential to gain an understanding of the essence of compassion in relation to humanity. The Dalai Lama, the spiritual head of Buddhism who is regarded as 'the ocean of compassion', has much to offer in his view that human nature is basically compassionate (Davidson and Harrington, 2002).

The terms compassion, empathy and altruism have sometimes been used interchangeably yet refer to different but sometimes overlapping phenomena (Monroe, 2002). Compassion is considered to be an essential component of nursing care, but what precisely is meant by compassionate care and the kinds of issues which arise in dealing with its application are often unclear (Dietze and Orb, 2000). Being a good nurse is a professional nurse who incorporates humanistic values, viewing the patient as a whole and an individual whilst striving for high-quality care (Burke and Harris, 2000; Watkins, 2000).

Interestingly, Bassett (2002) in her study of nurses' perceptions of care and caring suggested that although the humanistic aspects of care were important, the patients actually valued a high level of competency and skills in their nurse. She goes on to explain that perceptions of caring are context driven and that the acutely ill patient would understandably expect the correct drugs at the right time and so on, whereas the patient with the long-term condition would appreciate the psychological/emotional support. We can deliver compassionate care in small ways, such as simply applying lipstick for an ill patient before visiting time, knowing that she would feel 'undressed' without it. However, we can also deliver compassionate care in ways that can be detrimental to our own physical, psychological and spiritual health, and this is particularly relevant when dealing with patients who are dying or who have suffered trauma (Collins, 2003). If we return to the definition of compassion as a shared sense of suffering, compassionate nurses can endanger their own health in actually experiencing patients' pain and suffering, and it is that interaction between nurses' and patients' characteristics that identifies caring behaviour (Rafli et al., 2004). Pask (2001) discusses the nurse's capacity to see what is morally salient in the care setting and to understand their patients' needs and deliver care with compassion which she sees as a virtue of altruism.

This humanistic approach to caring has been characterised by Fry (1991) as a 'moral point of view' which encompasses respect and love for others and is lived in that person's (the nurse's) own life. The work of Wilkes and Wallis (1998) demonstrated that compassion was expressed throughout a three-year training programme for nursing students. First-year students expressed compassion in terms of being friendly and loving, whereas second-year students expressed compassion and enacted it through communication. The third-year students expressed compassion in a professional sense as well as a personal sense, and used conscience in a much more extended way to that of the first- and second-year students. Thus, compassion was seen to be at the centre of caring.

Compassion is quite difficult to cultivate, particularly in the face of death and disease, which of course is what a large proportion of nurses are involved with in their daily work. Boleyn-Fitzgerald (2003) argues that we are making unreasonable demands upon healthcare professionals, if it is claimed that compassion is an obligation within the professional roles. This is reflected in the work of Smith (1992), who suggests that some nurses behave the way they do in order to protect themselves from anxiety related to certain episodes of patient care. Labelling of patients such as 'the nuisance' or 'the pain' or 'difficult' conveniently places them into categories where nurses are able to objectify them and their symptoms. She suggests that these distancing strategies, including the 'seen it all before' attitude, help nurses to avoid the anxiety associated with patient care.

CASE STUDY

Working in an acute Trust, Sarah frequently encountered patients who had severe or life-threatening illnesses. Mandy was a young patient who was the same age as Sarah and had been diabetic all of her life. The complications of diabetes had manifested in all of her body systems, which meant that nursing her was particularly challenging. Sarah was involved in one particular aspect of her care, which was fracture management and wound care. Over a long period a relationship developed between the two young women as Mandy was admitted to and discharged from hospital, numerous times, as a result of a variety of diabetic complications. During this time wound care and fracture management became increasingly difficult as the wounds on her limb deteriorated and there was no evidence of fracture healing. Unable to weight bear and perform her activities of living, along with multi-system involvement, depression almost seemed inevitable for Mandy. Because of the mutual trust and respect for each other, Sarah became the sole provider of wound care and plaster cast management, which was an arrangement that worked well until Mandy started to develop problems outside of Sarah's normal working hours. Her clinical condition deteriorated and Sarah was called upon more and more to attend to her specialist needs with regards to wound care and fracture management. Being called by the hospital when Sarah was off duty became a regular occurrence, but because of the compassionate nature of Sarah and this shared sense of suffering, she found it impossible to refuse the patient's requests.

CONCLUSION

Compassion is an expression of altruism which is considered to be a moral virtue and one of the integral components of nursing practice. However, it is essential to protect the health and wellbeing of those who are engaged in compassionate care, and this needs to be achieved through education and also in clinical practice. The compassionate practice described in the case study is undoubtedly altruistic and was probably of great importance to the recipients of that care. Unfortunately, although the patients and relatives may have found comfort in such care, it was given to the detriment of the professional's health and wellbeing.

FURTHER READING

Davidson, R.J. and Harrington, A. (eds) (2002) *Visions of Compassion: Western Scientists and Tibetan Buddhists Examine Human Nature*. New York: Oxford University Press.

REFERENCES

Bassett, C. (2002) 'Nurses' perceptions of care and caring'. *International Journal of Nursing Practice*, 8: 8–15.

Bjorkstrom, M.E., Johansson, I.S. and Athlin, E.E. (2006) 'Is the humanistic view of the nurse role still alive in spite of an academic education?' *Journal of Advanced Nursing*, 54(4): 502–10.

Blum, L. (1980) 'Compassion', in A.M. Rorty (ed.), *Explaining Emotions*. Los Angeles: University of California Press, Berkley. pp. 507–17.

Boleyn-Fitzgerald, P. (2003) 'Care and the problem of pity'. *Bioethics*, 17(1): 1–16.

Burke, L.M. and Harris, D. (2000) 'Education purchaser's views of nursing as an all graduate profession'. *Nurse Education Today*, 20: 620–8.

Collins, S. (2003) 'Too tired to care? The psychological effects of working with trauma'. *Journal of Psychiatric and Mental Health Nursing*, 10: 17–27.

Davidson, R.J. and Harrington, A. (eds) (2002) *Visions of Compassion: Western Scientists and Tibetan Buddhists Examine Human Nature*. New York: Oxford University Press.

70tze, E. von and Orb, A. (2000) 'Compassionate care: a moral dimension of nursing'. *Nursing Inquiry*, 7: 166–74.

Fry, S.T. (1991) 'A theory of caring: pitfalls and promises', in D.A. Gaut and M. Leininger (eds), *Caring: The Compassionate Healer*. New York: National League for Nursing. pp. 161–72.

Monroe, K.R. (2002) 'Explicating altruism', in S.G. Post, L.G. Underwood, J.P. Schloss and W.B. Hurlbut (eds), *Altruism and Altruistic Love: Science, Philosophy and Religion in Dialogue*. New York: Oxford University Press. pp. 106–22.

Pask, E. (2001) 'Nursing responsibility and conditions of practice: are we justified in holding nurses responsible for their behaviour in situations of patient care'? *Nursing Philosophy*, 2(1): 42.

Prilleltensky, I. and Prilleltensky, O. (2003) 'Towards a critical health psychology practice'. *Journal of Health Psychology*, 8(2): 197–210.

Rafli, F., Oskouie, F. and Nikravesh, M. (2004) 'Factors involved in nurses' responses to burnout: a grounded theory study'. *BMC Nursing*, 3: 6 (accessed from www.biomedcentral.com/1_472-6955/3/6 on 13 Nov. 2004).

Smith, P. (1992) *The Emotional Labour of Nursing: How Nurses Care*. Basingstoke: Macmillan.

Watkins, M. (2000) 'Competency for nursing practice'. *Journal of Clinical Nursing*, 9: 338–46.

Wilkes, L.M. and Wallis, M. (1998) 'A model of professional nurse caring: nursing students' experience'. *Journal of Advanced Nursing*, 27: 582–589.

Cross-References *Caring, Competence, Confidence, Coping, Empathy, Nurturing, Respect, Value.*

11 Competence

Andrea McLaughlin

DEFINITION

Competence has often been described as difficult to define (Ashworth and Morrison, 1991; and Ashworth Saxon, 1990). Watson (2002) and Dolan (2003) agree, and add that competence is also poorly defined. The Manpower Services Commission (1985), focus on the ability of the individual to perform activities within their occupation. Jessop (1991) asserts that competence is the ability to perform to recognised standards, to maintain or improve quality, whereas While (1994) defines competence as what a person knows, and not how they perform. Both the United Kingdom Central Council for Nursing, Midwifery and Health Visiting (UKCC) (1999) and the Department of Health (1999) indicated their concerns that nurses should be fit for practice, award and purpose, and supported the use of competencies to assess fitness for registration as a nurse. This was extended by the Nursing and Midwifery Council (NMC) (2004a) and the Quality Assurance Agency for Higher

Education (QAAHE) (2001) when their proficiencies and benchmark statements for award of qualifications were published. Although the statements maintain that competence must be achieved, they remain broad with no indication of how assessment may be undertaken.

KEY POINTS

- Competence is difficult to define.
- Competence is mandatory for registration as a nurse.
- Competence must be maintained after registration.
- Competence should indicate the minimum level of safe practice.

DISCUSSION

There are a number of discreet elements embraced by the concept of competence, and these are discussed below.

Requirements for registration

The requirements for registration as a nurse are determined by the NMC, which states that: 'to practise competently you must possess the knowledge, skills and abilities required for lawful, safe, and effective practice without direct supervision' (NMC, 2004b: 9).

Protection of the public is a major factor when delivering healthcare (DoH, 1999; UKCC, 1999), and this has recently been emphasised by the NMC which states that 'registration is a licence to practice and is the prime means of protecting the public' (NMC, 2006: 11). When assessing students there is a need to ensure that they are prepared to the same minimum level. Based on guidance from *Fitness for Practice* (UKCC, 1999) student nurses have to complete two sets of competencies; one set at the end of the Common Foundation Programme and the second at the end of the two-year branch programme.

Level of performance

The main objective in assessing competence in nursing programmes is the assurance that the student is able to 'perform skills with due regard for safety and other factors pertinent to that skill' (DoH, 1999: 29). These may be factors such as a timescale, or predetermined conditions such as 'using aseptic technique' or 'according to an agreed protocol'.

The assessment of competence cannot occur unless there are conditions imposed which clearly state the minimum standard of performance. Within nursing programmes this is achieved by the provision of learning outcomes which define the students' minimum level of performance, such as 'the student will demonstrate dressing a surgical wound, using aseptic technique'. Therefore, failing to use aseptic technique indicates that competence has not been achieved.

Skills and Objective Structured Clinical Examinations (OSCE)

Skills and Objective Structured Clinical Examinations (OSCE) are divided into small sections, so that the student knows what they have to do, step by step, to pass the assessment. This is particularly useful for promoting inter-mentor reliability, as if a group of practitioners are asked to demonstrate a skill they may all perform it safely but differently, as individuals develop their own style with experience. Using a standard form itemising all the steps to be assessed may aid this process. Competence implies safety, capability and security, which may exist even if the skill is not performed as quickly or as smoothly as it would be by an expert. These factors will develop with practice and experience as the student becomes confident and able to execute the skill efficiently. Stipek (2002) reports that as students develop competence, they develop confidence and motivation. The key to competence is whether the skill is performed safely and linked to appropriate standards and not whether it was smooth and 'poetry in motion'.

Assessing competence

Within nursing, the Standards of Proficiency are stated by the NMC (NMC, 2004b), but these are somewhat broad and do not give distinct levels of competence. They are the standards that must be achieved at the end of the programme of education, whilst competence must be assessed throughout the programme at all levels. Cowan et al. (2005) promote a holistic approach, as competence can incorporate knowledge, skills, attitudes and performance, in complex combinations. Student nurses at the point of registration must be fit for practice and fit for award (UKCC, 1999); these are assessed via theoretical assessments and skills acquisition/inventory, but McManus et al. (1998) draw attention to the fact that achievement in theoretical work does not always mean competence in practice.

competence

Fitness for purpose is the third area identified by the UKCC (1999), and the assessment of this area is more complex. Fitness for purpose implies the integration of theory and practice which is enhanced and influenced by other factors such as attitudes, values, ethical principles and use of evidence to underpin practice, reflection, problem-solving and decision-making skills. This combination should produce a competent professional who can assess, plan, implement and evaluate care, and who has the ability to transfer knowledge and skills to a variety of situations. Assessment of competence in performing practical skills usually commences with simpler skills and progresses to more complex ones. Formative assessment is part of nursing programmes and may occur initially in a skills laboratory or other simulated situation, prior to the skill being performed in the 'live' setting. Formative assessment may aid both the development of confidence and the ability of the student to perform the skill smoothly and efficiently. Summative assessment confirms that the student has the ability to perform the skill unaided, safely, and to the required standard, and ideally should take place in the practice area, although simulation may be utilised if there is no opportunity to perform the skill when giving direct care. Wherever the assessment takes place, the NMC indicate that the practice-based mentor should be involved with assessment of competence (NMC, 2006). Practice assessment must also include the integration of relevant theory and evidence to underpin care delivery. As the student progresses through the programme, assessment of competence will focus on more complex skills. It is not sufficient for a student to achieve competency once only, and it is likely that rehearsals take place prior to the summative assessment.

Competence should not be seen as the ability to perform well on a single occasion, but the ability to repeat the performance to the same standard on a regular basis. This ensures that expertise develops and the student is able to progress to play an inherent role in the teaching and assessment of others – a far cry from the old process of 'see one' 'do one' 'teach one', where practice was not always discussed and questioned (Crouch, 2005). Students are now encouraged to review, assess and develop their skills post-qualification so that clinical credibility is maintained. The NMC require that practitioners maintain competence by a process of continuous updating and that this is declared at the renewal of registration that occurs on a three-yearly basis (NMC, 2004c).

Assessing competence is a complex issue as methods have to be practical, reliable, consistent, valid and accurate. The assessment tool must differentiate clearly between the student who is competent and the one who is not. Assessment tools may include learning outcomes, reflections on practice, critical incident analysis, observation, demonstration of skills and OSCEs. It is mandatory that programmes of nursing include a process to record and assess knowledge skills and attitudes (NMC, 2004a) which are linked to the NMC proficiencies. The assessment documents may vary between institutions but there is a common purpose, which is to enable the student to demonstrate attainment to the required standard prior to registration. Assessment tools may measure many factors, including students' performance at a specified level, confidence, use of skills, knowledge, understanding, motivation, analytical skills, learning from experience, and the ability to integrate theory into practice.

It may be argued that many practitioners could assess competence and all could reach differing conclusions, as individual definitions and expectations could be diverse, so mentor preparation is important to enable standardisation of assessment throughout the profession.

CASE STUDY

Janet was a student nurse who had worked as a healthcare assistant (HCA) prior to commencing nurse education. As an HCA she had observed venepuncture many times. She had on one occasion, under supervision, been allowed to take blood herself. At the beginning of her first placement on an acute surgical ward Janet asked her mentor to assess her in performing venepuncture as she was to complete an OSCE. The mentor confirmed that Janet had not yet learned about this at university, but a session on venepuncture was to be taught within the next few weeks. The mentor talked to Janet about the anatomy of blood vessels and gave her a copy of the ward policy on venepuncture. She arranged for Janet to work with the phlebotomist on a number of occasions to observe the skill of venepuncture and the safety aspects of working with blood. Janet worked with her assessor and practiced the procedure using a model and became used to handling equipment with due regard to safety. Janet then performed venepuncture over a few days, on a group of clients, under the direct supervision of her mentor. The mentor questioned Janet on aspects of practice and safety during this time. When the mentor was satisfied with Janet's performance, she arranged a time for the OSCE to be completed. Janet was not as quick at taking blood or as efficient at handling the equipment as the assessor, but she performed the procedure safely, using the correct equipment. She complied with all safety measures and gave correct and logical explanations to the client, and achieved a 'pass'. Janet had learned the skill logically from an expert and had time to consolidate her knowledge and explored practice. The mentor had observed her performing the procedure on a number of occasions and knew that her performance was repeatable.

CONCLUSION

Competence remains difficult to define, although it is a key issue in ensuring that the student is fit for award, practice and purpose. The mentor has the opportunity to be a key player in both the formative and summative assessment processes, but should be properly prepared for this role (NMC, 2006). In the event that a student is deemed 'not competent', there should be a support system in place within the practice area and linking with the Higher Education Institution (HEI) to help the student to achieve competence. Achieving competence is the key to delivering and maintaining quality care within nursing, and therefore it must not be under-estimated or allowed to erode.

FURTHER READING

Crouch, D. (2005) 'Proving your competency'. *Nursing Times,* 101(6): 22–4.
Dolan, G. (2003) 'Assessing student nurses' clinical competency: will we ever get it right?' *Journal of Clinical Nursing,* 12: 132–41.
Nursing and Midwifery Council (2004) *Standards of Proficiency for Pre-registration Nursing Education.* London: NMC.

REFERENCES

Ashworth, P. and Morrison, P. (1991) 'Problems of competence-based nurse education'. *Nurse Education Today,* 11: 256–60.
Ashworth, P. and Saxon, J. (1990) 'On "competence"'. *Journal of Further and Higher Education,* 14(2): 3–25.
Cowan, D.T., Norman, I. and Coopamah, V.P. (2005) 'Competence in nursing practice: a controversial concept'. *Nurse Education Today,* 25(5): 355–62.
Crouch, D. (2005) 'Proving your competency'. *Nursing Times,* 101(6): 22–4.
Department of Health (1999) *Making a Difference: Strengthening the Nursing, Midwifery and Health Visiting Contribution to Health and Healthcare.* London: DoH.
Dolan, G. (2003) 'Assessing student nurses' clinical competency: will we ever get it right?' *Journal of Clinical Nursing,* 12: 132–41.

Jessop, G. (1991) *Outcomes, NVQs, and the Emerging Model of Education and Training*. London: Falmer.

Manpower Services Commission (1985) *Guidance Notes for Two-Year Youth Training Schemes*. Sheffield: Manpower Services Commission.

McManus, C., Richards, P., Winder, B.C. and Sproston, K.(1998) 'Clinical experience, performance in final examinations and learning style in medical students'. *British Medical Journal*, 316: 345–50.

Nursing and Midwifery Council (2004a) *Standards of Proficiency for Pre-registration Nursing Education*. London: NMC.

Nursing and Midwifery Council (2004b) *Code of Professional Conduct: Standard for Conduct, Performance and Ethics*. London: NMC.

Nursing and Midwifery Council (2004c) *The PREP Handbook*. London: NMC.

Nursing and Midwifery Council (2006) *Standards to Support Learning and Assessment in Practice*. London: NMC.

Quality Assurance Agency for Higher Education (2001) *Benchmark Statement for Nursing*. London: QAAHE.

Stipek, D. (2002) *Motivation to Learn: Integrating Theory and Practice*, 4th edn. Boston, MI: Allyn and Bacon.

United Kingdom Central Council for Nursing, Midwifery, and Health Visiting (1999) *Fitness for Practice – The Peach Report*. London: UKCC.

Watson, R. (2002) 'Clinical competence: starship or straitjacket?' *Nurse Education Today*, 22(6): 476–80.

While, A.E. (1994) 'Competence versus performance: which is more important?' *Journal of Advanced Nursing*, 20(3): 525–31.

Cross-References *Accountability, Assessment, Confidence, Ethics, Holistic care, Problem solving.*

12 Confidence

Carole Capper

DEFINITION

Confidence within the context of nursing practice can be defined in two ways. First, it can be defined as a secret that is confided or entrusted to another (Wordnet Search, 2006), something which nurses deal with in their everyday practice. Alternatively, it can be defined as 'freedom from doubt; belief in yourself and your abilities', and it is this definition within the context of nursing practice that will be discussed in this chapter (Wordnet Search, 2006). Professional confidence is also defined as an internal feeling of self-assurance and comfort, as well as being tested and/or reaffirmed by other nurses, patients and friends (Crooks et al., 2005).

KEY POINTS

- Professional confidence is associated with clinical competence.
- Professional confidence is a dynamic process and is influenced by both personal and professional factors.
- Confidence affects performance.

DISCUSSION

Professional practice encompasses caring, compassion, competence, commitment, comportment and confidence (Roach, 1992), and professional confidence should, ideally, be nurtured within the nursing curriculum (Crooks et al., 2005) and throughout a professional career by means of clinical supervision, mentorship and peer support. For the nurturing of professional confidence it would be reasonable to assume that the teachers in nurse education should also be confident and competent both in practice and classroom settings; nurse lecturers should therefore have practical and recent experience of nursing (Nursing and Midwifery Council (NMC) (2002). This is supported further in Recommendation 26 of the *Fitness for Practice* document which states that 'service providers and Higher Education Institutes should support dedicated time in education for practice staff and dedicated time in practice for lecturers, to ensure that practice staff are confident and competent in teaching and mentoring roles and lecturers are confident and competent in the practice environment' (UKCC, 1999: 10).

The links between competence and confidence have been highlighted, not only by the NMC (2002) but also by post-registration nursing students (Farrand et al., 2006) and postgraduate medical students (Williams et al., 1997). However, Morgan and Cleave-Hogg (2002) argued that no direct relationship between confidence and competence has actually been established.

Pre-registration nursing programmes have two main aims. First, they enable the student to acquire the theoretical knowledge which underpins their practice, and second, they assist the student to acquire the competence in clinical skills associated with their practice (Farrand et al., 2006). In the past, student nurses articulated that upon qualifying from Project 2000 they lacked the confidence and experience to make clinical decisions (Last and Fullbrook, 2003).

'I need to develop more confidence' is a common refrain articulated by students of nursing, both pre- and post-registration. However, despite the importance of professional competence being acknowledged in the literature, there is surprisingly little written about its development and strategies to promote confidence. Professional confidence affects all aspects of nursing in terms of relationships with patients/clients, peers and other members of the multidisciplinary team, all of which will ultimately affect patient care. Other factors to consider are issues which affect confidence, and these include environmental factors, education and training, support and supervision.

Despite the paucity of research around confidence and pre-registration nursing students, Chesser-Smythe (2005) demonstrated how student nurses' confidence in their first clinical placement was higher in those who had previous work experience in healthcare, suggesting that familiarity with situations influences confidence levels. Moreover, the acquisition of knowledge has also been shown to have an impact on confidence levels (Neary, 1997).

Professional confidence has also been linked with professional and personal stress (Williams et al., 1997), so it is reasonable to assume that it is a complex, dynamic process affected by both professional and personal influences (Brown et al., 2003). With much of the literature being related to competence and the ability to carry out certain tasks, it is no surprise that research shows that despite significant increases in senior house officers' confidence for carrying out a range of activities, confidence remained low in several areas – the key area being related to technical skills (Williams et al., 1997). Acknowledgement of training and education techniques and their effects upon confidence have suggested that confidence affects performance (Byrne et al., 2005). Whilst there are many issues around training and education involving patients as teachers (Wykurz and Kelly, 2002), simulated clinical tasks (Byrne et al., 2005) and how they increase confidence, reduce anxiety and generate new insights, there is very little discussion about increasing confidence for lecturers in a practice context. However, Bentley and Pegram do suggest that 'credibility is dependent on context: knowledge of the clinical area, recency in practice and verification of practice by others are all context specific factors, which allow confidence and competence to be maintained' (2003: 177). This is particularly pertinent in view of the fact the Department of Health (1999) proposed the new programme of nurse education curriculum be founded upon outcomes-based competency principles. However, with the emphasis on clinical skills and the educational reforms within nurse education, one could argue that this may have been achieved at the expense of the theoretical underpinning knowledge of practice (Watson and Thompson, 2000). This is also supported by Gerrish, who questioned whether educational reforms have truly equipped nurses with the 'necessary knowledge, skills and confidence' (2000: 473).

Communication is another common theme referred to throughout the literature regarding confidence, as advanced communication skills enhance confidence in dealing with interpersonal relationships. This dynamic process is influenced by so many factors, both personal and professional, all of which can affect clinical and academic performance and ultimately patient care.

CASE STUDY

Jane was an extremely competent senior clinical nurse when, owing to life changes, it was necessary for her to leave the fast-paced, acute clinical environment that she had been working in for many years and change her professional direction to a slower-paced sphere of nursing. Her ability to perform the technical aspects of her new role was never in question and her clinical competence remained excellent. However, three months into the new job she started to experience anxiety. Upon questioning, it was apparent that the new team was not as cohesive and supportive as the one that she had previously left, and as a consequence her self-confidence was severely undermined in dealing with interpersonal relationships. This in turn affected her clinical expertise, as she did not feel empowered to question established working practices within her new environment and suggest methods of improving patient care with specific client groups. Ultimately, her anxiety increased as her autonomy was affected and she felt that she was unable to offer the best care to her patients. Confidence became a major issue for Jane in all aspects of her work, so much so that she resigned from her post in order to return to an area in which she felt adequately supported.

CONCLUSION

Although the above case study does not demonstrate confidence in the context of competence, it does convey an important message with regard to peer support, teamworking and communication and the effect that they have upon confidence, even in a skilled, experienced nurse. When the clinical experience is such an integral part of nurse education and is such an influencing factor in the professional development of student nurses, the support of new students and staff is of paramount importance. This can make a difference as to whether or not a new member of staff remains in a particular clinical environment, and it may influence the student in confirming their choice of nursing as a career.

FURTHER READING

Balzer-Riley, J. (2003) *Communication in Nursing*, 5th edn. London: Mosby.
Daly, J. (2002) *Contexts of Nursing: An Introduction*. Oxford: Blackwell Science.

REFERENCES

Bentley, J. and Pegram, A. (2003) 'Achieving confidence and competence for lecturers in a practice context'. *Nurse Education in Practice*, 3(3): 171–8.

Brown, B., O'Mara, L., Hunsberger, M., Love, B., Black, M., Crooks, D. and Noesgard, C. (2003) 'Professional confidence in baccalaureate nursing students'. *Nursing Education in Practice*, 3(3): 163–70.

Byrne, A.J., Blagrove, M.T. and McDougall, S.J.P. (2005) 'Dynamic confidence during simulated clinical tasks'. *Post Grad Medical Journal*, 81: 7885–8.

Chesser-Smythe, P. (2005) 'The lived experiences of general student nurses on their first clinical placement: a phenomenological study'. *Nurse Education in Practice*, 5(6): 320–7.

Crooks, D., Carpio, B., Brown, B., Black, M., O'Mara, L. and Noesgard, C. (2005) 'Development of Professional Confidence by post diploma baccalaureate nursing students'. *Nurse Education in Practice*, 5(6): 360–7.

Department of Health (1999) *Department of Health Making a Difference: Strengthening the Nursing, Midwifery and Health Visiting Contribution to Health and Healthcare.* London: The Stationary Office.

Farrand, P., McMullan, M., Jowett, R. and Humphries, A. (2006) 'Implementing competency recommendations into pre registration nursing curricula: effects upon levels of confidence in clinical skills'. *Nurse Education Today*, 26(2): 97–103.

Gerrish, K. (2000) 'Still fumbling along? A comparative study of the newly qualified nurse's perception of transition of student to qualified nurse'. *Journal of Advanced Nursing*, 32(2): 473–80.

Last, L. and Fullbrook, P. (2003) 'Why do students leave? Suggestions from a Delphi study'. *Nurse Education Today*, 23: 449–58.

confidence

Morgan, P.J. and Cleave-Hogg, D. (2002) 'Comparison between medical students' experience, confidence and competence'. *Medical Education*, 36: 534–9.

Neary, M. (1997) 'Project 2000 students' survival kit: a return to the practical room (nursing skills laboratory)'. *Nurse Education Today*, 17(1): 46–52.

Nursing and Midwifery Council (2002) *Standards for the Preparation of Teachers of Nursing, Midwifery and Health Visiting*. London: NMC.

Roach, M.S. (1992) *The Human Act of Caring: A Blueprint for the Healing Professions*. Ottawa: Canadian Hospital Association Press.

United Kingdom Central Council for Nursing, Midwifery and Health Visiting (1999) *Fitness for Practice: Report of the Commission for Education*. London: UKCC.

Watson, R. and Thompson, D.R. (2000) 'Recent developments in UK nurse education: horses for courses or courses for horses?' *Journal of Advanced Nursing*, 32(5): 1041–2.

Williams, S., Dale, J., Glucksman, E. and Wellesley, J. (1997) 'A Senior House Officers' work-related stressors, psychological distress and confidence in performing clinical tasks in accident and emergency: a questionnaire study'. *British Medical Journal*, 314: 713.

Wordnet Search (2006) wordnet.princeton.edu/perl/webwn?s=confidence (accessed 7 Dec. 2006).

Wykurz, G. and Kelly, D. (2002) 'Developing the role of patients as teachers: literature review'. *British Medical Journal*, 325: 818–21.

Cross-References *Communication, Nurturing, Role model, Teamwork.*

13 Coping

Tom Mason

DEFINITION

In defining coping there is always a relationship between a perceived stress and a personal response. Irrespective of the types of stress and the wide array of sources from which it is derived, as well as the wealth of individualised human responses to it, the pivot is the relation between action and reaction. This can be seen in what is possibly the most commonly used definition of coping by Lazarus and Folkman as 'the process of managing external or internal demands that are perceived as taxing or exceeding a person's resources' (1984: 24). Numerous terms have been employed to deal with the concept of coping from an overall generalist perspective to incorporate both behavioural and psychological responses to stress, such as 'coping responses', 'coping mechanisms' and 'coping strategies' (Grasha, 1983; Savickas, 1995). However, when coping is referred to from a psychiatric perspective, the term 'defence mechanism' is usually used to indicate the ways in which a person defends their ego (Gross, 2001).

KEY POINTS

- Coping strategies may be conscious or unconscious.
- Coping strategies can be considered healthy or unhealthy.
- Ways of coping may be behavioural or psychological.
- A person's ego is defended by coping strategies.

DISCUSSION

The study of coping in healthcare has focused on three main areas: (a) the mechanisms involved in coping; (b) the felt experience of coping; and (c) the different ways in which people cope. We are faced with stress in many areas of life and employ coping strategies to overcome them, for example, in healthcare settings (Baron et al., 2003; Zehnder et al., 2006), in facing abuse (Esteban, 2006), when in pain (Collen, 2005) or when managing catastrophic events (Menendez et al., 2006). Furthermore, it is argued that stress and coping feature large in the adolescent–parent stage of normal family relations (Bagdi and Pfister, 2006). Given the numerous ways that people can cope with stressful circumstances, a number of theoretical models have emerged in an attempt to account for this human characteristic. In this chapter we will briefly mention the three main frameworks of coping from (a) psychological, (b) behavioural and (c) psychiatric perspectives.

Psychological

Psychologists have produced a number of theoretical models of coping, and three will be outlined here. Cohen and Lazarus (1979) classified all the coping strategies that people employ when faced with stressful circumstances into the following framework:

- *Direct action response* – in which the person attempts to manage or alter their relationship with the stressor. For example, they may themselves escape from it or they may remove the stressor itself.
- *Information seeking* – this is a coping strategy that employs a deeper understanding of the problem being faced and allows the individual to make predictions about future problems, thus reducing the stress.
- *Inhibition of action* – basically this involves the person doing nothing, which may be the best strategy for short-term stressors.
- *Intrapsychic or palliative coping* – this involves the individual changing their internal response to the stress through mental defence mechanisms or changing their internal emotional state through drugs, alcohol, meditation, yoga, relaxation and so on.
- *Relating* – in which the individual turns to others for help and support.

The second psychological model of coping to be mentioned here is that by Taylor (1986). In this simple model Taylor argues that there is an assessment of the stressful situation in relation to the individual's abilities to challenge, change or overcome the problem being faced.

Later, Folkman and Lazarus (1988) developed a 'Ways of coping' questionnaire from which they further developed their theory of eight main coping strategies. They argued that there were two main perspectives on which people focus when in a stressful position, and these were: *problem-focused*, in which the person perceives something in the environment as troubling, and *emotion-focused*, where the person focuses on managing their internal feelings rather than the external environment. Within the problem-focused perspective they included the two coping strategies named 'confrontive' and 'planning to solve the problem'. In the emotion-focused perspective they highlighted the coping strategies of 'distancing', 'escape-avoidance', 'accepting responsibility', 'exercising self-control of the expression of feelings', 'seeking social support' and 'positive reappraisal'.

Behavioural

From a behaviouralist perspective, coping strategies are said to be either adaptive or maladaptive (Gross, 2001). Adaptive coping would involve such approaches as avoiding situations which bring back painful memories, working through stressful events and consequences, and coming to terms with painful circumstances. Maladaptive coping strategies, on the other hand, may include taking illicit substances, alcohol, engaging in histrionic behaviour, becoming aggressive and deliberate self-harm. However, it must be stated that there are many behaviours that could be placed within both adaptive and maladaptive coping strategies frameworks, and the distinction between overt behavioural responses and inner psychological processes is not always clear. For example, Grasha (1983) identified a number of behavioural and psychological strategies, which overlap, when people employ them in coping with stressful events:

- *Objectivity* – the separation of feelings from thoughts to assist us in understanding how we think and feel in relation to an objective assessment of our behaviours.
- *Logical analysis* – systematically evaluating our problems to assist explanation and make plans for solutions.
- *Concentration* – the ability to shelve, or bracket out, disturbing thoughts and feelings to help us focus on the task in hand.
- *Playfulness* – the ability to enhance the enjoyment of current situations through previous experiences, feelings or thoughts regarding a stressful event.
- *Tolerance of ambiguity* – involves the ability to function when others or ourselves are unable to make rational choices due to the stressful situation being perceived as complicated.
- *Suppression* – the ability to consciously inhibit an impulse, feeling or thought until a more suitable time or place is available.

Many therapeutic techniques used in psychology to help people cope with stress use a combination of behavioural and psychological approaches. For example, cognitive behavioural therapy (CBT) is based on 'changing people's beliefs, attitudes and attributions about their worlds, and so helping them to act more positively and change things for the better' (Banyard and Hayes, 1994: 97). This brings us to our third coping framework of mental defence mechanisms.

coping

Psychiatric

Mental defence mechanisms, also known as 'ego defence mechanisms', 'mental mechanisms' or 'dynamisms', are a part of normal healthy

Compensation	Inversion
Conversion	Projection
Denial	Rationalisation
Displacement	Reaction formation
Dissociation	Rechannelisation (sublimation)
Fantasy	Regression
Idealisation	Repression
Identification	Restitution
Incorporation	Substitution
Internalisation	Symbolisation
Introjection	Undoing

Figure 5   *Major mental defence mechanisms*

psychological functioning but can also be unhealthy and pathological (Laughlin, 1970). Their presence is pathological or normal depending upon the degree in relation to (a) how they are employed, (b) how psychologically efficacious they are as a defence, and (c) whether the net contribution they make to the individual's psychic functioning is constructive or destructive (Clark, 1998). There are around fifty such mental defence mechanisms that have been identified (with literally hundreds of ways in which they can be employed), and are divided into major, minor and combined. The major mental defence mechanisms can be seen in Figure 5.

The reader is directed to the further reading section in this text for a fuller explanation of all these mental defence mechanisms, and we will briefly outline one – that of *denial* – as it is possibly the most commonly understood by both professional and lay persons. Laughlin stated that 'psychologically, denial is a primitive and desperate unconscious method of coping with otherwise intolerable conflict, anxiety and emotional distress or pain' (1970: 57). Denial operates at a primitive level comparable with the psychology of the infant. A painful thought or feeling is denied conscious awareness and is driven into an unconscious state (which later can possibly cause psychological problems). Denial is a complete disavowal or negation of a painful event and is employed to resolve emotional conflict and allay consequent anxiety.

CASE STUDY

Helen, a middle-aged woman working as a paediatric nurse on a children's intensive care ward, was promoted to Ward Sister shortly after a series of deaths on the ward were identified as being the result of an infectious outbreak. She found the increased pressure of responsibility and the children's suffering to be a heavy stress upon her and began drinking alcohol heavily in the evenings. This worsened and she began taking alcohol at work and even stopping her car on the way into work in the mornings to have a drink to steady her nerves. This continued for several months until she was stopped by the police for drink-driving and banned from driving for two years. She was seen by a counsellor and was said to be in denial that her new responsibility was too much for her and was the main cause of her drinking. Following treatment she returned to work in a more junior, non-clinical, post and her consumption of alcohol ceased at work and reduced to a more socially acceptable level in off-duty time.

CONCLUSION

Humans have ways of coping with stressful events, and these can be either consciously or unconsciously derived. The number of ways in which we can respond to stress is only limited by our human imagination, and the array of human behaviours available to us is testimony to this wealth of responses. All sports, hobbies and pastimes may well be employed as coping mechanisms, amongst other things, as can socialising, relaxing and going on holiday. Coping mechanisms can be healthy, physically and psychologically, as well as becoming unhealthy and dangerous. They exist by their nature to defend ourselves, and in effectively doing so they are often difficult for us to identify, as in the case example above. Although we can change our coping mechanisms, we cannot abandon them altogether, as to do so would make us vulnerable to all manner of random thoughts about the bad things that may befall us. Without coping strategies we could not cope.

coping

FURTHER READING

Cramer, P. (2006) *Protecting the Self: Defense Mechanisms in Action*. New York: Guilford Press.

Gross, R. (2001) *Psychology: The Science of Mind and Behaviour*, 4th edn. London: Hodder & Stoughton.

REFERENCES

Bagdi, A. and Pfister, I.K. (2006) 'Childhood stressors and coping actions: a comparison of children and parents perspectives'. *Child & Youth Care Forum*, 35(1): 21–40.

Banyard, P. and Hayes, N. (1994) *Psychology: Theory and Application*. London: Chapman & Hall.

Baron, S.E., Morris, P.K., Goulden, V., Dye, L. and Fielding, D. (2003) 'The relationship between perceived stress and coping mechanisms with treatment outcome in new adult patients with atopic eczema'. *British Journal of Dermatology, Supplement*. 149: 36–7.

Clark, A.J. (1998) *Defense Mechanisms in the Counselling Process*. London: Sage.

Cohen, F. and Lazarus, R.S. (1979) 'Coping with the stresses of illness', in G.C. Stone, F. Cohen and N.E. Ader (eds), *Health Psychology: A Handbook*. San Francisco, CA: Jossey Bass.

Collen, M. (2005) 'Life of pain, life of pleasure: pain from the patients' perspective'. *Journal of Pain and Palliative Care Pharmacotherapy*, 19(4): 45–52.

Esteban, E. (2006) 'Parental verbal abuse: culture-specific coping behaviour of College Students in the Philippines'. *Child Psychiatry & Human Development*, 36(3): 243–59.

Folkman, S. and Lazarus, R.S. (1988) *Manual for the Ways of Coping Questionnaire*. Palo Alto, CA: Consulting Psychologists Press.

Grasha, A.F. (1983) *Practical Applications of Psychology*, 2nd edn. Boston, MD: Little, Brown & Co.

Gross, R. (2001) *Psychology: The Science of Mind and Behaviour*, 4th edn. London: Hodder & Stoughton.

Laughlin, H.P. (1970) *The Ego and its Defenses*. London: Butterworth.

Lazarus, R.S. and Folkman, S. (1984) *Stress, Appraisal and Coping*. New York: Springer.

Menendez, A.M., Molloy, J. and Magaldi, M.C. (2006) 'Health responses of New York City firefighter spouses and their families post September 11, 2001 terrorist attacks'. *Issues in Mental Health Nursing*, 27(8): 905–17.

Savickas, M.L. (1995) 'Work and adjustment', in D. Wedding (ed.), *Behaviour and Medicine*, 2nd edn. St. Louis, MO: Mosby-Year Book.

Taylor, S. (1986) *Health Psychology*. New York: Random House.

Zehnder, D., Prchal, A., Vollrath, M. and Landolt, M. (2006) 'Prospective study of the effectiveness of coping in pediatric patients'. *Child Psychiatry & Human Development*, 36(3): 351–68.

Cross-References *Guilt, Problem solving, Reflection, Sense of humour.*

14 Crisis management

Janet Barton

DEFINITION

Crisis occurs when a person is confronted with a critical incident or stressful event that is perceived as overwhelming despite the use of traditional problem-solving and coping strategies. The events may happen both in a person's private life or their professional arena. A crisis can also cross over from the private to the professional as well as the reverse if the person cannot contain it or is under immense prolonged stress. Often it is not one single event that triggers a crisis but a series of smaller stressors coming together to overwhelm the person. When a crisis does occur it may trigger physiological, affective and/or behavioural responses (Lalonde, 2004).

KEY POINTS

- By its very nature life will bring a person a crisis.
- The older we get or the more time we spend at work, the greater the chances of us facing a crisis.
- The more crises we face, the more able we become to deal successfully with the next one. Each crisis we experience makes us a stronger and more capable person.
- A crisis is a subjective issue.
- Crises can be prioritised.
- There are ways of managing a crisis through coping strategies.
- The ability to manage a crisis comes with professional and personal experience.

DISCUSSION

According to Parsons (1996) there are three types of crises. The first is *immediate*, with little warning of their arrival, probably with no time to research the problem and no plan of action in place. Second is *emerging*, in which they may be slow to form but are, again, unpredictable with particular difficulty in terms of identifying the issues. Third is *sustained*, and these last a long time, possibly weeks and months, and they are usually maintained by speculation, gossip and rumour.

Adversity is a good teacher, and a crisis can teach us a lot about life in general and about ourselves. The key question is how well can we learn from the experience. Dealing with and living through a crisis can be extremely unpleasant, and certain personal qualities will help us cope better, and these include self confidence, humour and resilience.

The idea of managing a crisis within healthcare is a little researched phenomenon and is usually more associated with the worlds of business and politics. There is little in the literature which discusses how to manage a crisis within healthcare. Because of this, the findings of other professions will be drawn upon to transfer the knowledge and utilise the results (Sheaffer and Mano-Negrin, 2003). However, in one healthcare study reporting on the testing of a model to prevent the crisis of medical disputes, Tzeng claims that in-service training should feature large in healthcare organisations and that 'one of the main purposes of offering on-job training related to crisis management is to build an atmosphere which promotes quality of nursing care through preventing the incidences of medical errors and medical disputes' (2006: 560).

When talking about a crisis, it immediately brings to mind such concepts as stress, chaos, a problem requiring immediate resolution and at the very least immediate considerations to correct something. A crisis is a very subjective experience, as what one individual perceives as a problem to be solved in a methodical manner and at speed, another may think of it as a problem which although may require a methodical approach to rectify, may take time to come to an optimal outcome. In all cases there is one common denominator, that is, that a problem has arisen that requires action to rectify. There are many types of crises which a person may wish to prioritise. For example, a person may view a crisis as not being able to join friends on an evening out as they are working the late shift, yet whilst working on that shift there is a life-threatening incident to a patient when they suffer a cardiac arrest. Under these circumstances the first perceived crisis falls into its rightful place as a low priority, as the life-threatening incident rises to the top of the list for managing a crisis. The ability to manage a crisis comes through the experience of the individual, both professionally and through life experiences. These experiences can be utilised through the process of reflecting (Gibbs, 1988), thus enabling the person to bring these experiences to the forefront should a crisis emerge. Crisis management does not follow a rigid set of rules (Hwang and Lichtenthal, 2000).

Factors

1. A stimulus that sets off an action, process or series of events.
2. The individual dealing with the crisis experiences distress.
3. There is a probability of there being a loss, danger or humiliation to a person or property, or both.
4. The person involved has little control of the factors influencing the crisis.
5. The event feels unexpected and so the person has not had time to plan.
6. There is a disruption to the routine.
7. The outcome is initially unknown.
8. A crisis can be a short or long duration.

Principles of crisis management

- *Step 1*: Validate the problem; get as much information as possible that may influence decision making on how to react. This can be done through communication skills.
- *Step 2*: Evaluate the severity of the crisis.
- *Step 3*: Ensure the safety of those involved in the crisis management, including oneself.
- *Step 4*: Explore all options for dealing with the crisis and develop a specific action plan. Obtain commitment and support from the appropriate people. Use appropriate coping strategies. Focus on strengths and confidence, use these to learn from them and adapt them to the current situation.
- *Step 5*: Follow up the outcome when the crisis is resolved to evaluate and reinforce actions where appropriate.

crisis management

Although it is difficult to foresee the specifics of a future crisis, which makes it difficult to formulate a specific plan, we can be forearmed by organising a general outline plan of action. Sapriel (2003) outlined the components of a business contingency plan of action, which includes risk identification and evaluation, assessment of severe or minor losses to be incurred, and a set of plans to include crisis management, business continuity and business recovery. The general plan may also include such aspects as accessing managing resources, dealing with communication including media, next of kin and both up and down management levels. Plans may also include operationalising legal teams if there are legal implications, dealing with emotional reactions of those involved, and how to respond in order to provide support and stabilise the event. The more one can get right from the outset, the better the chance of effective crisis management.

CASE STUDY

Julie, a staff nurse, has been qualified for six months. She is based on a 36-bedded surgical ward. One day she went on late duty to the ward to be told by the Sister in charge that the senior nurse had telephoned in sick and that she would have to take charge. Furthermore, she would only have two care assistants to support her. Julie did think that it was wrong to have been put in that situation and did have some concerns, which she kept to herself. However, she did feel that she could cope. After the early shift went off duty a crisis developed. A patient began to deteriorate, which demanded Julie's attention, whilst in the meantime a patient fell out of bed and one of the carers became ill. Julie felt very stressed and started to feel that she was not coping. Using her problem-solving abilities she knew she needed help and support if the crisis was to be resolved without further deterioration. Julie telephoned the Matron, who sent her some trained staff to help. The crisis was resolved and Julie learnt from the experience. Julie learnt to be assertive the next time a similar scenario occurred, and insisted on acquiring trained staff help before the early shift went off duty. She also documented her concerns if assistance was not forthcoming.

CONCLUSION

People are individuals, and how they approach and manage a crisis will vary. It is important that we maintain a sense of perspective and be objective. We need to act in order to bring a crisis to an end. A sense of humour can be invaluable in times of great stress. Remember that a crisis will come to an end even if when it is happening it appears unresolvable. Be positive and have confidence in yourself, and do not worsen the situation by overstating the problem. Treat a problem as a problem before it turns into a crisis. Many people have been through worse, and it may be that we have to face worse in the future, but face it and come through it a stronger and more confident person. Do not merely survive a crisis, but thrive on it as well.

FURTHER READING

Sapriel, C. (2003) 'Effective crisis management: tools and best practice for the new millennium'. *Journal of Communication Management*, 7(4): 348–55.

Tzeng, H.-M. (2006) 'Model testing on the crisis interventions and actions to prevent medical disputes: a Taiwanese nursing perspective'. *Journal of Clinical Nursing*, 15(5): 554–64.

REFERENCES

Gibbs, G. (1988) *Learning by Doing. A Guide to Teaching and Learning Methods Further Education Unit*. Oxford: Oxford Polytechnic.

Hwang, P. and Lichtenthal, J.D. (2000) 'Anatomy of organizational crises'. *Journal of Contingencies and Crisis Management*, 8(3): 129–38.

Lalonde, C. (2004) 'In search of archetypes in crisis management'. *Journal of Contingencies and Crisis Management*, 12(2): 76–88

Parsons, W. (1996) 'Crisis management'. *Career Development International*, 25(2): 43–6.

Sapriel, C. (2003) 'Effective crisis management: tools and best practice for the new millennium'. *Journal of Communication Management*, 7(4): 348–55.

Sheaffer, Z. and Mano-Negrin, R. (2003) 'Executives' orientations as indicators of crisis management policies and practices'. *Journal of Management Studies*, 40(2): 573–606.

Tzeng, H.-M. (2006) 'Model testing on the crisis interventions and actions to prevent medical disputes: a Taiwanese nursing perspective'. *Journal of Clinical Nursing*, 15(5): 554–64.

Cross-References *Communication, Coping, Problem solving, Sense of humour.*

15 Data, information, knowledge

Adam Keen

DEFINITIONS

The term 'data' is defined as a unit (or units) of fact without any understanding of how one fact may relate to another. Consequently, data are symbols open to interpretation, but existing without meaning. Information is defined when data is formatted, structured and named (Desrosières, 1998). In simple terms, information is data with an associated understanding of context that leads to the identification of meaning. As a result, information is a dynamic concept dependant on an individual's ability to understand data. Knowledge is defined as the understanding required for the use of information in order to bring about action (Desrosières, 1998). Subsequently, knowledge is complex (Hebda et al., 2005) and has associations with learning; for example, where data and information can be easily transferred, knowledge must be learned. Keen's (2007) model of data information and knowledge hierarchy is illustrated in Figure 6.

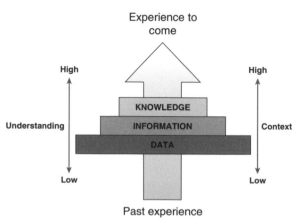

Figure 6   *The data information and knowledge hierarchy (adapted from Keen, 2007)*

KEY POINTS

- Data and information can be readily transferred, whereas knowledge must be learned.
- Movement up the data, information and knowledge hierarchy requires an increased level of understanding of context within the individual.
- Any profession seeks to distinguish itself from other professions through the development of a body of knowledge.
- The concepts of information and knowledge are associated with issues of power and responsibility.
- Health informatics is the study and processing of information related to healthcare.

DISCUSSION

The title of this chapter may at first appear odd within a text on key concepts in nursing. Surely data, information and knowledge are three separate concepts and deserve individual attention? Yet, when defining any one concept it is necessary to consider how it is bordered by those related to it (Gerring, 2001). It should be noted that of the three, knowledge represents the concept attached to the greatest degree of uncertainty. The nature of knowledge represents an ongoing philosophical debate beyond the scope of this chapter. However, in examining individual definitions of data, information and knowledge, it is possible to identify a bond that fuses each concept together within a hierarchy (Desrosières, 1998; Georgiou, 2002).

Figure 7 shows the relationship that exists between the concepts of data information and knowledge. The diagram illustrates that by increasing an understanding of context, data is interpreted and information is formed. Furthermore, by widening contextual understanding of information it becomes possible to learn how information can be used to bring about action, thus generating knowledge. Such a hierarchy is not a new concept (Georgiou, 2002), and Desrosières (1998) described the origin of the hierarchy as a consequence of the social need to share knowledge. Through the sharing of knowledge, new actions can take place, and consequently through the creation and classification of new data, new knowledge can be generated. In this sense, data originates from a knowledgeable action; information originates from the classification and naming of data; and knowledge and learning result from the logical development of past information into new actions (Desrosières, 1998). Hence an 'action–data–information' cycle can facilitate the classification and storage of new knowledge (see Figure 7) (Desrosières, 1998).

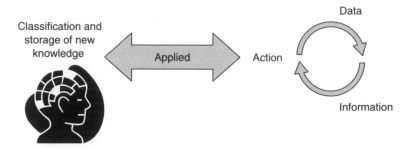

Figure 7   *The action–data–information cycle*

Given that a number of philosophical theories exist relating to the nature of knowledge, it is perhaps unsurprising that numerous classifications of 'nursing knowledge' can be found within literature. Of the many classifications in use, it is possible to identify a degree of overlap existing between types. For example, Edwards (2002) identified two broad categories of nursing knowledge: propositional and practical. Propositional knowledge (also referred to as declarative knowledge) represents the ability to describe how data and information may be used to carry out an action, whereas, practical knowledge is the know-how required for using this propositional knowledge to carry out the action for real. For example, it is possible to learn how the nursing process is used to deliver individualised care by reading a text book; this is an example of developing propositional knowledge. However, to utilise the nursing process in a practice setting requires the additional knowledge of how to apply a linear description of care delivery in a non-linear reality; this is an example of practical knowledge. It should be stressed that Edward's classification of nursing knowledge into two types is somewhat limited. Where propositional knowledge relates to questions of 'what to do', and practical knowledge relates to questions of 'how to do it', a third category of knowledge 'conditional' can be argued to exist relating to the fundamental questions of 'when', 'where' and 'why' a nurse should act. This third category of knowledge relates specifically to the nurse's ability to think strategically (Anderson, 1983), and to apply this strategic thinking into action.

The concepts of propositional knowledge and practical knowledge can be shown to relate to Benner's (1984) model for the development of clinical competence. According to Benner, a novice nurse has dependence on generalised theoretical rules of conduct (propositional knowledge). As the novice acquires experience, learning occurs through action, and the nurse begins to make sense of situational data to form information. This is then used to form knowledge for future actions (practical knowledge), thus facilitating the development of competence through experiential learning. Experiential learning theories, such as that of Benner's, are well acknowledged within education (Gibbs, 1988; Kolb, 1984; Quinn, 2000), and have come to represent a cornerstone of nurse education. It is possible to trace the historical roots of the perceived need for nursing knowledge. According to Nightingale (1860), it is recognised as the knowledge which everyone ought to have, as distinct from medical knowledge, which only a professional can have.

Nightingale's emphasis relates to nursing knowledge as a practical everyday reality, common to all, and consequently akin to the concept of common sense. Such a notion is obviously at odds to the emphasis given today on nursing as a profession developing specialist practitioners. Indeed, Edwards (2002) argued that the development of a nursing body of knowledge is perceived as a major contributor to the recognition of nursing as a profession. In comparing these two perspectives it becomes possible to identify two polar identities which can be related to the concept of power as described by the theories of Postman (1993) and Bauman (2002), and can be seen in Figure 8.

Consider as an example an intensive care unit. Within this highly technical environment there is, for patients and their families, an utter reliance on the specialised skills of those providing care. To the novice, the plethora of data that is generated as a result of the various treatments can be intimidating. The ability to interpret data into meaningful information

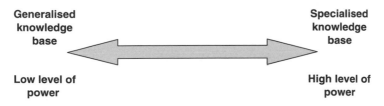

Figure 8   *Generalised versus specialised knowledge continuum*

which can be used to inform care requires specialist knowledge. Nurses in possession of this knowledge assume an authority for the social, psychological and moral affairs of those in their care. Patients and their families are alienated from a generalised view of their illness and treatment as a consequence of the restricted specialist knowledge of the nurse. This triggers a subsequent reliance on additional specialists to 'fill in the gaps', and as patient care progresses, a fragmentation of power occurs. By retaining expertise, the specialised organisation denies an individual the right to action by alienating them from any other source of information. In effect, the organisation (acting as a bureaucracy) has a monopoly on information and therefore can control its application.

By accepting the notion that data, information and knowledge are connected to the concept of power, it becomes important to recognise that an inherent responsibility not to abuse this power is placed on the nurse. This is in part recognised within the United Kingdom by statutory law through acts such as the Nursing and Midwifery Order (2001), responsible for the creation of the Nursing & Midwifery Council, the Data Protection Act (1998) and the Freedom to Information Act (2000). Although these measures go some way to protect individuals accessing healthcare systems (and similar bureaucracies), it can be argued that they are insufficient to prevent the alienation and disempowerment of patients. Indeed, the presence of statutory law can become a useful defence for bureaucracies to defend their monopoly on access to information.

In tandem with the responsibility to ensure that a position of power is not abused, the nurse has an obligation to ensure that patient-specific data is well managed. In healthcare the study of how information can be managed and applied is defined under the umbrella term of *health informatics* (Abbott et al., 2004). The term *information governance* is given to the narrower focus of how information is held, obtained, recorded, shared and used ethically (Cayton, 2006). Given the central role of the nurse in the collection, interpretation and use of patient data, it can be argued that information governance is already a concern to nurses, and therefore health informatics is deserving of specific emphasis within nurse education programmes.

CASE STUDY

Percy is 76 and has been unwell for some time. Experiencing weight loss, a lack of appetite and some central back pain, he is finding coping alone in his bungalow quite difficult and has to rely increasingly on the help of his family. After seeing his general practitioner he was sent to hospital for an urgent scan and met with a consultant surgeon the same day. Percy was worried that the diagnosis was not going to be good news, and asked his daughter to speak with the surgeon on his behalf. He stressed that he did not want to know anything about the diagnosis just yet. The surgeon respectful of Percy's wishes offered to refer Percy to the community nursing team for support in the coming weeks.

On meeting Percy in his home, the community nurse explained that she had received some details from the surgeon and had compiled a set of case notes. She used her professional knowledge to collect and document assessment data from Percy. She then interpreted this data to form information as to Percy's specific needs. In implementing knowledge she formulated a plan of care and carefully documented this. As part of the plan it was agreed that the nurse would visit again in two week's time. The nurse explained that it was normal for patients to keep hold of their case file between visits, and Percy agreed to do this. When looking at the file some time after the nurse had left, Percy read his diagnosis of primary pancreatic cancer with lung and liver metastases. He later contacted his daughter expressing concern at his diagnosis and wanting information his daughter could not provide.

In this case study the nurse can be seen to use knowledge to generate new data which is then interpreted to form information. This in turn is used to design a plan of care, demonstrating an additional use of knowledge. Thus the action–data–information cycle (Desrosières, 1998) is seen to repeat. The patient's inadvertent discovery of diagnosis highlights the need to manage patient information carefully. Here no breach of confidentiality has been made; however, the information held by the caring team had not been used in concordance with the patient's wishes. This arguably represents an unethical use of information resulting in the isolation of the patient. The mismanagement of information illustrated in this scenario could have occurred for numerous reasons; it should therefore be stressed that the responsibility for the management of patient information involves all those who have access.

CONCLUSION

It is only through the development of a contextual understanding of data existing within our environment that we can hope to form meaningful information. By learning how to apply this information to generate action, we can be said to acquire knowledge. Whereas data is factual, information and knowledge represent dynamic concepts dependant on the level of understanding held by the individual. Closely associated to the concept of knowledge is the associated notion of power. Power associated to specialist knowledge is inherent within nurse–patient relationships, and consequently nurses must recognise a responsibility not to abuse this level of trust.

FURTHER READING

Edwards, S. (2002) 'Philosophy, nursing and knowledge', in J. Daly, S. Speedy, D. Jackson and P. Darbyshire (eds), *Contexts of Nursing: An Introduction*. Oxford: Blackwell.

Georgiou, A. (2002) 'Data, information and knowledge: the health informatics model and its role in evidence-based medicine'. *Journal in Evaluation in Clinical Practice*, 8(2): 127–30.

REFERENCES

Abbott, W., Blankley, N., Bryant, J. and Bullas, S. (2004) *Current Perspectives: Information in Healthcare*. Swindon: British Computer Society Health Informatics Committee.

Anderson, J.R. (1983) *The Architecture of Cognition*. Cambridge, MA: Harvard University Press.

Bauman, Z. (2002) *Modernity and the Holocaust*. Oxford: Blackwell.

Benner, P. (1984) *From Novice to Expert: Excellence and Power in Clinical Nursing Practice*. Menlo Park, CA: Addison-Wesley.

Cayton, H. (2006) *Information Governance in the Department of Health and the NHS*. Crown Copyright: Department of Health. www.connectingforhealth.nhs.uk/crdb/information_governance_review.pdf (accessed 19 Jan. 2007).

Data Protection Act (1998) *Chapter 29*. Crown Copyright. www.opsi.gov.uk/acts/acts1998/19980029.htm (accessed 19 Jan. 2007).

Desrosières, A. (1998) *The Politics of Large Numbers: A History of Statistical Reasoning*. London: Havard University Press.

Edwards, S. (2002) 'Philosophy, nursing and knowledge', in J. Daly, S. Speedy, D. Jackson and P. Darbyshire (eds), *Contexts of Nursing: An Introduction*. Oxford: Blackwell.

Freedom of Information Act (2000) *Chapter 36*, Crown Copyright. www.opsi.gov.uk/acts/acts2000/20000036.htm (accessed 19 Jan. 2007).

Georgiou, A. (2002) 'Data, information and knowledge: the health informatics model and its role in evidence-based medicine'. *Journal in Evaluation in Clinical Practice*, 8(2): 127–30.

Gerring, J. (2001) *Social Science Methodology; A Criterial Framework*. Cambridge: Cambridge University Press.

Gibbs, G. (1988) *Learning by Doing. A Guide to Teaching and Learning Methods.* Oxford: Further Education Unit, Oxford Polytechnic.

Hebda, T., Czar, P. and Mascara, C. (2005) *Handbook of Informatics for Nurses and Health care Professionals.* New York: Pearson Prentice Hall.

Keen, A. (2007) 'Health informatics', in R. Hogston and B. Marjoram (eds), *Foundations of Nursing Practice,* 3rd edn. Basingstoke: Palgrave McMillan.

Kolb, D.A. (1984) *Experiential Learning: Experience as the Source of Learning and Development.* New York: Prentice-Hall.

Nightingale, F. (1860) *Notes on Nursing: What it is and What it is Not.* New York: D. Appleton and Company. http://digital.library.upenn.edu/women/nightingale/nursing/nursing.html (accessed 17 Jan. 2007).

Nursing and Midwifery Order (2001) *Statutory Instrument 2002 Number 253,* Crown Copyright. www.opsi.gov.uk/si/si2002/20020253.html (accessed 19 Jan. 2007).

Postman, N. (1993) *Technopoly: The Surrender of Culture to Technology.* New York: Vintage Books.

Quinn, F.M. (2000) *Principles and Practice of Nurse Education,* 4th edn. Cheltenham: Stanley Thorns.

Cross-References *Accountability, Feedback, Managing technology, Record keeping.*

16 Dignity

Victoria Ridgway

DEFINITION

When defining dignity it is important to examine its origins within healthcare and especially nursing. Dignity is cited in models of care, standards and professional codes. The Nursing and Midwifery *Code of Professional Conduct* (2004) states that all registered nurses should respect the patient as an individual, by promoting and protecting their dignity. Furthermore, the *Essence of Care* (DoH, 2001a) document identifies factors relating to privacy and dignity for health practitioners to benchmark against.

Although the term has entered our popular vocabulary, it has to be questioned whether nurses fully understand the term. This is somewhat hindered and reinforced within healthcare literature, as the concept of dignity or its meaning is not always made clear. It is widely accepted within healthcare that in providing and maintaining a client's dignity they will potentially receive better care; those who experience a lack of dignity conversely then may encounter poorer health interventions and have less positive outcomes in relation to care received (Walsh and Kowanko, 2002).

The word 'dignity' is derived from the Latin meaning worthy. *The Oxford Dictionary* (1983) suggests dignity can be used in three ways; first, defining the concept as 'a calm and serious manner or style showing suitable formality or indicating that one deserves respect'. The second entry draws upon the concept of 'worthiness', and the third refers to an individual's rank or position. Furthermore, the word 'honour' is used in many definitions (*Webster's International Dictionary*, 1986). Therefore, dignity is a state, quality or manner worthy of esteem, respect and self-respect, so dignity refers to care in any setting which supports and promotes, and does not undermine, a person's self-respect regardless of any difference. Thus, this definition of dignity is based upon the moral requirements to respect all human beings, irrespective of individual differences (Dignity and Older Europeans Project, 2006). Pullman (1999) concurs with this and philosophically refers to basic human dignity as being recognised to all irrespective of colour, class or creed. Thus dignity is not a quality of being highly valued, but is the highest human value (wikipedia.org).

KEY POINTS

- Characteristics of dignity are varied and vast.
- Nurses are exhorted to maintain a client's dignity.
- Individuals expect that their dignity will be preserved.
- Lack of dignity may lead to poorer health outcomes.
- Patient dignity is highly valued by patients.

DISCUSSION

The concept of dignity within healthcare draws upon elements of respect and the nature of clients' healthcare needs, and illustrates the relevance of the three dictionary definitions. First, we refer to formality. To a certain degree this exists between a client and a nurse and serves to protect the individual, allowing the nurse to provide essential care in close proximity which in other circumstances would be unacceptable. Second, worthiness or respect, where each person has a fundamental right to be respected, despite the literature strongly suggesting that respect should be earned. Third, the dictionary refers to rank or position. Here, by the very nature of our roles as nurses and clients, a certain hierarchy in the relationship exists. Hospitals in particular can depersonalise an individual; for example, routines maintained at home are different in a hospital environment, and illness and disability can remove a person's ability to self-care. Therefore, with the removal of normal roles and behaviours a person's dignity may be important to maintain. This relates to the Human Rights Act (1998). Conversely, Oxtoby (2003) suggested that this can present risks to a person maintaining their dignity, and Birrell and Jones (2006) concur with this. Thus, dignity is care in any setting that supports, promotes, and does not undermine a person's self-respect regardless of any difference. Furthermore, if dignity is viewed in this manner, consideration must be given to an infant who we may presume has less dignity (wikipedia.org).

Mairis (1994), in attempting to clarify a definition of dignity, categorised the concept into: maintenance of self-respect, maintenance of self-esteem, and appreciation of individual standards. Furthermore, Mairis demonstrated that there are four basic prerequisites that are necessary for dignity to exist. First, 'dignity as an human quality'. This could refer to person worthiness or respect; however, Mairis argues that it can solely be a human quality. Furthermore, Saner (1980), cited in Walsh and Kowanko (2002), referred to dignity as an innate human freedom. Second, self-advocacy promotes dignity; this could refer to informed consent, individual choice and information receiving, all ensuring an individual's dignity is maintained. Third, Mairis states that 'dignity may be demonstrated by behaviour, speech, conduct and dress'. This concept is discussed widely within health literature, drawing upon a person's behaviour as an outward sign of personal standards and opinions. Finally, Mairis referred to dignity being developed by individual life experiences. This can be cross-referenced with the third concept and has a direct correlation with behaviour, dress, conduct and speech, which in turn are informed by role modelling, values, beliefs, attitudes and persons' responses to life experience. So, people learn to preserve their dignity as a number of finite measurable qualities, merits and achievements because people around them will constantly estimate, evaluate and appreciate them. George (1998) concurs with this, referring to dignity being bestowed on individuals within their social environment.

Characteristics of dignity can be vast and varied (Walsh and Kowanko, 2002), ranging from a positive self-image, with an individual being described as composed, self-controlled, to an individual experiencing feelings of value, worth, confidence and pride. When dignity is lost, self-image may be lacking or poor, and literature refers to loss of pride, worth and value. Furthermore, Mairis (1994) refers to feelings of ridicule, embarrassment, shame, foolishness, degradation, humiliation and distress. In addition, patients refer to their emotional response when they experience a lack of dignity, which includes anger, anxiety and embarrassment (Walsh and Kowanko, 2002).

Themes relating to dignity in relation to the role and duty of a nurse include providing privacy and private space, consideration of a client's emotions and feelings, giving time, treating the client as an individual/person and providing respect, advocacy and control towards the client (Walsh and Kowanko, 2002). However, qualifying these actions and behaviours is difficult owing to the problems involved in the measurement of emotional support and respect and the demonstration of value. Furthermore, patients' perceptions of dignity emphasise being exposed, being acknowledged, the nurse showing discretion, consideration, not being rushed, or seen as an object, being given time to decide and make choices and, most importantly, being seen as a person (Walsh and Kowanko, 2002).

Factors that have been held responsible for the absence of dignity are many. Birrell and Jones (2006) cited mixed-sex wards, mixing tablets with food, derogatory labels and exposure of body parts. Furthermore, work by Cooper and Coleman (2001) reported that nurses perceive patients according to their mental capacity and physical appearance, citing that a disfigured person may be viewed as less human.

The Department of Health (2006) has recently published guidance aimed at improving dignity in care and draws upon lack of respect for an individual's dignity in care, stating that this can take many forms and the experience will, and may, differ from person to person. Examples include having to eat with their fingers; being rushed and not listened to; having their privacy neglected, for example, having to use a commode in the hospital ward rather than being wheeled to the toilet. Many other guidelines exist, including the *National Service Framework for Older People* (DoH, 2001b), which refers to dignity in care, and Help the Aged (1999), which has raised the issue of older people's dignity.

CASE STUDY

A student nurse during her first clinical experience is instructed by her mentor, a qualified nurse, to feed Mary at lunch. The student is aware that Mary is a new resident, who was transferred from an acute ward following a stroke. The student collects the appropriate tray and proceeds to Mary who is seated at the table with three other residents. The student introduces herself and then commences the skill of feeding Mary using a spoon. Mary opens her mouth chews and swallows the food. However, during the process tears fall down her cheeks. The student, disturbed by this, stops and wipes Mary's face, then continues with the task until the food has been consumed. Following the procedure the student reflects upon the experience, trying to understand why Mary had cried. She decides to read Mary's assessment details and discovers Mary is capable of feeding herself. The next day when instructed by her mentor to feed Mary, instead of performing the skill, the student gives Mary the fork. Mary smiles and says, 'Thank you'.

CONCLUSION

Dignity for patients and clients involves elements of respect, privacy, control, advocacy and time. Dignity is an inherent characteristic of human beings, coming from within; for example, personal attributes and individual behaviours coupled with respect conferred towards others are key attributes (Jacelon et al., 2004). Furthermore, dignity is a learnt behaviour.

Therefore, to maintain an individual's dignity takes many forms and differs according to that particular person. Walsh and Kowanko (2002) observed that nurses and patients have different perceptions of dignity. This presents a challenge to nurses as an individual persona is influenced by experience, upbringing, education, rank and role. Consequently, ensuring dignity is to treat an individual as an equal, ensuring respect, privacy and confidentiality, providing choice, making a person feel accepted and ensuring a quality service (Policy Research Institute on Ageing and Ethnicity, 2001).

dignity

FURTHER READING

Department of Health (2006) *Dignity in Care, Practice Guide*. London: Department of Health Publications.

REFERENCES

Birrell, J. and Jones, C.A. (2006) 'Promoting privacy and dignity for older patients in hospital'. *Nursing Standard*, 20(18): 41–6.

Cooper, S.A. and Coleman, P.G. (2001) 'Caring for the older person: an exploration of perceptions using personal construct theory'. *Age and Ageing*, 30(5): 399–402.

Department of Health (2001a) *Essence of Care: Patient Focused Benchmarking for Clinical Governance*. London: HMSO.

Department of Health (2001b) *National Service Framework for Older People*. London: The Stationary Office.

Department of Health (2006) *Dignity in Care, Practice Guide*. London: Department of Health Publications.

Dignity and Older Europeans Project (2006) www.cf.ac/dignity

George, L.J. (1998) 'Dignity and quality of life in old age'. *Journal of Gerontological Social Work*, 29: 39–52.

Help the Aged (1999) *The Views of Older People on Hospital Care: A Survey*. London: Help the Aged.

Human Rights Act (1998) www.pfc.org.uk/node/300

Jacelon, C.S., Connelly, T.W., Brown, R., Proulx, K. and Vo, T. (2004) 'A concept analysis of dignity for older adults'. *Journal of Advanced Nursing*, 48(1): 76–83.

Mairis, E.D. (1994) 'Concept clarification in professional practice-dignity'. *Journal of Advanced Nursing*, 19: 947–53.

Nursing Midwifery Council (2004) *The NMC Code of Professional Conduct Standards for Conduct, Performance and Ethics*. London: NMC.

The Oxford Paperback Dictionary (1983), 2nd edn. Oxford: Oxford University Press.

Oxtoby, K. (2003) 'Preserving patients privacy and dignity'. *Nursing Times*, 99(48): 18–21.

Policy Research Institute on Ageing and Ethnicity (PRIAE) (2001) *Dignity on the Ward, Policy Research Institute on Ageing and Ethnicity*. Bradford: University of Bradford.

Pullman, D. (1999) 'The ethics of autonomy and dignity in long-term care'. *Canadian Journal of Ageing*, 18: 24–46.

Saner, H. (1980) 'The dignity and rights of the patient'. *Bulletin Der Schweizer Akademie Der Medizinischen Wissenschaften*. 36: 235–47.

Walsh, K. and Kowanko, I. (2002) 'Nurses' and patients' perceptions of dignity'. *International Journal of Nursing Practice*, 8: 143–51.

Webster's International Dictionary (1986) *Webster's Third New International Dictionary of the English Language, Unabridged. With Seven Language Dictionary*. Chicago, IL: Encyclopaedia Britannica.

Wikipedia.org/wiki/Dignity

Cross-References *Advocacy, Autonomy, Caring, Communication, Compassion, Empowerment, Reflection.*

17 Diversity

Julie Bailey-McHale

DEFINITION

In recent years diversity and difference have become key concepts in political, social and cultural theory. The changing nature of the world we live in, particularly with increasing cultural diversity, has led to changing perceptions of the nature of society. The concept of diversity is particularly difficult to define. It is closely associated with concepts such as difference and equality. Its use has grown recently and it is now common for organisations to have a diversity statement. The concept implies an acceptance of the uniqueness of each individual and the recognition of difference. Kandola and Fullerton (1998) defined diversity as the range of visible and non-visible differences that exist between people. They further considered that managing diversity harnesses these differences to create a productive environment in which all individuals feel valued, where talents are fully utilised and organisational goals are met. It is the acceptance of the presence of a wide variety of characteristics that help to define an individual, including: race, ethnicity, gender, sexual orientation, socio-economic status, age, ability and faith.

KEY POINTS

- Diversity acknowledges the intrinsic worth and uniqueness of each individual.
- It refers to a range of characteristics that may or may not be labelled as deviant within a culture.
- Diversity is closely linked with concepts such as equality, prejudice, discrimination and anti-discriminatory practices.

DISCUSSION

The concept of diversity is an important consideration for health and social care professionals. Arguably, it is inconceivable to think about a

diversity

person without being aware of differences. We tend to think of others in terms of female/male, black/white, gay/straight and so on, defining them as either/or. The Nursing and Midwifery Council (2004) insist that nurses should protect the interests and dignity of patients regardless of their gender, age, race, ability, sexuality, economic status, lifestyle, culture and religious or political beliefs. While some nurses are convinced that they do treat everyone the same, this perception in itself displays a lack of awareness and understanding of the complex nature of diversity. We would not expect a woman to provide a urine sample in a bottle, nor would we offer a lamb chop to a vegetarian! Offering the same treatment to all is not acceptable, as care should be established on the basis of individual need and not on the assumption of sameness. An understanding of diversity and difference can help to highlight these issues. Nytanga (2001) argued that understanding cultural diversity is important for three reasons: it provides an opportunity to learn about different ways of understanding the world; it enables an appreciation of the commonalities amongst cultures; and it demonstrates ways of interacting with each other. Recognising and celebrating equality, diversity and rights is fundamental to caring.

The concept of diversity needs to be understood in relation to a number of other important concepts, particularly the impact of prejudice, stereotypes and discrimination. Giddens (2006) described prejudice as opinions or attitudes held by one group about another. Prejudice is often based on stereotypes. The power of a stereotype cannot be underestimated. Chryssochoou (2004) noted that a stereotype could be classified as the grouping of particular characteristics which form a psychological representation of the individual or group. Discrimination is often the result of stereotyping and refers to actual behaviours towards an individual or a group (Giddens, 2006). Thompson (2006) adds that discrimination takes place on three levels:

- *Personal level*: individual thoughts, feelings and actions.
- *Cultural context*: common values and shared ways of thinking.
- *Structural level*: the accepted social order and accepted social divisions.

An individual can have prejudiced beliefs and opinions based on stereotyped views. However, discrimination only occurs when those beliefs are translated into negative behaviours.

Stereotypes, prejudice and discrimination can lead to oppression, which can become internalised. Oppression can be understood in terms of the systematic subjugation of a group of people by another group of people; this subjugation is often maintained by social beliefs and practices. When oppressed group members believe the messages relayed to them they can internalise those messages, leading to internalised oppression. If individuals accept those beliefs, then the original stereotypes are perpetuated and this reinforces the prejudice. The sociological theory of labelling is useful here to understand how difference can be labelled as bad or not normal. Labelling theory suggests that the social categories created within a society are a reflection of the power structure evident in that society. What is important is to examine which groups in society have the power to label others as different. Howard Becker is a sociologist mostly associated with labelling theory. Becker argued that deviant behaviour only becomes deviant when it is labelled as such, and his theory starts from the assumption that no act is intrinsically deviant (Giddens, 2006).

The concept of multiple oppressions is also worth considering. The importance of this can be demonstrated if the experience of a young woman who identifies as a lesbian with a psychiatric diagnosis of bipolar disorder is considered. She may experience discrimination at a number of levels on the basis of her gender, sexual orientation and psychiatric diagnosis. Her experiences will be different to a heterosexual male with the same diagnosis. Thompson (2006) would argue that the structure of the oppression is the same for all oppressed groups. However, the oppression would be experienced differently. Therefore, it is important for nurses to acknowledge their own values and beliefs when caring for another; racism, ageism, sexism and heterosexism are examples of prejudice that may be held by a nurse. By an individual acknowledging their own prejudice and challenging taken-for-granted assumptions, acts of discrimination can be prevented.

The concept of diversity is not entirely unproblematic. Often the idea of diversity is seen as being in opposition to social unity. A consideration of the concept of multiculturalism in relation to diversity can highlight difficulties. Three approaches have been suggested to describe ethnic integration: assimilation, the melting pot theory and cultural pluralism (Hartmann and Gerteis, 2005). Assimilation reflects the notion that immigrants should abandon their cultural norms in favour of the values and norms of the society they have entered. The concept of 'the melting pot society' suggests that cultural differences are merged and become blended to make up new values and norms. Cultural pluralism recognises the equal validity of a range of subcultures, therefore ethnic differences are respected and celebrated.

There is much investigation into the effects of various cultural differences on health and well being. The idea that health and illness are socially patterned and not random phenomena is widely accepted (Nettleton and Gustafsson, 2002). The debate concentrates on the causes of these differences. Understanding cultural norms and values will inevitably impact on the quality of care a nurse can offer patients. Inequalities in health on the basis of gender, socio-economic status and ethnicity are well established (Acheson, 1998). The effects of sexuality on health and well being have also been the subject of research. Dean et al. (2000) referred to some healthcare workers feeling uncomfortable providing healthcare for lesbian, gay and bisexual people. Mackereth (1995) highlighted the impact of heterosexism and homophobia on healthcare provision. Robertson (1998) and Cant (2005) revealed the reluctance of gay men to disclose their sexuality in healthcare settings. Acknowledging and respecting difference and diversity in the people we care for is essential for effective healthcare.

CASE STUDY

Trevor is a 52-year-old man who has been suffering with cholecystitis for the past six months. He is being admitted to hospital for planned surgery. Trevor has enjoyed a long-term relationship with his male partner, Ted, for twenty-two years. They have recently entered into a civil partnership. Although Trevor is 'out' with certain close friends, he is worried about telling the nurse about his sexuality. On a previous admission to hospital ten years ago his partnership was completely ignored and he was told that his partner could not be his next of kin. Whilst in the waiting room Trevor notices that all of the posters and leaflets have images of heterosexual couples and there is no literature that refers to lesbian, gay, bisexual or transgender issues. On being admitted to the ward the nurse refers to Trevor's partner as his 'friend'. Whilst completing the admission paperwork the nurse asks Trevor if he is married. Trevor panics at the questions and tells the nurse he lives alone. When asked for next of kin details, Trevor gives his brother's name. The nurse completes the admission and leaves Trevor worrying that he has not given accurate details about his circumstances. He also feels guilty at denying his partnership. Ted is also concerned that the information may affect Trevor's care and discharge arrangements, and that should anything happen to Trevor he will not be informed.

After a couple of days on the ward Trevor feels able to talk to his primary nurse about the information he gave to her on admission. He explained how the lack of visibility of lesbian, gay, bisexual and transgender issues can create a sense of otherness and exclusion. He also told the nurse that her assumptions about his partner and the language that she used during the admission immediately put him in a position where he had to decide whether to 'come out' to the nurse or not. At a particularly stressful time this could have been avoided. The nurse was able to reflect on the assumptions she had made and particularly the heterosexist assumptions present within the admission paperwork of the ward and the unnecessary stress this had placed on Trevor.

CONCLUSION

Diversity is a difficult concept to define. It involves a number of other important themes to make sense of its meaning and importance in nursing. It can be problematic for nurses, as it involves an honest appraisal of one's own values and possible prejudice. Embracing the importance of diversity also means that individual nurses must be willing to speak out when they are confronted by discriminatory practices. Respecting diversity suggests the recognition of the intrinsic worth and uniqueness of the self and others and is a fundamental pre-requisite to caring.

FURTHER READING

Thompson, N. (2006) *Anti-discriminatory Practice*, 4th edn. London: Palgrave Macmillan.

REFERENCES

Acheson, D. (1998) *Independent Inquiry into Inequalities in Health*. London: HMSO.
Cant, B. (2005) 'Exploring the implications for health professionals of men coming out as gay in healthcare settings'. *Health and Social Care in the Community*, 14(1): 9–16.
Chryssochoou, X. (2004) *Cultural Diversity: Its Social Psychology*. Oxford: Blackwell.
Dean, L., Meyer, I., Robinson, K., Sell, R., Sember, R., Silenzio, V., Bowen, D., Bradford, J., Rothblum, E., White, J., Dunn, P., Lawrence, A., Wolf, D. and Xavier, J. (2000) 'Lesbian, gay, bisexual and transgender health: findings and concerns'. *Journal of the Gay and Lesbian Medical Association*, 4: 102–51.
Giddens, A. (2006) *Sociology*, 5th edn. Cambridge: Polity Press.

diversity

113

Hartmann, D. and Gerteis, J. (2005) 'Dealing with diversity: mapping multiculturalism in sociological terms'. *Sociological Theory*, 23: 2.

Kandola, R. and Fullerton, J. (1998) *Diversity in Action: Managing the Mosaic*, 2nd edn. London: Institute of Personnel and Development.

Mackereth, P. (1995) 'HIV and homophobia: nurses as advocates'. *Journal of Advanced Nursing*, 22: 670–6.

Nettleton, S. and Gustafsson, U. (2002) *The Sociology of Health and Illness Reader*. Cambridge: Polity Press.

Nursing and Midwifery Council (2004) *Code of Professional Conduct*. London: NMC.

Nytanga, B. (2001) 'Celebrating cultural diversity'. *International Journal of Palliative Nursing*, 7: 2.

Robertson, A.E. (1998) 'The mental health experiences of gay men: a research study exploring gay men's health needs'. *Journal of Psychiatric and Mental Health Nursing*, 5: 35–40.

Thompson, N. (2006) *Anti-discriminatory Practice*, 4th edn. London: Palgrave Macmillan.

Cross-References *Caring, Dignity Reflection, Respect.*

18 Educator

Jean Mannix and Annette McIntosh

DEFINITION

The term 'educator' comes originally from the latin 'educare' meaning to lead out, signifying the giving of intellectual, moral, and/or social instruction and is defined as one who gives training in, or information on, a particular subject (Oxford Dictionary 2006). However, this definition implies that learning is a passive process requiring little effort on behalf of the individual.

There are two widely held theories of learning employed within nurse education, cognitivism and humanism, which espouse learning and education as active processes. The cognitivist school of thought considers that learning is an internal, purposive process concerned with thinking, perception, organisation and insight. The learner is seen as being actively involved in seeking out new information, problem solving and referring to past experience, and thus understanding is developed. Bruner (1966) considered that the aim of education was to instil a general understanding of the whole structure of a subject, while Ausubel (1968) advocated a method of expository teaching, linking new knowledge to students' previous experience. Humanism concerns the feelings and experiences that lead to the personal growth and fulfilment of an individual.

KEY POINTS

- Nurse educators must promote lifelong learning and the development of reflective, analytical and critical thinking skills.
- Supporting learning in practice is essential, necessitating the integration of theory with practice.
- The role of service users is an important element in nurse education.
- The nurse has a key role in educating patients in healthcare.

DISCUSSION

When considering the concept of educator from a nursing perspective, the role can be seen to be interchangeable between nurses, nurse educationalists, students and service users. These will be discussed in relation to: the context of nurse education; education within a Higher Education Institution (HEI); education in practice; nurses as patient educators; and service users as educators.

The context of nurse education

The educational preparation of nurses has undergone several changes since the 1970s, in tandem with the growth of nursing as a profession and developments in the National Health Service (NHS). In the 1980s, the United Kingdom Central Council for Nursing, Midwifery and Health Visiting (UKCC) recommended that students should have supernumerary status and become responsible to educationalists rather than to service managers (UKCC, 1986). This heralded a move from service-led to education-led preparation of students. This model, Project

2000 (P2000), was implemented from 1989 onwards with the curriculum based on a health-orientated paradigm, placing greater emphasis on the social and psychological aspects of care. The notion of professional accountability, by which nurses were expected to take increased responsibility for their care delivery through a commitment to research-based practice and an ability to analyse and change practice, also received greater emphasis.

From the mid-1990s, nurse education was situated within HEIs. A commission in the late-1990s identified that, while there were significant strengths within the P2000 programme, there were concerns about the fitness for practice of newly registered nurses, particularly with regard to practical skills (UKCC, 1999). A new curriculum model, addressing the acquisition of practical skills, was developed for implementation, in line with the Department of Health's (DoH) plans to modernise the NHS and improve the public's health (DoH, 1999).

Educating within an HEI

Nurse educators today face the challenge of utilising teaching and learning strategies that will ultimately produce nurses who are fit for purpose, practice and award. Nurse education has to provide an holistic and student-centred approach to learning, promoting self-reflection, lifelong learning and competence and confidence in delivering high-quality, evidence-based care. The education of students necessitates the acquisition of knowledge simultaneously with clinical skills, thus requiring the integration of theory and practice. Nurse authors support the need to situate the two elements closely together and for knowledge to inform practice through a framework of reflection (for example, Burnard, 1989; Burns and Glen, 2000). In line with the recommendations of the DoH (1999), outcome competencies are used as the standards for registration, portfolios of experience demonstrate fitness for practice and experiential, and problem-based and interprofessional learning are required to be embedded within the curriculum. It is also essential for HEIs and healthcare providers to work in partnership on a range of aspects, including student support and mentorship and ensuring the quality of clinical placements as learning environments.

Educating in practice

Quinn (2000) stated that learning which takes place in the clinical environment can be argued to be much more meaningful than that gained in the classroom, but noted that exposure to practice does not equate to learning in practice. Professional learning in practice is seen by a number of authors to come from systematic analysis and reflection upon experience and requires an environment conducive to learning and support from skilled practitioners and educationalists (for example, Pollard and Hibbert, 2004). Studies from researchers such as Dunn and Hansford (1997), Jackson and Mannix (2001) and Papp et al. (2003) support the notion that qualified staff are key in creating the right environment and acting as role models, with the ward manager being particularly influential.

The learning environment also influences the ability of students to embrace their own learning needs and undertake the role of educators themselves. Aston and Molassiotis (2003) established that peer support from student educators was an under-utilised resource within the clinical environment. Often senior students assume the role of educator with junior students. This can be a powerful learning relationship; at its simplest it is a form of role modelling which, if formally channelled, could provide a rich and meaningful learning experience. To promote this educator role, the supportive relationship could be formalised and provide a robust mechanism to reduce anxieties for junior students and develop teaching skills and confidence for senior students for their future mentoring and assessing role (NMC, 2006).

Educating clients/patients

The role of the nurse as an educator is widely accepted as an essential component of nursing. Unfortunately, health education is often viewed as disease orientated, whereas health promotion is considered more as all-encompassing of the wider context of health. Whitehead (2001) suggests that there are two different educator roles within nursing: traditional and radical. The traditional nurse educator is often viewed as the expert, frequently using persuasion and manipulation within a medical model, which can lead to a victim-blaming approach. In contrast, the radical health educator embraces personal health beliefs and needs by engaging in partnership with clients, and thus enables health promotion through education. This can empower clients to become involved in community development and, ultimately, other health-enhancing activities (Whitehead, 2001). The role of educator within health promotion should not be distinguished as different from any other educator roles within nursing. Whitehead recommends that for nurses to successfully undertake this role, there needs to be a shift from the traditional disease orientated framework; a more pragmatic approach that gives consideration to the wider determinants of health within a bio-psychosocial model may be more effective.

When engaging in health education and health promoting activities, learning also takes place between student nurses and patients; this is a distinct phenomenon. Whilst educating and promoting health, the student will be exposed to a variety of behaviours and lifestyles which may well enable them to better understand the complexity of the educator role within nursing. This relationship between patient and student can be an exploration of learning that is influential to both contributors. This binary approach to learning can achieve collaboration and partnership through mutual respect and benefit.

The patient/service user as educator

While patients have been a focal point in nurse education, they historically have had relatively passive and understated roles as educators. More recently, service user involvement in education is gaining momentum, driven by both political and professional imperatives (Warne and McAndrew, 2005). Many authors (for example, Abma and Widdershoven, 2005) have addressed the involvement of service users in relation to the planning, delivery and evaluation of services, including education, in line with the NHS plan (DoH, 2000). This entails placing the service user at the centre of all aspects of healthcare, through activities such as panel membership and involvement in the development and delivery of nurse education programmes. As Bennett and Baikie (2003) note, within clinical practice service users can educate students from their perspective and contribute to the student learning experience by informing the development of professional attitudes, knowledge and behaviours.

CASE STUDY

Tom is a student nurse on a busy surgical ward. His mentor, Mary, is an experienced practice educator and facilitates Tom's learning through working with him, using his clinical learning outcomes and portfolio as a guide. Tom is keen to be as skilled as Mary, and observes her professional and personal behaviour within the ward environment through working alongside her. Mary helps Tom to spend time with patients discussing their experiences and feelings, as encouraged by his HEI lecturers. He is also required to work with other healthcare professionals to achieve his learning outcomes. Tom found this more difficult to fulfil due to lack of opportunities and his workload. Tom confided his difficulties to Mary at their weekly reflection meeting and, in conjunction with the ward manager, a planned schedule of activities was put into place, allowing Tom to fulfil his clinical learning outcomes.

Reflecting on his learning experiences, Tom noted the different influences within his clinical placement. In particular, Tom considered that the interaction with patients had provided a rich and fulfilling educational experience. Mary had proved to be a sound role model and educator and, even when it was not possible to be on the same shift together, had ensured that Tom had been guided in his learning. Her intervention to ensure that he had the benefit of interprofessional learning was important, as was the supportive response from the ward manager. Tom considered that this experience had been a positive one and had facilitated his learning and development.

CONCLUSION

The role of an educator is a key concept in nursing. Nurse education takes place in both HEI and clinical settings, with educators required to promote lifelong learning and academic skills within a student-centred approach. The development of evidence-based practical skills requires that theory and practice are integrated and that the clinical learning environment is supportive and conducive to learning, including robust systems of mentorship. The notion of service users as educators is an increasingly important element of nurse education, while nurses have a key role in educating patients in healthcare.

FURTHER READING

Quinn, F.M. (2000) *The Principles and Practice of Nurse Education*. Cheltenham: Stanley Thornes.
Warne, T. and McAndrew, S. (eds) (2005) *Using Patient Experience in Nurse Education*. London: Palgrave Macmillan.

educator

REFERENCES

Abma, T.A. and Widdershoven, G.M. (2005) 'Sharing stories: narrative and dialogue in responsive nursing evaluation'. *Evaluation and the Health Professions*, 28(1): 90.
Aston, L. and Molassiotis, A. (2003) 'Supervising and supporting student nurses in clinical placements: the peer support initiative'. *Nurse Education Today*, 23: 202–10.

Ausubel, D.P. (1968) *Educational Psychology: A Cognitive View.* New York: Holt, Rinehart & Winston.

Bennett, L. and Baikie, K. (2003) 'The client as educator: learning about mental illness through the eyes of the expert'. *Nurse Education Today,* 23(2): 104–11.

Bruner, J. (1966). *Towards a Theory of Instruction.* Cambridge, MA: Balknap Press.

Burnard, P. (1989) 'Experiential learning and andragogy – negotiated learning in nurse education: a critical appraisal'. *Nurse Education Today,* 9: 300–6.

Burns, I. and Glen, S. (2000) 'An educational model for preparation for practice?', in S. Glen and K.Wilkie (eds), *Problem-Based Learning in Nursing.* London: Macmillan.

Department of Health (1999) *Making a Difference: Strengthening the Nursing, Midwifery and Health Visiting Contribution to Health and Health Care.* London: The Stationary Office.

Department of Health (2000) *The NHS Plan: A Plan for Investment, A Plan for Reform.* London: The Stationary Office.

Dunn, S.V. and Hansford, B. (1997) 'Undergraduate nurses' perceptions of their learning environments'. *Journal of Advanced Nursing,* 25(6): 1299–306.

Jackson, D. and Mannix, J. (2001) 'Clinical nurses as teachers; insights from students of nursing in their first semester of study'. *Journal of Clinical Nursing,* 10: 270–7.

Nursing and Midwifery Council (2006) *Standards to Support Learning and Assessment in Practice.* London: NMC.

Oxford Dictionary (2006) www.askoxford.com (accessed 20 Nov. 2006).

Papp, I., Markkanen, M. and von Bonsdorff, M. (2003) 'Clinical environment as a learning environment: student nurses' perceptions concerning clinical learning experiences'. *Nurse Education Today,* 23(4): 262–8.

Pollard, C. and Hibbert, C. (2004) 'Expanding student learning using patient pathways'. *Nursing Standard,* 19(2): 40–3.

Quinn, F.M. (2000) *The Principles and Practice of Nurse Education.* Cheltenham: Stanley Thornes.

UKCC (1986) *Project 2000. A New Preparation for Practice.* London: UKCC.

UKCC (1999) *Fitness for Practice: Report of the Commission for Education.* London: UKCC.

Warne, T. and McAndrew, S. (eds) (2005) *Using Patient Experience in Nurse Education.* London: Palgrave Macmillan.

Whitehead, D. (2001) 'Health education, behavioural change, social psychology: nurses' contribution to health promotion'. *Journal of Advanced Nursing,* 34(6): 822–32.

Cross-References *Mentoring, Problem solving, Professional development, Reflection, Role model, User involvement.*

19 Empathy

Tom Donovan

DEFINITION

Empathy is the capacity to experience the emotions of another person and is widely accepted as a crucial element of therapeutic and supportive relationships. Empathy has been described as ability, attitude, an interpersonal process, a trait, sensitivity and perceptiveness (Kunyk and Olson, 2001). The principal elements of empathy constitute seeing the world as others see it; being non-judgemental; understanding another's feelings and communicating this understanding (Wiseman, 1996).

The use of empathy as a therapeutic intervention is attributed to Carl Rogers (1902–1987), who described the ability to empathise as:

> to assume, in so far as he [sic] is able, the internal frame of reference of the client, to perceive the world as the client sees it, to perceive the client himself as he is seen by himself, to lay aside all perceptions from the external frame of reference while doing so and to communicate something of this empathic understanding to the client. (1951: 29)

KEY POINTS

- Empathy is the vicarious experience of the feelings, thoughts or attitudes of another person.
- Empathy is distinct from sympathy.
- Empathy as a concept and a skill is a fundamental component of the nurse–patient relationship.
- The application of an empathic approach to clinical care yields tangible benefits to patients and for health professionals.
- Nurses and other health professionals often fail to demonstrate empathy in everyday clinical practice.
- The skill of empathy can be acquired through training.

DISCUSSION

Nursing is an art and a science that seeks to understand the human consequences of ill-health. An understanding of an individual's experience can furnish nursing with invaluable insights to advance the development of strategies to support patients, carers and others. If the need to be acknowledged and understood is a fundamental human trait and a close understanding of patient's experiences can inform patient care, then empathy must be a key element in the way that nurses communicate and fully engage with their patients.

The art of nursing is exemplified in the (sometimes ephemeral) nature of the nurse–patient relationship, in which the development of empathy, effective communication and supportive interventions are crucial factors. As a core element of nursing practice, the relationship that evolves between a nurse and a patient represents a defining aspect of nursing. Crucially, the nature and quality of such relationships retains the potential to enhance or diminish clinical care.

Mok and Chiu (2004) found that when relationships of trust are formed, nurses were not only regarded as health professionals, but also became part of a family or a good friend. The nurses in this study demonstrated and communicated understanding of their patients' suffering. They were aware of their patients' unspoken needs and provided comfort without actually being asked. The quality of these relationships significantly enhanced their patients' physical and emotional state, supported their adjustment to their illness and eased physical symptoms. A significant factor in this study appears to be the capacity of the nurses to attune to their patients' situations. The use of empathy in this instance not only improved the nurse–patient relationship, but also contributed positively to clinical care and outcomes.

Sympathy or empathy?

Although conceptually distinct, empathy and sympathy are central to caring relationships and retain similar characteristics. Both reside within a beneficent desire to help and to acknowledge the feelings or distress of others.

Sympathy, and thus to sympathise or have sympathy for, connotes an appreciation of another person's difficulties, sorrow or troubles and usually describes 'feeling sorry for someone'. It is a reflexive, affective response to another's plight. Sympathy is a feeling of understanding and a desire to support a person in need. It arises involuntarily and reactively and tends to be concerned with feelings of compassion, pity and tenderness. However, sympathy and being sympathetic may also imply a collusive and somewhat judgemental relationship in which the sympathiser supports the position of the distressed person.

Empathy transcends this position and implies a more complex and intense level of human engagement and understanding. In an empathic relationship, the empathiser consciously attempts a psychical engagement to sense another person's situation, feelings, and motives. Thus, empathy is a deliberate attempt to perceive an experience from the perspective of another person. It entails trying to understand another's experience 'as if' one were that person.

Rogers (1975) further developed this concept and suggested that the state of 'being empathic' has several facets. For Rogers, being empathic meant entering the private perceptual world of another and experiencing that world and its flow of emotions. Rogers saw empathy as a way of being. Yet, unlike sympathy, the empathiser is also required to move within this world without making judgements. Being with another in this way and laying aside personal judgements and prejudice allows the empathiser to lay aside themselves and become 'a confident companion to a person within their inner world' (1975: 4).

Yet to some, the distinctions between empathy and sympathy remain unclear. Even in sympathy one is drawn to the distress of another person, and in offering sympathy there is an inevitable sharing of pain. Black (2004) suggests that both terms are commonly used to describe three distinguishable things:

- A capacity to put us in touch with the emotional state of another.
- The use of 'trial identification' to discover, consciously or unconsciously, the emotional state of another.
- The affect of compassion.

However, whilst semantic and conceptual arguments over the distinctions persist, it is hard to doubt that demonstrating genuine compassion and understanding for another is an affirming human trait and a beneficent and therapeutic intervention.

The application of empathy in clinical practice

Nursing scholars suggest that empathy is a necessary constituent of care and that nurses need to 'get in the skin' of patients to truly appreciate their needs (Henderson, 1978). This implies that empathy should form

empathy

part of the skills repertoire of nurses and is a skill that can be acquired and used in clinical practice.

Evidence suggests that when empathic approaches are absent or diminished, quality of care and nurse–patient relationships are compromised. Reynolds and Scott (2000) concluded that many recipients of clinical care may not feel that their situation is understood by health professionals. This is particularly evident when patients are emotionally vulnerable. In a study of patients undergoing chemotherapy, for example, Farrell et al. (2005) found that experienced nurses could not identify their patients' chief concerns. This failure to elicit concerns has been associated with later development of anxiety and depression (Parle et al., 1996). Sadly, many of the issues identified by patients yet missed by nurses in this study could have been addressed, reduced or alleviated.

Health professionals sometimes worry that exploring sensitive issues will unleash strong emotions that they will be unable to manage. Yet, if patients are encouraged to talk about their concerns and feelings they are more likely to put things in a better perspective and cope more effectively. Some health professionals also believe that engaging emotionally with patients will engender difficult questions such as 'Why hasn't this treatment worked?' or 'Am I dying?' They are also concerned that if they allow patients to talk about their worries they will empathise with the patient's situation too closely and become upset. They may then become concerned about their own emotional survival (Maguire and Pitceathly, 2003). However, demonstrating empathy and understanding need not engender significant personal costs to the listener.

Reflection as a tool

Reflection is a skill that nurses can use to demonstrate empathy. Reflection is the skill of communicating back to the patient that their words and feelings have been heard and acknowledged. This usually consists of reflecting back some of the words that the patient uses. It is an effective way of keeping the focus of a conversation within the patient's frame of reference whilst demonstrating that concerns have been heard and understood. Consider the example below:

Patient: I just couldn't believe it when the doctor said it was cancer.
Nurse: You couldn't believe it?
Patient: No, it just came out of the blue. I'd always been so well. I've never been ill before.

Nurse:	It must have been quite a shock for you then, because you had been so well.
Patient:	Yes, it was. A terrible shock. My world just seemed to fall apart from that moment.
Nurse:	Your world fell apart. That sounds awful.
Patient:	It was awful ... it was terrible

The nurse's responses here were clearly focused upon the patient's perspective and the emotional content of the conversation. Even this very short extract demonstrates:

- That the patient has been heard (*You couldn't believe it?*)
- Acknowledgement (*It must have been quite a shock for you.*)
- Understanding (*Your world fell apart. That sounds awful.*)

Engaging empathically with others implicitly imposes a cost to the empathiser. By feeling the experiences of others, the empathiser will experience, in a real way, their emotional pain. Yet healthcare work inevitably engenders a degree of emotional labour, and recognition of this factor may be a determinant in developing effective empathic relationships. Some research suggest that health professionals actually benefit and become more effective when they acknowledge such emotional labour and engage in the process of empathy (Halpern, 2007; Larson and Yao, 2006).

Can nurses learn to be empathic?

Empathy is a skill that may be acquired through effective training. Approaches to teaching empathy usually encompass interpersonal skills training workshops, but innovative approaches such as combined literature and medicine courses have also been used to foster an appreciation and application of empathy in practice (Shapiro et al., 2004). However, evidence suggests that some courses do not help nurses or other professionals to offer empathy. Factors such as the optimum length and effective components of empathy training remain unknown, and most studies of empathy education have been methodologically weak and have not explored the evaluation of recipients (Reynolds et al., 1999).

empathy

CASE STUDY/EXERCISE

Watching a distressing report in the news, reading a powerful story or watching a dramatisation on television can sometimes be quite upsetting, even though the events do not relate to you. Think about a recent event that did not involve you directly, but caused you to become emotional.

- Why did this event or story touch you in this way?
- Did you put yourself in the shoes of another person?
- Did you try to imagine what life would be like for that person?
- What did you experience – sympathy or empathy?
- Can 'feeling' the emotions of other people help us to become better practitioners?

CONCLUSION

Empathy underpins the humanistic elements of clinical practice. Although it may be challenging to apply, in most instances it remains a critical factor in developing and nurturing effective therapeutic relationships. 'The gentle and sensitive companionship of an empathic stance … provides illumination and healing. In such situations, deep understanding is, I believe, the most precious gift one can give to another' (Rogers, 1975: 9).

FURTHER READING

Nelson-Jones, R. (2003) *Practical Counselling and Helping Skills*, 4th edn. London: Sage.

REFERENCES

Black, D.M. (2004) 'Sympathy reconfigured: Some reflections on sympathy, empathy and the discovery of values'. *International Journal of Psychoanalysis*, 85(3): 579–95.

Farrell, C., Heaven, C., Beaver, K. and Maguire, P. (2005) 'Identifying the concerns of women undergoing chemotherapy'. *Patient Education and Counselling*, 56: 72–7.

Halpern, J. (2007) 'Empathy and patient–physician conflicts'. *Journal of General Internal Medicine*, 22(5): 696–700.

Henderson, V. (1978) *Principles and Practice of Nursing*, 6th edn. New York: Macmillan.

Kunyk, D. and Olson, J.K. (2001) 'Clarification of conceptualizations of empathy'. *Journal of Advanced Nursing*, 35(3): 317–25.

Larson, E. and Yao, X. (2005) 'Clinical empathy as emotional labor in the patient–physician relationship'. *Journal of the American Medical Association*, 293: 1100–06.

Maguire, P. and Pitceathly, C. (2003) 'Managing the difficult consultation'. *Clinical Medicine*, 3(6): 532–7.

Mok, E. and Chiu, P.C. (2004) 'Nurse–patient relationships in palliative care'. *Journal of Advanced Nursing*, 48(5): 475–83.

Parle, M., Jones, B. and Maguire, P. (1996) 'Maladaptive coping and affective disorders in cancer patients'. *Psychological Medicine*, 26: 735–44.

Reynolds, W. and Scott, B. (2000) 'Do nurses and professional helpers normally display much empathy?' *Journal of Advanced Nursing*, 31(1): 226–34.

Reynolds, W., Scott, B. and Jessiman, W.C. (1999) 'Empathy has not been measured in clients' terms or effectively taught: a review of the literature'. *Journal of Advanced Nursing*, 30(5): 1177–85.

Rogers, C.R. (1951) *Client-Centered Therapy*. London: Constable and Robinson.

Rogers, C.R. (1975) 'Empathic: an unappreciated way of being'. *The Counselling Psychologist*, 5(2): 2–10.

Shapiro, J., Morrison, E. and Boker, J. (2004) 'Teaching empathy to first year medical students: evaluation of an elective literature and medicine course'. *Education for Health (Abingdon)*, 17: 73–84.

Wiseman, T. (1996) 'A concept analysis of empathy'. *Journal of Advanced Nursing*, 23: 1162–7.

Cross-Reference *Caring, Communication, Compassion, Competence, Coping, Holistic care, Nurturing, Reflection.*

20 Empowerment

Ann Bryan

DEFINITION

One of the main issues when considering the term 'empowerment' is the complexity of the definition itself. It has become a familiar term used within a variety of social policy and welfare contexts, each bringing differing interpretations. This makes it difficult to define as it manifests itself differently in each setting. A number of commentators state that no consensual definition exists in relation to the concept of empowerment (Hage and Lorenson, 2005; Hanson and Bjorkman, 2005; Nyatanga and Dann, 2002). Roberts (1999) has even suggested that the concept should be based on individuals' own definitions. However, perhaps it is best described by Nyatanga and Dann, as representing 'both a process and an outcome involving the individual or group's ability to pull from within themselves the power to influence or control significant events in their lives' (2002: 235). Therefore, the essence of empowerment is that it cannot be given but must be acquired by those who desire it. This acquisition is dependent on the facilitation of the necessary conditions which make it possible.

KEY POINTS

- Empowerment is found at different levels – organisational, individual and community.
- The definitive aspiration of empowerment is wellbeing.
- For patients to be empowered, healthcare practitioners must be empowered.
- Empowerment is a dynamic psychological process which necessitates a reciprocal patient–practitioner interaction.

DISCUSSION

Various philosophical and psychological theoretical approaches, including Menon (2002), Freire (2000) and Kanter (1979), have been used in the literature (Hage and Lorenson, 2005; Hanson and Bjorkman, 2005; Kuokkanen and Leino-Kilpi, 2000) to give a greater understanding of the concept of empowerment within the healthcare setting. These approaches will be discussed in this chapter at the macro, micro and meso levels, which equate to the organisational, individual and community. The levels will be viewed in the context of their dialectical relationship with each other.

Organisational

Democratic management theory is mainly responsible for determining concepts of empowerment at the organisational level. For an organisation to be empowered it needs to be democratically managed (Kanter, 1979). This, in turn, requires its members to share information and have control over decisions while being involved in devising strategic objectives. As Wallerstein maintains, 'In an empowering organisation, individuals assume genuine decision-making roles and hence become empowered through their work' (1992: 201).

Within the healthcare setting in the United Kingdom empowerment is seen as a key determinant of health, and this ideology has become established as a way of promoting patients' control over their wellbeing. It is reflected in many government policies and communications including the

Patient's Charter (DoH, 1991), *The NHS Improvement Plan* (DoH, 2004b) and *Better Information, Better Choices* (DoH 2004a). However, these documents can be regarded as visionary frameworks (Nyatanga and Dann, 2002), which in their own right will not empower individuals unless the healthcare system itself is a truly empowered organisation.

Lewis and Urmston (2000) see a contradiction between the healthcare objective of empowerment and the hierarchical structure of the NHS. The notion that empowerment can be dictated by policy is directly opposed to the goal of providing a healthcare environment in which staff and, subsequently, patients can develop power and autonomy. Nursing staff cannot be empowered by the downward dictation of policy in the organisational hierarchy of the NHS, which has a long history of authoritarianism. Indeed, Rodwell (1996), Roberts (1999) and Kuokkanen and Leino-Kilpi (2000) advocate that staff empowerment will significantly increase with a reduction in the hierarchical and authoritarian elements within the organisation.

For the government policy of empowerment to be achieved, Lewis and Urmston (2000) argue that a comprehensive reappraisal of attitude and culture is needed within the NHS. Changing the management structure is not enough on its own to facilitate it. Nurses must be encouraged to develop the personal qualities which will enable them to participate to a much greater extent in the wider decision-making process.

Individual

At the individual level definitions of empowerment are psychological in nature. This power-from-within is acquired by achieving a sense of self-knowledge, self-discipline and self-esteem, resulting in a 'feeling of greater control' over one's life (Rissel, 1994: 42). Individuals are able to determine the outcome they desire. Nyatanga and Dann (2002) state that the ultimate goal of empowerment is wellbeing. In health and healthcare settings the patient must experience wellbeing in coping with disease, disability, treatment and making healthy living choices. Evidence suggests that individuals who take control of their health improve the quality of their lives (Hage and Lorenson, 2005; Roberts, 1999; Shearer and Reed, 2004).

One of the major issues concerning patient empowerment is the term 'patient' itself. The continued use of this label by healthcare professionals helps to maintain their superiority and control over the patient. This is because historically patients have been expected to fulfil the sick role, where they passively adjust and conform (Parsons, 1950). Caring for the sick inevitably involves the related concepts of control and paternalism (Laverack, 2005), and these are at variance with patient empowerment which necessitates an equal partnership between the healthcare recipient and the healthcare provider.

For an equal partnership to become a reality there has to be a meaningful patient–practitioner interaction which facilitates a reciprocal understanding of health-related needs. This interaction is a process based on active patient participation and can only be realised when individuals are allowed to make free and conscious choices related to their own lives (Freire, 2000). However, there is a contradiction between patient choice and the enforcement of policies and care delivery by healthcare professionals. It is only by considering the individual's unique perspective and experience that practitioners are able to effectively empower the patient. This means that patients who articulate their needs instead of passively accepting health provision should not be regarded as demanding and difficult.

Community

Humans are social beings. Freire (2000) argues that they can only exist collectively within communities and do not function independently of each other. Community empowerment is closely linked with individual and organisational empowerment. Laverack (2005) maintains that there is a synergistic interaction between the micro, macro and meso levels and that community empowerment is an ongoing dynamic process between the three levels. Roberts (1999) supports this view by asserting that each of the levels of empowerment is in a dialectical relationship with the other.

Community empowerment has been perceived in the literature mainly as a continuum comprising the following elements:

1. Personal action
2. The development of small mutual groups
3. Community organisations
4. Partnerships
5. Social and political action
   (Jackson et al., 1989)

The continuum model shows how individual action can develop into effective community empowerment which has the potential to change the power base (French, 1990). It is through working in partnerships that individuals are able to acquire the necessary support and resources which will enable them to obtain outcomes favourable to the community as a whole. The role of healthcare practitioners is to facilitate the movement of people along the five-point continuum. They accomplish this objective by working as equal partners alongside various individuals, groups and community organisations.

CASE STUDY

Mary is a 64-year-old spinster with chronic obstructive pulmonary disease and cardiac disease. She lives alone and is fiercely independent. Last winter she was taken into hospital on a number of occasions owing to increased periods of breathlessness. Following her latest admission, she was visited by a community matron who reviewed her care. Community matrons are autonomous practitioners who have advanced clinical practice skills. Their role has recently been developed within the NHS to co-ordinate services and empower patients with long-term conditions to self-manage their care.

A major issue identified during the initial assessment by the community matron was that Mary did not understand her medication. In discussing this with her it became apparent that she had little comprehension of how the diseases were affecting her health, so the community matron suggested to Mary that she enrol on an expert patient programme. Completing this course has not only increased Mary's knowledge of her condition, but has also given her the confidence to become an expert patient facilitator. She has improved the quality of her own life and is now enabling other individuals with long-term conditions to empower themselves.

CONCLUSION

Empowerment occurs at the organisational, individual and community levels within the healthcare setting. To understand the concept fully, each level cannot be viewed in isolation but must be seen as part of a complex relationship. In this relationship the role of the healthcare practitioner is of vital importance in promoting conditions in which individuals can make their own informed choices. As long as health professionals expect patients passively to accept medical decisions,

empowerment

patients will never be able to assume control over their own feelings of wellbeing. Empowered individuals are regarded as equal and respected partners within the healthcare environment.

Nurses have a key role in enabling patient empowerment. However, to fulfil this role effectively they also need to be empowered, which will involve fundamental changes in the hierarchical and authoritarian structure of the healthcare organisation. Without this realisation, it is unlikely that the necessary reciprocal patient–practitioner interaction will take place to facilitate the dynamic process of empowerment.

FURTHER READING

Laverack, G. (2005) *Public Health Power, Empowerment and Professional Practice*. Basingstoke: Palgrave Macmillan.

REFERENCES

Department of Health (1991) *Patient's Charter*. London: HMSO.

Department of Health (2004a) *Better Information, Better Choices*. London: Department of Health Publications.

Department of Health (2004b) *The NHS Improvement Plan*. London: Department of Health Publications.

Freire, P. (2000) *Pedagogy of the Oppressed*. New York: Continuum.

French, J. (1990) 'Boundaries and horizons, the role of health education within health promotion'. *Health Education Journal*, 49(1): 7–9.

Hage, A.M. and Lorenson, M. (2005) 'A philosophical analysis of the concept of empowerment; the fundament of an education-programme to the frail elderly'. *Nursing Philosophy*, 6: 235–46.

Hanson, L. and Bjorkman, T. (2005) 'Empowerment in people with mental illness: reliability and validity of the Swedish version of an empowerment scale'. *Scandinavian Journal Caring Science*, 19: 32–8.

Jackson, T., Mitchell, S. and Wright, M. (1989) 'The community development continuum'. *Community Health Studies*, 8(1): 66–73.

Kanter, R.M. (1979) 'Power failure in management circuits'. *Harvard Business Review*, 57(4): 64–75.

Kuokkanen, L. and Leino-Kilpi, H. (2000) 'Power and empowerment in nursing: three theoretical approaches'. *Journal of Advanced Nursing*, 31(1): 235–41.

Laverack, G. (2005) *Public Health Power, Empowerment and Professional Practice*. Basingstoke: Palgrave Macmillan.

Lewis, M. and Urmston, J. (2000) 'Flogging the dead horse: the myth of nursing empowerment?' *Journal of Nursing Management*, 8: 209–13.

Menon, S. (2002) 'Toward a model of psychological health empowerment: implications for healthcare in multicultural communities'. *Nurse Education Today*, 22(1): 28–39.

Nyatanga, L. and Dann, K.L. (2002) 'Empowerment in nursing: the role of philosophical and psychological factors'. *Nursing Philosophy*, 3(3): 234–9.

Parsons, T. (1950) *The Social System*. New York: Free Press.

Rissel, C. (1994) 'Empowerment: the holy grail of health promotion'. *Health Promotion International*, 9(1): 39–47.

Roberts, K.J. (1999) 'Patient empowerment in the United States: a critical commentary'. *Health Expectations*, 2(2): 82–92.

Rodwell, C.R. (1996) 'An analysis of the concept of empowerment'. *Journal of Advanced Nursing*, 23(2): 305–13.

Shearer, N.B.C. and Reed, P.G. (2004) 'Empowerment: reformulation of a non-Rogerian concept'. *Nursing Science Quarterly*, 17(3): 253–9.

Wallerstein, N. (1992) 'Powerlessness, empowerment and health: implications for health promotion programmes'. *American Journal of Health Promotion*, 6(3): 197–205.

Cross-References *Communication, Coping, Equality, Reflection, Respect.*

21 Environment

Elizabeth Mason-Whitehead

DEFINITION

Students studying nursing today soon realise that they are tapping into a number of discreet disciplines. These fields of expertise include sociology, psychology, public health and economics, which bring together the specific bodies of knowledge that are the essential components for nursing in a holistic manner. Each of these areas has a different interpretation as well as a common understanding of what the environment means to individuals and societies. Defining the environment in relation to nursing is summarised in Figure 9.

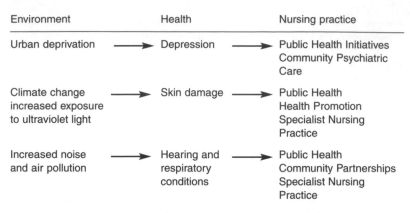

Environment		Health		Nursing practice
Urban deprivation	⟶	Depression	⟶	Public Health Initiatives Community Psychiatric Care
Climate change increased exposure to ultraviolet light	⟶	Skin damage	⟶	Public Health Health Promotion Specialist Nursing Practice
Increased noise and air pollution	⟶	Hearing and respiratory conditions	⟶	Public Health Community Partnerships Specialist Nursing Practice

Figure 9   *Examples of how the environment influences health and nursing practice*

At a fundamental level, our environments are the spaces we occupy and they can mean something different to each individual person, whether we are considering the survival of the planet or the security of our own homes. Critical to this chapter is exploring the impact our environments have on the physical, social and emotional wellbeing of individuals and societies.

KEY POINTS

- An overview of the breadth of environmental issues which pose a threat to populations and communities is an important prerequisite for nurses working in clinical practice. For example, the module content for common foundation programmes might include the effects on health from global threats. Such an example is the spread or rise in malaria from global warming. Pollution of air and water together with food contamination are associated with significant health problems and risks.
- The environment is a significant component in forming our experiences and memories. For example, the children's ward in a hospital can influence whether or not children requiring intermittent long-term care wish to return to hospital.
- Nurses can be influential in shaping the environments in which they work. For example, working with colleagues to ensure that patients have pleasant waiting rooms with access to toilets and refreshments.
- Nurses go to the environments wherever their patients/clients live and work, such as a hospital, inner city, rural community, war zone,

factory, holiday resort and prison. For example, a community psychiatric nurse visiting a mother living on a remote farm could be a critical line of communication for the mother and her family.

- The environment can affect a patient/client's wellbeing in a negative or positive way. For example, a negative effect could be having men and women on a hospital ward sharing the same wash and toilet facilities, resulting in a lack of privacy and increased embarrassment. A positive effect may be offering a range of alternative treatments, for example aromatherapy and reflexology, to patients on an oncology ward.
- Nurses have an important role to play in working towards a safer and greener environment. For example, nurses can work with agencies in advising on bio-degradable nappies which do not add to the burden of landfill sites.
- A knowledge of environmental public health is essential for nurses to develop (with other agencies) and deliver appropriate health promotion strategies. For example, understanding the effect of ozone depletion through the release of chlorofluorocarbons (CFCs) and the effects this has on the skin. Nurses have a substantial public health role in informing their clients about the dangers of being exposed to sunlight (Mason and Whitehead, 2003).
- Nurses can work towards improving the safety and wellbeing of their community clients. For example, being a member of relevant policy committees to campaign for safer streets, such as a reduction in air pollution from factory chimney omissions, increasing the safety of pelican crossings and increased play areas.

DISCUSSION

The following five significant areas provide a starting point for discussion and debate.

The context of environments within time and place

There is a general agreement that the role of a person's environment in shaping their lives must not be underestimated. The memories we have of our physical, social and emotional environments can be likened to connecting rooms which we pass through across years and decades. Our memories are often so vivid that in our mind's eye we can go back in time and remember events and locations with great clarity. It is difficult to find a more disturbing account than that provided by Primo Levi as he recorded his first days in Auschwitz. Primo Levi, an Italian Jewish chemist, was transported to Auschwitz in 1943. His account of this vile and unspeakably cruel environment has made a profound contribution to our understanding of every aspect of the world's humanity:

> This is hell. Today, in our times, hell must be like this. A huge, empty room: we are tired, standing on our feet, with a tap which drips while we cannot drink the water, and we wait for something which will certainly be terrible, and happens and nothing continues to happen. What can one think about? One cannot think any more, it is like being already dead. Someone sits down on the ground. The time passes drop by drop. (1987: 28)

Almost ten years after Levi's account, 1000 miles from Auschwitz and a distance in humanity that cannot be calculated, two social researchers, Michael Young and Peter Willmott, wrote a now famous account of their three-year research project. *Family and Kinship in East London* was a poignant record, which revealed that despite the immense poverty and deprivation that existed in Bethnal Green, there existed a community overcoming all the odds with human kindness, kinship and resilience. Here is an example of one of their most significant findings, the strength of the mother and daughter relationship:

> The daughter continues to live near her mother. She is a member of her extended family. She receives advice and support from her in great personal crisis and on the small domestic occasions. They share so much and give such help to each other because, in their women's world, they have the same functions of caring for home and bringing up children. (Young and Wilmott, 1957/1986: 61)

Clean environments: traditional nursing practices and rituals addressing new healthcare challenges

This chapter is being written at a time when the environment of the nurse, her/his colleagues and patients has never been under greater scrutiny. The birth of MRSA has been the wake-up call to all those who work in health. MRSA thrives in environments where there is infection and dirt. Nurses are now bombarded with all manner of books, DVDs, videos, training programmes, skills days, leaflets, policy documents, notices, reports, lectures and seminars dedicated to improving cleanliness; the cleanliness of ourselves, our patients and our clinical environments. As a consequence of MRSA, cleanliness, a traditional skill of nursing practice, is now enjoying somewhat of a revival. Florence Nightingale may well have stated the seminal word on the importance of a clean environment when in 1859 she wrote: 'It cannot be necessary to tell a nurse that she should be clean or she should keep the patient clean, seeing that the greater part of nursing consists in preserving cleanliness (1859: 72).

The anthropologist Mary Douglas examined the meanings of what it is to be unclean in different cultures. She asserted that the rules of hygiene alter with changes in our state of knowledge (Douglas, 1966). The relationship between cleanliness religion and charity is illustrated by St Catherine of Sienna who, when she felt revulsion from tending wounds, reproached herself by drinking a bowl of pus (Douglas, 1966). New students of nursing may be surprised at the rituals that nurses engage in as they attempt to shape and control their environments (Mason and Whitehead, 2003). Even today nursing is interwoven with a combination of traditional and evidence-based practices combining old rituals and new procedures.

Inequalities in health: old problems looking for new solutions

The harsh realities of nursing practice in many inner city and poor rural areas of the United Kingdom today remain echoes of the landmark reports of the 1980s and 1990s. The *Independent Inquiry into Inequalities in Health* (Acheson, 1998) was one report that analysed the effects of the environment on our physical, social and emotional wellbeing. The inequalities of the physical environment, poor housing, inadequate public transport, lack of access to green spaces and fresh air are associated with mental and physical illnesses. In collaboration with colleagues, nurses are ideally placed to work towards safer and healthier environments through the strengthening of community health and social policies. Nurses working in some of the most disadvantaged areas in the United Kingdom frequently report that there are not enough resources. Tudor-Hart's 'inverse care law' (1971) may still have resonance with the most deprived areas not always having the most resources.

Global threats: challenges to contemporary nursing practice

Students entering nursing today will be familiar with many of the global changes that now threaten our environment (see Figure 10). There are a growing number of public health consequences from these global threats that are now evident in nursing practice. One such example is the rise in morbidity and mortality, particularly in the young, old and sick, from the increased number of heatwaves which occur in various parts of the world. The rising temperatures can also lead to other health problems, such as a growth in the spread of infectious diseases. With the growth of evidence accumulating in establishing the relationship between ill health and climate changes, nursing education, policy and practice are preparing to meet the challenges ahead.

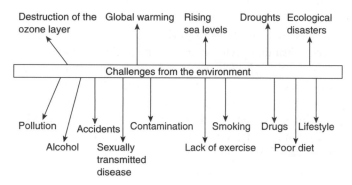

Figure 10   *The breadth of environmental challenges faced by nursing practice today*

Working towards positive environments: the nurse's role in developing healthy environments

The role of the nurse in whatever environment, irrespective of status, grade or speciality, has a recognised and expansive role to play in shaping the environments of her or his patients and clients, and this is demonstrated in Figure 11.

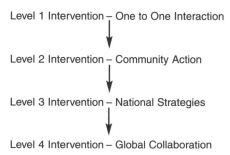

Figure 11   *The nurse's role in working towards positive environments*

CASE STUDY

This case study demonstrates how the environments of four generations of one family are influenced by their surroundings and the work of the nurses who are involved in their care.

Sally Timpson is 87 years old. She has lived, worked and raised her children in the inner city of Liverpool all her life. Five years ago Sally moved to sheltered accommodation. With the help of various members of the primary healthcare team, including the district nurse, Sally enjoys a relatively comfortable and contented life. Recently, however, Sally and her family became very anxious and worried when they heard that Sally's daughter Claire was involved in a serious car accident. The treatment and care Claire subsequently received involved a wide range of health professionals. Once Claire returned home the therapy and nursing care continued and Claire, with support, is learning again to live in her own environment. Claire's son, James, is a lone parent who lives with his twin sons on an out-of-town housing estate. The health visiting service provides James and his family with health promotion, support and access to meeting new friends who share similar experiences to James. Like his mother and grandmother, James is dependent upon the understanding and support from a range of specialities within nursing to enable him and his sons to live and thrive within their own home environments, irrespective of how varied and different they may be.

CONCLUSION

Nurses continue to work positively to enhance the environments of their patients, clients and colleagues. Whatever our role is, whether it is attending to the personal hygiene of a patient, presenting a policy on handwashing to a nursing conference, or writing this chapter, we all share the common belief that it ought to be done to the best of our ability.

FURTHER READING

Baggott, R. (2000) *Public Health and Politics.* Basingstoke: Macmillan.
Mason, T. and Whitehead, E. (2003) *Thinking Nursing!* Maidenhead: Open University Press.

REFERENCES

Acheson, D. (1998) *Independent Inquiry into Inequalities in Health Report* (1998). London: The Stationary Office.

environment

139

Douglas, M. (1966) *Purity and Danger: An Analysis of the Concepts of Pollution and Taboo*. London: Routledge.

Tudor-Hart, J. (1971) 'The Inverse Care Law'. *Lancet*, 27 February, 405–12.

Levi, P. (1987) *If This Is A Man – The Truce*. London: Abacus.

Mason, T. and Whitehead, E. (2003) *Thinking Nursing!* Maidenhead: Open University Press.

Nightingale, F. (1859/1980) *Notes on Nursing*. Edinbugh: Churchill Livingstone.

Young, M. and Willmott, P. (1957/1986) *Family and Kinship in East London*. London: Penguin.

Cross-References *Diversity, Empowerment, Equality, Holistic care, Inequalities in health, Realism, User involvement, Value.*

22 Equality

Mary Malone

DEFINITION

The general principle of equality asserts that in all public matters, such as the provision of healthcare, individuals should be treated identically (for example, Rawls, 1999). The principle of equality is associated with the belief that, by virtue of their shared humanity, all people should enjoy equal satisfaction of certain basic common rights and needs. These include the right to be healthy and the need to have adequate food, sanitation and accommodation. In the United Kingdom, the Equality Act (The Stationary Office, 2006) aims to ensure that individuals have equal opportunities to achieve their full potential in life and that they are unhindered by prejudice or discrimination. Equality and 'achievement' are, therefore, closely linked with each other.

Ensuring equality is complicated by the fact that people are not equal in terms of their characteristics and attributes. Individuals differ in terms of their physical, mental and emotional capacities and also in terms of the financial resources upon which they can draw. If identical health promoting interventions were offered to all, then differences between the most and least advantaged would increase rather than diminish; in such a situation *inequality* rather than equality of health outcome would be the final result. In order to prevent this, interventions which differ both in nature and in degree are required.

KEY POINTS

- Equality is linked to basic human rights and to concepts of fairness and social justice.
- The principle of equality recognises the right to health and to the satisfaction of health-related needs.
- In the United Kingdom, government policy is committed to removing unfair barriers to individual health and achievement and to harnessing the skill and potential of every member of society whatever their background. Health promotion is central to this.
- The discipline of health promotion is a fundamental element within 21st century nursing.
- The concept of 'equity' recognises the health impact of differences between individuals and population groups.
- Equitable healthcare provision identifies the role of various interventions, which recognise and make provision for these differences.
- In recognising and providing for individual and group differences, equitable healthcare provides equal opportunities for the achievement of health and wellbeing.
- Equity is a fundamental goal of health promotion, and nurses have an important role in providing an equitable healthcare service.

DISCUSSION

In order to understand how nurses can contribute to an equitable health service, it is important to identify the main causes of health *inequalities* and to identify what is known about effective interventions to tackle these. Poverty is a major cause of health inequalities and of ill health. Poorer children and adults are disproportionately exposed to risk factors for illness and disease, and this, in turn, makes it difficult for them to achieve health outcomes which are equal to those in more affluent groups (DoH, 2005). Whilst life circumstances at every age influence health, those experienced in childhood are particularly important. Childhood is a period of rapid development and children have a raised sensitivity to environmental influences. Poor nutrition and strained family relationships, for example, have the potential to affect a child's physical and mental health both during childhood and in their adult years (DoH, 2005). Childhood and adolescence are also those times in life when adult health behaviours such as cigarette smoking are initiated. Health behaviours such as these have a major impact on adult health (Graham and Power, 2004).

Not only poverty but also inequalities in living standards have a major impact on health expectations. Societies where standards of living are generally more equal have fewer incidences of disease and lower morbidity rates than those societies in which there are major differentials between the living standards of the rich and the poor (Wilkinson, 1986). In addition, race, ethnicity, culture and educational achievement all have an impact upon living standards. Inequalities between different societal groups in relation to children's birth weight, child development, body shape and size as well as in disease, disability and death have been described as the physical manifestation and embodiment of such inequalities (Graham, 2007).

Attitudes to health and different patterns of health information seeking exist among different social, economic and cultural groups (Graham, 2007). New forms of information sharing, in particular those dependent on emergent technologies such as the Internet, have added to the complexity. The World Wide Web has made new and hitherto unknown levels of health information available, but concerns for inequality between different groups in the use of this information have been expressed (Castells, 2003). The 'digital divide', or the gap between those who have access to the new technologies and those who do not, may serve to increase pre-existing inequalities between people who were already health 'information rich' and others who are 'information poor'. Such a divide can serve only to make equality in terms of health outcomes between the rich and the poor even more difficult to achieve.

All nurses, irrespective of their location or clinical field, have a duty to contribute to equality in healthcare provision. This contribution is made at one or more than one of the following levels: the individual level; the organisational level; and at social policy-making level.

Working at an individual level to promote health equality

Health information giving occurs at the individual level and it promotes health equality in a variety of ways, including:

- The adoption of healthier behaviours.
- Promoting access to health and social services.
- Increasing confidence among service users, both in terms of gaining access to necessary services and in adopting behavioural change.
- Helping disadvantaged individuals and groups identify the types of service which is most appropriate to their health needs.

Giving health information in a variety of practice settings is a well-established nursing role, and numerous studies illustrate how effective this can be (for example, Whitehead, 2004).

Nurses also work at an individual level to help vulnerable people identify health needs, to develop self-esteem and, in addition, to enhance the skills and competencies which facilitate behaviour change. Nursing interventions such as therapeutic listening and non-directive counselling incorporate these elements and have been particularly effective in work with parents and young children (Davis et al., 2004). In addressing health behaviours, these interventions make an important contribution to child and family health promotion and, thereby, to promoting equality of health outcomes in future generations.

Working at an organisational level to promote health equality

All nurses have a responsibility to ensure that their organisations promote equality of service access through non-discrimination of service users in terms of their race, language or levels of physical or mental ability. In practical terms this may mean ensuring availability of language and interpretation services and providing means of physical access to service premises for those with a disability. An example of this would be ensuring the provision of ramps for wheelchair users in a primary healthcare setting.

Tones and Green (2004) identify a more holistic approach to organisational health promotion, which they call a 'settings' approach. The settings approach aims to harness the health-promoting potential of organisations (Kickbush, 1998) and to utilise the practical opportunities which many settings offer for promoting health and reducing health inequalities. It incorporates the principle that: 'Health is created and lived by people within the settings of their everyday life: where they learn, work, play and love' (WHO, 1986).

The key feature of the settings approach is that the ethos of the setting and all the activities that occur within it must incorporate an element of health promotion. Examples include healthy schools, healthy cities, health promoting hospitals, health in prisons and workplace health promotion. Specialist community nurses working with school-age children may find the settings approach particularly supportive in their efforts to influence the school environment. The settings approach to health promotion is applicable to all fields of nursing as the potential to reduce inequalities and to promote health equality is related to the ethos and orientation of the organisation rather than to its physical location or particular client group (Tones and Green, 2004).

Working at a policy-making level to promote health equality

Most nurses will promote equality in health outcomes through their health education work and health information giving to individuals, families and communities. In order to be effective, however, work at the individual and the organisational level must acknowledge the wider socio-political determinants of health (Robinson and Hill, 1998). Effective nurse health educators acknowledge that health education programmes can only be effective if they are delivered within and enhanced by the supportive framework of healthy public policy. The most effective health education programmes are those that are conducted in the context of overall health planning and in conjunction with a wide range of health-promoting activities (Dougherty, 1993).

CASE STUDY

Janice is a community staff nurse working in a district nursing team. She visits Mrs D weekly for palliative care. Mrs D is 38 years old and has terminal lung cancer. She lives in local authority accommodation; she has worked hard for many years at a local supermarket and has smoked cigarettes since she was 13 years old. At each visit Janice meets with Mrs D's husband and their two daughters. They all smoke cigarettes. Janice is mindful of the tension within the family and the stresses they are all experiencing. She knows that smoking may be a way of dealing with these difficulties, and that it may also be an activity that the family share. Smoking cigarettes together may be the family's way of facing the impending sadness of Mrs D's death. Janice is also aware that cigarette smoking is a major cause of ill health and that it causes inequality of health outcomes between different social groups. Janice does not want to deny the family the opportunity to improve their chances for future good health, nor does she want to contribute to the inequalities in health expectations they already experience by denying them information and support in smoking cessation.

Janice continues to visit the family and strengthens her relationship with them. As Mrs D becomes weaker, Janice increases her contacts and provides practical help and pain relief for Mrs D. Janice suggests that the family might find it helpful to talk with someone about their experiences, and puts them in touch with the counsellor at the local GP practice. Janice resolves to raise the issue of smoking with the family at a time that seems appropriate and to offer them the chance to think about what they might want to do as a family or individually in relation to this. Janice resolves to help the family make contact with the most appropriate sources of help at the time that is right for them.

CONCLUSION

It is accepted that people have a right to healthcare which is fair and equitable. Moreover, the health service should be equitable in terms of its clinical provision and in terms of the health outcomes produced. Nurses contribute to equitable healthcare through: (i) their work with individuals; (ii) organisational-level work ensuring equal access to services and also by influencing the nature of the organisations in which they work; and (iii) through both influencing and working purposively within the context of local and national government policy.

FURTHER READING

Department of Health (2005) *Tackling Health Inequalities: A Programme for Action Status Report*. London: Department of Health.

REFERENCES

Castells, M. (2003) *The Internet Galaxy Reflections on the Internet, Business and Society*. Oxford: Oxford University Press.

Davis, H., Day C. and Bidmead, C. (2004) *The Parent Adviser Training Manual: Working in Partnership with Parents*. London: Psychological Press.

Department of Health (2005) *Tackling Health Inequalities: A Programme for Action Status Report*. London: Department of Health.

Dougherty, C.J. (1993) 'Bad faith and victim blaming: the limits of health promotion'. *Healthcare Analysis*, 1: 111–9.

equality

Graham, H. (2007) 'Poverty and health: global and national patterns', in J. Douglas, S. Earle, S. Handsley, C.E. Lloyd and S. Spurr (eds), A *Reader in Promoting Public Health Challenge and Controversy*. London: Sage.

Graham, H. and Power, C. (2004) *Childhood Disadvantage and Adult Health: A Lifecourse Framework*. London: Health Development Agency. Available online at www.had.nhs.uk/evidence

Kickbush, I. (1998) 'Health promotion for the 21st century: an era of partnerships to achieve health for all'. Press Release (WHO/47). Geneva: World Health Organization.

Rawls, J. (1999) *A Theory of Social Justice*. Oxford: Oxford University Press.

Robinson, S. and Hill, Y. (1998) 'The health promoting nurse'. *Journal of Clinical Nursing*, 7: 232–8.

The Stationary Office (2006) *Equality Act*. London: The Stationary Office.

Tones, K. and Green, J. (2004) *Health Promotion Planning and Strategies*. London: Sage.

Whitehead, D. (2004) 'A concept analysis of health promotion and health education: advancing and maturing the concepts'. *Journal of Advanced Nursing*, 47(4): 15–24.

Wilkinson R.G. (ed.) (1986) *Class and Health: Research and Longitudinal Data*. London: Tavistock.

World Health Organization (1986) *Ottawa Charter for Health Promotion*. Geneva: WHO.

Cross-References *Advocacy, Caring, Dignity, Diversity, Empowerment, Ethics, Inequalities in health, Nurturing, Reflection, Respect, User involvement.*

23 Ethics

Alison Hobden

DEFINITION

Have you ever been in a situation where you simply did not know what the 'right thing' was to do? Maybe you were asked to carry out a procedure that was against the regulations but was thought to be for the good of the patient. For example, administering a medicine on the verbal request of a doctor, or being asked to carry out a procedure unsupervised. Such situations are sometimes called 'ethical dilemmas'. Professional practice is conducted within a framework of rules (such as The Nursing and

Midwifery Council *Code of Professional Conduct: Standards for Conduct, Performance and Ethics*, 2004) and principles that underpin those rules. Nurses have a legal and professional duty to work within those rules; however, a rule does not always provide us with an answer when we are faced with a difficult question. We often only think of ethics in terms of high-profile cases, such as should a baby live or who should get an intensive care bed. However, all practice is guided by ethics. The underpinning principles of practice are normally based on ethical theories. Ethical theories have been developed over many years from moral philosophy and have been adapted to form the basis of healthcare ethics. There are a number of different ethical theories:

- Deontology
- Consequentialism
- Principalism
- Virtue ethics

All aim to systemise and generalise decision making, but fail. However, each theory has its own strengths and weaknesses.

KEY POINTS

- Practice is bound by legal and professional duties.
- Professional duties are underpinned by moral philosophy.
- There are a number of different ethical principles that can be used to guide our decision making.

DISCUSSION

Ethical theory is there to consider the moral choices that people make. It is analysing a moral argument and looking at what should happen and not necessarily at what is happening. It has its grounding in the values that people live by and provides a framework to analyse the reasons given for the choices people make and the implications of those choices. The different theories will also provide a language to describe those choices.

ethics

147

Deontology

This is derived from the work of Kant (1785), who viewed moral life as being bound up with 'doing one's duty'. Therefore, a moral act is carried out from a sense of duty rather than for any gain. Kant asserted that some duties were absolute and unconditional, such as truth telling and never killing anyone, regardless of what the consequences might be. For an action to be moral, the underlying principle must be universal, which would apply to anyone in similar circumstances. So at the centre of this philosophy lies the idea that you treat someone only in a way that you would want the whole of society to be treated. This is known as Kant's 'categorical imperative'. If we are faced with a difficult decision, we can therefore ask 'would I treat the next patient in this way, or am I making some exception to the rules?' If you were not willing to treat everyone in this way, the deontological approach would suggest that this is not a moral choice

Consequentialism

Consequentialism, or utilitarianism, describes ethical theories that judge an action in terms of the consequences of that action. Here the outcome of the action is more important than the act itself. Important consequentialists/utilitarians were Jeremy Bentham (1748–1832) and John Stuart Mill (1808–73), who stated that an action could be considered just if it resulted in the greatest good or least amount of harm for the greatest number of people. Thus, probable consequences of possible alternative actions must be examined in the assessment of a just action. However, in healthcare it is not always easy to determine the consequences of individual actions, and who decides what the best outcome is. On occasions the deontologist and consequentialist approach can oppose one another, as one centres on the rights of the individual while the other asserts the rights of the larger society.

Principalism

More recently, healthcare practitioners have sought to find formulas to help us solve our dilemmas. Beauchamp and Childress (2001) have suggested that there are four major ethical principles that need to be considered in healthcare:

- Respect for autonomy
- Non-maleficence
- Beneficence
- Justice and veracity

Their system is commonly referred to as principalism. Respect for autonomy refers to people's capacity to choose freely for oneself and to be able to direct one's own life. '...The personal rule of the self that is free from both controlling interferences by others and from limitations, such as inadequate understanding, that prevent meaningful choice' (Beauchamp and Childress, 2001: 58).

Autonomy permits an individual to choose whether they wish treatment in accordance with their own plans. Respect for autonomy recognises an individual's right to make judgements and decisions for themselves, and so caution must be applied if for any reason an autonomous decision taken by a patient is overruled. Respect for autonomy, therefore, underpins the need for informed consent regarding all aspects of care.

At the heart of the principle of non-maleficence is the notion of not knowingly causing harm to someone. The principle is expressed in the Hippocratic oath: 'I will use treatment to help the sick according to my ability and judgement, but I will never use it to injure or wrong them' (Beauchamp and Childress, 2001: 113). This principle is often discussed when looking at the doctrine 'double effect', that is, one act can have two possible effects: one good effect (intended) and one harmful effect (unintended). The harmful effect is allowed if proportionally it is less than the good effect. This is often related to drug therapies where the treatment has harsh side-effects (such as bone marrow suppressions from chemotherapy) but the intended outcome is good – that is, the cure of the underlying cancer.

Beneficence is the principle of doing good and refers to the obligation to act for the benefit of others that is set out in Clause 1 of the NMC *Code of Professional Conduct* (2004). Finally, Beauchamp and Childress (2001) look at justice and veracity. Justice is about having fairness and transparency in our actions. This is most commonly considered when we look at the distribution of resources within healthcare, and both Beauchamp and Childress and Gillon (1986) insist that this should be governed by equity and fairness. Veracity considers openness in our professional conduct, centering on the principle of truth telling, which again is at the heart of informed consent.

Virtue ethics

Over recent years we have witnessed a rising interest in the arena of virtue ethics. Dating back to Aristotle, this approach takes the view that it is not so much the action that is important but the character or motivation of the agent. Virtue ethics proposes that a good (virtuous) person will always make the right choice in a difficult situation. This is distinct from other theories where carrying out the right act is what makes the person a good practitioner. Virtue ethics is underpinned by certain characteristics (or virtues) that we expect a virtuous agent to have. Although not proponents of virtue ethics themselves, Beauchamp and Childress (2001) suggested: compassion, discernment, trustworthiness, integrity and conscientiousness. This can be quite an abstract concept to grapple with, but consider the case of Harold Shipman. Many patients described him as being the model GP, giving time and attention to his patients. However, with hindsight, it is now clear that his motivation for doing this was dubious. Could we say he was putting his patient needs first, or was he satisfying his own needs? Whilst his technical skills were often impeccable, the fact that he was convicted of the multiple murders would now cause us to question his status as a professional. Virtue ethics provides us with an ethical model that allows us to do just that.

CASE STUDY

Sally is a student nurse on a busy surgical ward. It is the end of a long shift and all the staff are keen to get home. One of the patients, Mr Jones, needs to go to the toilet and requests a commode. Mr Jones needs hoisting onto the commode, however, the staff nurse working with Sally states that this will take too long and so instead asks Sally to help her lift Mr Jones onto the commode. Sally refuses to do this and goes to get the hoist, despite the protest of the staff nurse. Using the different ethical theories, Sally can construct an argument to support her actions. Sally has a duty of care to Mr Jones and he has a right to expect a safe level of care (deontology). Not using the hoist would be unsafe and could potentially cause harm to both Sally and Mr Jones (consequentialism, beneficence and non-maleficence). If this was an emergency situation and there was not time to get the hoist to move Mr Jones, you would then be using beneficence to analyse if the potential harm outweighed the good.

CONCLUSION

We have now explored some of the main schools of thought within modern biomedical ethics and you will have seen that opinions differ as to which one provides you with the elusive 'right answer'. The application of ethical theory helps to ensure that we have ethical decision making. Such theories are applied all the time, everywhere, and are not limited to a number of high-profile cases as is sometimes thought. The NMC *Code of Professional Conduct* (2004) provides a useful guide for practice and is based on ethical principles, and also Beauchamp and Childress' (2001) model can be of particular use when considering professional practice.

FURTHER READING

Edwards, S.D. (1996) *Nursing Ethics*. Basingstoke: Macmillan.
Gillon, R. (ed.) (1994) *Principles of Health Care Ethics*. Chichester: John Wiley.
Hope, T., Savulescu, J. and Hendrick, J. (2003) *Medical Ethics and Law, the Core*. London: Churchill Livingstone.

REFERENCES

Beauchamp, T.L. and Childress, J.F. (2001) *Principles of Biomedical Ethics*, 5th edn. Oxford: Oxford University Press.
Gillon, R. (1986) *Philosophical Medical Ethics*. Chichester: John Wiley.
Kant, I. (1785) *Groundwork of the Metaphysic of Morals*. London: Hutchinson and Co. Ltd.
Nursing and Midwifery Council (2004) *The NMC Code of Professional Conduct: Standards for Conduct, Performance and Ethics*. London: NMC.

Cross-References *Accountability, Advocacy, Equality, Respect.*

24 Evidence-based practice

Margaret Edwards

DEFINITION

It has been estimated that the volume of medical papers alone doubles every ten to fifteen years (Hook, 1999). Given the exponential growth in the availability of information relating to healthcare, it might be expected that knowledge should be greater and practice more effective (Dawes et al., 2005). The reality, however, as these authors have pointed out, is that there is often a gap between best evidence and practice. The evidence-based practice (EBP) movement has evolved and grown in response to the recognition of that gap. It has been a worldwide phenomenon. In Canada, it was led by David Sackett and his colleagues at McMaster University. In the United Kingdom, initiatives such as the Cochrane Collaboration (the international not-for-profit organisation preparing, maintaining and promoting the accessibility of systematic reviews of the effects of healthcare) have provided the impetus for its growth. The EBP movement has not been without its critics, though much of the criticism has arisen from a misunderstanding of the basic principles.

Over the years a number of definitions of EBP have been proffered. Early definitions related specifically to the practice of medicine, where it was increasingly acknowledged that many treatments did not work. The benefits of an approach to practice that involves using the best possible evidence for the care of patients and other users of health services has become apparent to other healthcare professionals, especially nurses. Evidence-based medicine and evidence-based nursing now form part of the wider evidence-based practice movement. In order to promote the principles, teaching and implementation of evidence-based practice, a consensus statement was agreed by delegates at the second international conference of Evidence-Based Healthcare Teachers and Developers held in Sicily in September 2003. The group agreed that 'evidence-based practice (EBP) requires that decisions about healthcare are based on the best available, current, valid and relevant evidence. These decisions should be made by those receiving care, informed by the tacit and explicit knowledge of those providing care, within the context of available resources' (Dawes et al., 2005: 1).

KEY POINTS

- Evidence-based practice ideally involves the use of good quality research.
- In the selection and application of 'best evidence', the practitioner combines critical appraisal skills with their own clinical experience.
- The recipient of care is best placed to determine the applicability of evidence to their own situation.

- Evidence-based practice is affected by the available financial resources.

DISCUSSION

Early negativity and misgivings surrounding the concept of evidence-based practice centered around two seemingly contradictory arguments: that it was 'old hat' or that it was a dangerous innovation, a cookbook approach to practice that would result in the loss of individualised and compassionate approaches to care (Di Censo et al., 1998; Greenhalgh, 2001; Sackett et al., 1996). In relation to medicine, Sackett et al. (1996) have pointed out that the notion that 'everyone already did it' failed to hold water in face of the variations in practice and in the patient outcomes that were being observed.

A powerful criticism of evidence-based medicine was that it diminished the value of practice experience. Greenhalgh (2001), writing from a mainly medical perspective, has pointed out that experience, though very valuable, must by definition have limits. The clinician's experience is limited to those patients whom he or she has encountered. What might have been learnt from all the other patients in the world whose cases are unknown to the particular clinician remains forever a mystery. The other cases can, however, be known through the accumulation of good quality research that is rigorous enough to be able to transfer assumptions from samples to populations. In nursing where research and research training have a more recent history and there is a long-standing professional ideology that reifies practice experience (Di Censo et al., 1998), lessons from medicine regarding the blind acceptance of 'expert' opinion may be illuminating. Vetter (1995) tells the tale of Archie Cochrane, the inspiration for the Cochrane Collaboration and the first president of the Faculty of Public Health Medicine, who shared early findings from a trial testing the effectiveness of care at home versus care in hospital with a group of eminent cardiologists. The cardiologists expressed the view that the trial should be stopped immediately when they saw that there was a high mortality rate in one of the groups. Cochrane then revealed that the deaths were occurring in the hospitalised group of patients!

Scepticism towards research in both nursing and medicine may be related to the fact that research findings have sometimes appeared to bear little resemblance to what is observed by practitioners in their daily work. The uncritical acceptance of research findings from poorly designed and executed studies may have fuelled resistance to the concept in some quarters. The emphasis therefore in the EBP movement is on high-quality research.

In looking at questions of effectiveness of treatments or other interventions systematic reviews where the results of good quality randomised controlled trials are pooled are held to provide the 'best evidence'. The randomised controlled trial is considered the gold standard design in questions of effectiveness because variables both known and unknown can be accounted for and controlled or be assumed to be occurring in a chance or random fashion amongst the sample. Randomised controlled trials cannot provide answers for all clinical questions and the 'best' evidence may be provided by other designs such as cohort or case control studies. In the former, two or more groups are followed up, often over very many years, to observe the development of disease. One of the most famous cohort studies that has followed up subjects for more than forty years has provided some of the strongest evidence for the harmful effects of smoking (Doll et al., 1994). In studying rare diseases, the case control study (where patients with a particular disease are paired and matched with another person who acts as a control) is often used to establish the cause of a disease, but it is difficult to control for unknown variables. What is important is that a chosen design is the most appropriate one to answer the question that is being asked.

Not all clinical questions or concerns can be answered through quantitative research designs. Local clinical audit may provide evidence of good practice and suggest further areas for enquiry. Research developed from the results of clinical audit is likely to seem more relevant to practitioners as it has arisen from the reality of practice. Best evidence may also come from rigorously executed qualitative studies that seek to elicit the patient's views and/or experiences of health and/or illness. The Sicily definition of EBP stresses the importance of the patient's perspective, views and preferences in the clinical decision-making process. The early exponents of EBP also recognised the centrality of the individual patient in the process, and early definitions of the concept spoke of the 'judicious' use of evidence for the interests of the individual patient (Sackett et al., 1996). Instead of rejecting clinical expertise, EBP demands that the practitioner uses judgement that comes from clinical experience in their application of best evidence for the benefit of the individual patient. That clinical decision making will also include the application of ethical principles to the patient situation as treatments though found to carry some benefit may be so expensive as to deprive a large number of other patients of care.

CASE STUDY

The early discharge of older patients from acute hospitals to intermediate care services has been likened to 'nothing less than a firm step backward into the neglectful Dark Ages of geriatric medicine' (Steiner, 2001: 433). Collective wisdom has often suggested that older carers will be over-burdened at home. However, when randomised controlled trials of nurse-led intermediate care facilities and district-nurse-led hospital at home teams have been conducted, patient outcome measures have not been found to differ. Evidence-based practice would require that the new service could be afforded as well as being safe. If patients require more services in another setting, and for longer, there may be no advantage to the NHS as a whole, and finite resources may be taken from another needy area. The principles of EBP would also demand that patient preference would be taken into account in deciding on place of care. Studies have consistently found that older medical patients tend to prefer care to be provided in their own homes (Edwards, 2004; Marks, 1991; Shepperd et al., 1998). A Cochrane review of hospital-at-home trials (Shepperd and Iliffe, 2003) did not find evidence of increased carer burden amongst carers of elderly medical patients. Armed with this knowledge, a nurse working in the arena of intermediate care or who is discharging an older patient to a community-based service might have some confidence in the ethical components of his or her actions because of the research evidence. Nonetheless, the disposition of the patient and his or her particular resources as well as the capacity and willingness of an elderly relative to deliver care at home would need to be assessed so that a 'judicious' decision could be made. A failed discharge with early readmission to the acute hospital might result from a thoughtless and blanket application of 'available' evidence.

CONCLUSION

From the Sicily consensus statement and from the above discussion, it is apparent that the concept of evidence-based practice involves more than just the application of research evidence to clinical practice. Evidence-based decision making involves the coming together of the four spheres that have been discussed above. Clinical decision making is informed by research or other best evidence, but the application of that evidence depends on clinical expertise to use research findings in the interest of the individual patient and in the interest of the wider society.

FURTHER READING

Craig, J.V. and Smyth, R.L. (2002) *The Evidence-based Practice Manual for Nurses.* London: Churchill Livingstone.

Greenhalgh, T. (2001) *How to Read a Paper: The Basics of Evidence-based Medicine,* 2nd edn. London: BMJ Publishing.

REFERENCES

Dawes, M., Summerskill, W., Glasziou, P., Cartabellotta, A., Martin J., Hopayian, K., Porzsolt, F., Burls, A. and Osbourne, J. (2005) 'Sicily statement on evidence-based practice'. *BMC Medical Education,* 5: 1. Available online at www.biomedcentral. com/1472-6920/5/1 (last accessed 25 Jan. 2007)

DiCenso, A., Cullum, N. and Ciliska, D. (1998) 'Implementing evidence-based nursing: some misconceptions'. *Evidence-Based Nursing,* 1: 38–9.

Doll, R., Peto, R., Wheatley, K., Gray, R. and Sutherland, I. (1994) 'Mortality in relation to smoking: 40 years' observations on male British doctors'. *BMJ,* 309: 901–11.

Edwards, M. (2004) *A Study to Determine the Appropriate Case-mix for a District Nurse-led Elderly Hospital at Home Team.* Unpublished PhD, King's College. London: University of London.

Greenhalgh, T. (2001) *How to Read a Paper: The Basics of Evidence-Based Medicine,* 2nd edn. London: BMJ Publishing.

Hook, O. (1999) 'Scientific communications: history, electronic journals and impact factors'. *Scandinavian Journal of Rehabilitation Medicine,* 31: 3–7.

Marks, L. (1991) *Home and Hospital Care Redrawing the Boundaries.* London: King's Fund Institute.

Sackett, D.L., Rosenberg, W.M., Gray, J.A., Haynes, R.B. and Richardson, W.S. (1996) 'Evidence-based medicine: what it is and what it isn't'. *BMJ,* 312: 71–2.

Shepperd, S. and Iliffe S. (2003) *Hospital at Home versus In-patient Hospital Care (Cochrane Review).* Oxford: Update Software.

Shepperd, S., Harwood, D., Jenkinson, C., Gray, A., Vessey, M. and Morgan, P. (1998) 'Randomised controlled trial comparing hospital at home with inpatient hospital care. I: three month follow up of health outcomes'. *BMJ,* 316: 1786–91.

Steiner, A. (2001) 'Intermediate care more than a "nursing thing"'. *Age and Ageing,* 30; 433–5.

Vetter, N. (1995) *The Hospital, From Centre of Excellence to Community Support.* London: Chapman & Hall.

Cross-references *Clinical governance, Data, information, knowledge, Researcher.*

25 Feedback

Irene Cooke

DEFINITION

There are many definitions of feedback. Some consider the mechanistic feedback which is experienced in the field of electronics; others define it as a sound distortion; feedback has also been considered as a biological response which occurs within the body due to the regulation of hormones and chemicals (Oxford English Dictionary, 2007). However, Menachery et al. have defined feedback within the context of effective learning as 'a process involving observation, problem identification, providing information, goal development and solution by trial and error' (2006: 440). This definition clearly links feedback to teaching and learning domains, and Eraut (2006) clarifies this concept further by relating feedback to other people's opinions, feelings and thoughts about individual performance.

Consequently, feedback can be considered from a variety of perspectives. However, as a concept used within nursing, it is probably best known as part of an educational process assessing individual performance. In this context, Menachery et al. have suggested that feedback can provide insight into the actions and consequences 'highlighting the dissonance between the intended result and the actual result' (2006: 440), which is linked to enhanced clinical performance. Students need feedback on their clinical performance so they can improve the level of skill acquisition (Glover, 2000), and this leads to increased confidence and subsequently enhanced patient care delivery. It is documented, however, that in order to be effective, feedback needs to be structured and constructive in the process of skill acquisition, and immediate feedback appears to be of particular benefit (Reece and Walker, 1998).

feedback

KEY POINTS

- Feedback is a fundamental component of teaching, learning and academic achievement.

- Feedback contributes to an individual's personal and professional development by enhancing knowledge, attributes and skills which contribute to lifelong learning.
- Feedback facilitates the assessment of the extent to which information has been successfully received and with what impact.
- Feedback should be structured, constructive and emotionally sensitive, using specific examples to reinforce areas of both strength and development.
- Feedback should be contemporaneous and timely – given as close to the event as possible.

DISCUSSION

Most people have a basic need to know how well they are doing, and the expectation of success is fundamental to motivation and effort (Atkinson, 1957). This is the case for nursing practice. As individuals, nurses need to know how well they are performing, and during clinical practice, feedback is given to the nurse from a variety of sources, which may include peers, colleagues, mentors, other health and social care professionals, patients and their families (Glover, 2000). The feedback may be communicated via a variety of mechanisms, such as individual or group discussions, presentations, written and verbal communication, web-based contact and patient surveys or questionnaires, which inform the individual or group of their strengths and limitations. This process may indeed act as a catalyst or motivator to identify areas of further development resulting in enhanced professional practice. In order for feedback to be successful, it is essential that there is mutual understanding between the parties involved, with a shared meaning acknowledged (Dickson, 1999). The respectful consensus of opinion subsequently forms the basis for the constructive interaction between the student and teacher (Glover, 2000). It has been found that the relationship between the feedback provider and recipient is an integral component as to whether feedback is valued and respected (Ward, 2003), and may determine whether the recipient considers the feedback to be valid. Feedback is considered to be emotionally sensitive (Eraut, 2006) and is strongly related to interpersonal relationships. Within healthcare environments, giving feedback to patients is a fundamental aspect of nursing practice in order to enable individuals to consider their own health-related progress and to realise opportunities for their health potential. Most people have developed sophisticated accounts of health and illness and wish to participate in interactions with healthcare workers (Nettleton, 2003), a trend that is increasingly evident in practice. Feedback is crucial in facilitating this process, in order to inform, empower and liberate patients to feel confident to work in partnership with health professionals (DoH, 2001). It is well known that giving comprehensive feedback to patients results in improved levels of concordance with treatments and medications (National Prescribing Centre, 2004), so consequently the patients' views should always be explored in healthcare interventions to optimise partnership working. Consideration of the impact of feedback on the patient will not be considered within this chapter. However, further reading in this area is identified below. Following a review of the literature, this chapter will explore feedback from two perspectives: patients' feedback to nurses, and student feedback.

Patients' feedback to nurses

It is documented that feedback from patients is an important component in the design and delivery of quality healthcare initiatives (Anderson et al., 2004), and there is increasing emphasis on patient and service user involvement in health and social care services (DoH, 2005, 2006a). A number of key health policy documents generated by government agencies encourage and report on patient and service user involvement (DoH, 2006b; Healthcare Commission, 2006). More research is now undertaken to explore the patients' views of healthcare provision and in particular the nursing contribution to care. The overall findings of research studies and health policies are:

- Patients value nurses working in partnership with them.
- Patients lack a clear understanding of professional nursing roles and responsibilities.
- Patients like having one nurse care for them rather than a number of nurses.
- Patients want their views to be acknowledged.
- Patients want to be treated with respect.

feedback

The above findings indicate that patients wish to enter into partnerships with nurses, and that they particularly value having one nurse to manage their overall care. This facilitates trust and confidence in the nurses' abilities (Mok and Chiu, 2004). Having a number of different nurses involved in the delivery of their care may contribute to the reported lack of clarity in determining individual nursing roles and, fundamentally, whom to contact when an issue arises. Patients have also requested that their views and beliefs are respectfully acknowledged when care is organised (Nettleton, 2003). In order to improve the quality of care, feedback from the patients' perspective is an essential part of this process (Coulter, 2002), which may make a positive contribution to the identification of continuing professional development requirements of nursing and service staff. In this context, feedback should be considered as a dynamic process which may actively reinforce key aspects of a quality service and also identify areas requiring further development and training. It is usual for patients to participate in this process in a number of ways, such as individual one-to-one feedback, participation in surveys (Gavin, 1997), group meetings, telephone interviews, post-hospital questionnaires and via the Internet. There are a number of patient websites which are primarily designed to facilitate this process, such as www.dipex.org.uk and www.patientopinion.org, where patients can share experiences of health-related conditions, which not only contributes to the knowledge base of patients and their families but also to health professionals.

Student feedback

Students receive feedback in a variety of formats and from a number of perspectives. Feedback may be given by patients and families, peers, colleagues, clinical mentors and academic lecturers at various times during a programme of study. However, student feedback is usually expressed as being either formative or summative, and usually related to the individual's clinical and academic performance whereby the acquisition of knowledge, skills and attributes are assessed. Feedback provides the mechanism to assess the extent to which information has been successfully received and with what impact, to demonstrate understanding. Students are advised to obtain feedback in respect of academic achievement (Whitehead and Mason, 2003), as this too can provide the stimulus for further learning. Glover (2000), in a study with third-year students, found that immediate and timely feedback in clinical practice enhanced student performance by promoting confidence. This in turn is directly linked to enhanced patient care and clinical competence (Menachery et al., 2006). Additionally, Butler and Winnie (1995) found that giving appropriate feedback to students helps them rate their own clinical practice in a realistic way. This strategy will facilitate self-awareness in students, contribute to reflective practice

(Menachery et al., 2006) and lead to deeper and more meaningful learning. As Eraut comments, '… feedback shapes learning futures … [students'] very sense of professional identity, is shaped by the nature of the feedback they receive' (2006: 118).

CASE STUDY

Ellie Smith is a 62-year-old lady who is about to be discharged home from hospital following an exacerbation of her chronic obstructive pulmonary disease (COPD). Whilst Ellie is waiting for her family to collect her from the ward, her primary nurse, Catherine, hands her a questionnaire which she explains is a survey to capture an insight into the quality of care which Ellie has experienced recently as an in-patient. Catherine explains that the questionnaire completion is optional, and is also anonymised. She explains that all patients have the opportunity to complete the form, and that the results of the completed questionnaires are used to inform the ward staff of their strengths and limitations. Ellie completed the form and posted it in the box at the end of the ward as she went home. The ward manager collected the completed patient surveys and identified that there was a need for staff to undertake additional updates in the treatment regimes of patients who have COPD. This information was communicated to the whole ward team, and this resonated with Catherine as she too had felt that she needed updating in some of the recent advances in the management of patients with COPD. This educational need was communicated to the ward manager during a feedback session, and Catherine was able to access further support in this area.

CONCLUSION

This chapter has determined that feedback is an essential concept in the education of nurses, as it facilitates learning both in practice and in academic achievement. Feedback also provides the essential mechanism to improve patient care by its contribution to reflective practice, which leads to the enhancement of clinical competencies. The concept of feedback also features highly in respect of quality in healthcare initiatives. Patient feedback makes a significant contribution to service delivery by informing staff of their own experiences of care, which may ultimately inform and shape future health strategies.

FURTHER READING

Cleary, M., Horsfall, J. and Hunt, G.E. (2003) 'Consumer feedback on nursing care and discharge planning'. *Journal of Advanced Nursing,* 42(3): 269–77.

Suikkala, A. and Leino-Kilpi, H. (2001) 'Nursing student–patient relationship: a review of the literature from 1984 to 1998'. *Journal of Advanced Nursing,* 33(1): 42–50.

Weiner, B. (1984) 'An attribution theory of achievement and emotion'. *Psychological Review,* 92: 548–75.

REFERENCES

Anderson, C., Blenkinsopp, A. and Armstrong, M. (2004) 'Feedback from community pharmacy users on the contribution of community pharmacy to improving the publics' health: a systematic review of the peer reviewed and non-peer reviewed literature 1990–2002'. *Health Expectations,* 7: 191–202.

Atkinson, J.W. (1957) 'Motivational determinants of risk taking behaviour'. *Psychology Review,* 64: 365.

Butler, D. and Winnie, P. (1995) 'Feedback and self-related learning: a theoretical synthesis'. *Review of Educational Research,* (65): 245–81.

Coulter, A. (2002) 'After Bristol: putting patients at the centre'. *BMJ,* 324: 648–51.

Department of Health (2001) 'The expert patient: a new approach to chronic disease management for the 21st century'. Available online at www.dh.gov.uk/en/Publicationsandstatistics/Publications/PublicationsPolicyAndGuidance/DH_4006801 (accessed 3 May 2007).

Department of Health (2005) 'Creating a patient-led NHS: delivering the NHS improvement plan'. Available online at www.dh.gov.uk/en/Publicationsandstatistics/Publications/PublicationsPolicyAndGuidance/DH_4106506 (accessed 29 April 2007).

Department of Health (2006a) 'A stronger local voice: a framework for creating a stronger local voice in the development of health and social care services'. Available online at www.dh.gov.uk/en/Publicationsandstatistics/Publications/PublicationsPolicyAndGuidance/DH_4137040 (accessed 29 April 2007).

Department of Health (2006b) 'Choice matters: increasing choice improves patients' experiences'. Available online at www.dh.gov.uk/en/Publicationsandstatistics/Publications/PublicationsPolicyAndGuidance/DH_4135541 (accessed 30 April 2007).

Dickson, D. (1999) 'Barriers to communication', in A. Long (ed.), *Interaction for Practice in Community Nursing.* Basingstoke: Macmillan.

Eraut, M. (2006) 'Feedback'. *Learning in Health and Social Care,* 5(3): 111–8. *BMJ,* 314: 227.

Glover, P.A. (2000) 'Feedback. I listened, reflected and utilised: third-year nursing students' perceptions and use of feedback in the clinical setting'. *International Journal of Nursing Practice,* 6: 247–52.

Healthcare Commission (2006) 'Variations in the experiences of patients using the NHS services in England'. Available online at www.healthcarecommission.org.uk/_db/_documents/Surveys_Variations_Report_200612211042.pdf (accessed 1 May 2007).

Menachery, E.P., Knight, A.M., Kolodner, K. and Wright, S.M. (2006) 'Physician Characteristics Associated with Proficiency in Feedback Skills'. *Journal of General Internal Medicine*, 21(5): 440–6.

Mok, E. and Chiu P.C. (2004) 'Nurse–patient relationships in palliative care'. *Journal of Advanced Nursing*, 48(5): 475–83.

National Prescribing Centre (2004) 'Saving time, helping patients: a good practice guide to quality repeat prescribing': *National Prescribing Centre*. Available online at www.npc.co.uk/repeat_prescribing/repeat_presc.htm (accessed 5 May 2007).

Nettleton, S. (2003) *The Sociology of Health and Illness*, 7th edn. Cornwall: Polity Press.

Oxford English Dictionary (2007) Available online at http://dictionary.oed.com/entrance.dtl (accessed 25 April 2007).

Reece, I. and Walker, S. (1998) *Teaching and Learning: Practical Guide*. Sunderland: Business Education Publishers.

Ward, D. (2003) 'Self-esteem and audit feedback'. *Nursing Standard*, 17(37): 33–6.

Whitehead, E. and Mason, T. (2003) *Study Skills for Nurses*. London: Sage.

Cross-References *Communication, Competence, Reflection, User involvement.*

26 Guilt

John Struthers

DEFINITION

Guilt is an emotion usually linked to the feeling of having done something wrong. Guilty feelings may be triggered by comparing one's thinking, actions or feelings before, during or after an event against an internal set of beliefs, values or rules. If the comparison violates an internal moral code, guilt feelings can be generated. The guilty feeling may prevent the considered action. However, if the event has already taken

163

guilt

place, remorse linked to blame can prevail. Guilt feelings can be healthy, when appropriate to the situation, in helping to motivate socially acceptable behaviour. On the other hand, the absence of guilt in a person may result in self-centred manipulation of others (Beck et al., 1993). However, excess guilt can become debilitating, due to the intrusiveness and persistence of the recurring guilt thoughts. The continual experience of guilt can sometimes become an intolerable, painful experience for the person to live with.

KEY POINTS

- Guilt is an emotion resulting from judging one's own behaviour against an internal standard, often resulting in blame.
- Guilt can be both supportive or destructive to wellbeing of self, others and society.
- Early childhood experiences shape our internal moral code.

DISCUSSION

Guilt is an extremely significant concept within healthcare but is not always an obvious component of a person's initial presentation. Differing theoretical approaches have focused on psychological and sociological explanations of guilt relating to a person's health state. Excessive guilt is often linked to mental ill health.

Psychological

Transactional analysis (TA) provides a model offering a psychological explanation as to the creation of the internal value system which individuals use to judge their own feelings, thoughts and actions. When the individual feels they are failing to live up to such internalised standards, guilt may result. The terms 'parent, adult, child' in TA explain the states of mind which form the personality, and are co-existent in everybody. These terms are not to be confused with their more frequent use linked to age and maturity: 'The "parent" is a huge collection of recordings in the brain of unquestioned or imposed external events perceived by a person in his early years' (Harris, 1995: 18). Information provided by significant parental figures is absorbed without question, for example, 'Don't do that it's wrong', 'God is watching you all the time'. Since the youngster does not contest these sayings, they become accepted as truths and are reinforced when the infant pleases its seniors by doing as requested. This embeds the 'contaminated' thought into the child's internal value system (Stewart, 1994). Contaminated thinking can then be replayed throughout life 'as if logical' without evidence to such questions as 'whether God can really see every action?' The replayed voice of significant others, often that of the parent or teacher, can be heard subconsciously repeating rules of the stored moral code. Both pleasant and unpleasant experiences are stored in the infant's memory during this dependent period. Later in life when these rules are not adhered to, feelings of guilt may result.

In TA the term 'child' refers to the manner in which the youngster sees, hears and understands the world. As infants have very few words, most reactions are feelings. All their desires to explore and carry out bodily functions wherever they are become socialised into accepted behaviours. Such actions reflect the dominant values of their parents, relating to culture, customs and spiritual beliefs. This process often results in many chastisements, therefore the developing youngsters begin to feel they are not acting correctly, unless they seek approval from the seniors by conforming to their expectations.

Irrespective of how old people are, they can return to their 'child' state of curiosity and desire to explore new experiences. However, as a person matures, their enthusiasm and ability to make lifestyle choices can be tempered with the repetitious 'critical voice' of the internalised 'parent' (Rayner et al., 2005). The person is trapped in a cycle of self-judgement, shame, and fear of disapproval or punishment. Such is the power of guilt from lingering past parental influences (Stewart, 2000). Health and life potentials remain untapped, creativity stifled, resulting in missed life opportunities. The depreciating effect of excessive guilt on a person's self-worth can lead to mental health problems.

The third part of the personality in TA is the 'adult', and it offers the hope required to break the cycle of the imposed guilt. The 'adult' part of the personality helps the person to develop their ability to think rationally: 'Through the "Adult" the little person can begin to tell the differences between life as it was taught and demonstrated to him (Parent), life as he felt it or wished it or fantasised it (Child), and life as he figures it out by himself (Adult)' (Harris, 1995: 30).

Sociological

Guilt is not all bad; it can also prompt useful social behaviour. Guilt can motivate relationship behaviour (Beck et al., 1993) and strengthen family ties. For instance, you may visit your granny, whom you haven't seen for over a year, when she sends you money to help with your studies.

Or you may return to study to complete your assignment. Guilt can assist in social control in respecting universal principles of right or wrong, such as respecting others' property, or not stealing. Those who break such principles or laws are often found 'guilty' in a legal sense and 'punished' (Giddens, 2003). To add a further dimension to the concept of guilt, its existence in some experiences enhances the excitement potential. This is most evident when one is doing something which might risk social embarrassment if caught. Experimenting with one's emerging sexuality can add to the desired tension and anticipatory excitement when challenging socially created taboos (Stainton Rogers and Stainton Rogers, 2001).

Mental health

Persistent guilt feelings are linked to presentations of depression and obsessive-compulsive disorders. Pathological guilt can become life threatening (Gamble and Brennan, 2006).

Many psychological therapies assist people to replace or 'decontaminate' the unhelpful thoughts which underlie the guilt. Suicide may appear as a final punishment and release from the guilt-ridden torture for some individuals (Hawton et al., 2006).

Therapies such as transactional analysis (Lister-Ford, 2002), cognitive therapy (Sanders, 2005) and solution-focused therapy (O'Connell, 2005) use different therapeutic approaches to assist the individual to challenge the 'truths' absorbed into the unconscious mind when an infant. The rational, logical thinking of the 'adult' part of the personality is developed to strengthen the person's ability to make their own assertive choices about life. Often the achievement of the long-term goal of experiencing appropriate levels of guilt through such therapies can initially generate more stress. Individuals may be required to test out new behaviours which in the past may have generated guilt to gain new evidence that they are alright, thus counteracting the old belief. For a person who has been told from early days that all 'dancing' is the work of the devil, having a first dance is likely to be a very emotional event. Shedding some inhibition releases the guilt, enabling the person to make up their own mind.

CASE STUDY

Peter escaped from a car crash with minor abrasions, while his son Billy was taken to hospital to be X-rayed for a possible neck injury. Peter had been larking about with Billy and forgot to check that his son's seat belt was securely fastened. As he waited, voices reminiscent of his parents ran through Peter's mind: 'More haste, less speed', 'Always check your own work', 'What sort of parent will you make if you still can't look after yourself?' Guilt related to not checking the seat belt created self-recrimination and overshadowed all Peter's previous conscientious parenting. Peter started to think: 'People will think I am a bad father. They would be right, I was careless, I should have known better'. New rules generated in Peter's mind further embed the guilt and its control over his behaviour. For example, 'I'll never do that again', 'I'll always double check things from now on' and 'My son won't trust me again'. Peter's persistent guilt led to depression. His doctor referred Peter to a mental health professional who assisted him to recognise and value his positive attributes as a father. Such awareness allowed Peter to value all aspects of his parental skills and counteract the guilt linked to this one event.

CONCLUSION

Guilt is an emotion which can drive socially cohesive behaviour and on occasions add a bit of spice to life. However, persistent unrelenting thoughts of guilt can threaten life itself. The emotional climate in which children grow and develop sets the scene for their response towards how they value themselves. Understanding guilt from a transactional analysis perspective not only assists healthcare practitioners to gain an understanding of others' behaviour, but can also lead to insights of one's own behavioural drivers. Regaining choice over one's thinking empowers individuals to be true to themselves and assists in maximising their own potential. 'It is a natural human tendency to feel guilt when we hurt another person or behave poorly. If we can calmly examine the guilt, we can grow and improve. Then 'guilt has done its work, and can be released' (Schiraldi, 2002: 86).

FURTHER READING

Harris, T.A. (1995) *I'm OK – You're OK*. Berkshire: Arrow Books.

REFERENCES

Beck, C., Rawlins, R.P. and Williams, S.R. (1993) *Mental Health Psychiatric Nursing: A Holistic Life-Cycle Approach*. St Louis, MO: Mosby.

Gamble, C. and Brennan, G. (2006) *Working with Serious Mental Illness: A Manual for Clinical Practice*, 2nd edn. Edinburgh: Elsevier.

Giddens, A. (2003) *Sociology*, 4th edn. Oxford: Polity.

guilt

Harris, T.A. (1995) *I'm OK – You're OK*. Berkshire: Arrow Books.

Hawton, K., Rodham, K. and Evans, E. (2006) *By Their own Hands: Deliberate Self-Harm and Suicidal Ideas in Adolescence*. London: Jessica Kinsley.

Lister-Ford, C. (2002) *Skills in Transactional Analysis, Counselling and Psychotherapy*. London: Sage.

O'Connell, B. (2005) *Solution-Focused Therapy*. London: Sage.

Rayner, E., Joyce, A., Rose, J., Twyman, M. and Clulow, C. (2005) *Human Development: An Introduction to the Psychodynamics of Growth, Maturity and Ageing*. London: Routledge.

Sanders, D. (2005) *Cognitive Therapy: An Introduction*, 2nd edn. London: Sage.

Schiraldi, G.R. (2002) *The Anger Management Sourcebook*. Chigaco, IL: Contemporary Books.

Stainton Rogers, W. and Stainton Rogers, R. (2001) *The Psychology of Gender and Sexuality*. Buckingham: Open University Press.

Stewart, I. (1994) *Eric Berne*. London: Sage.

Stewart, I. (2000) *Transactional Analysis Counselling in Action*, 2nd edn. London: Sage.

Cross-References *Autonomy, Coping, Reflection.*

27 Holistic care

Kay Byatt

DEFINITION

The concept of holism has been around since earliest history, its root 'holos' is derived from the Greek meaning' whole', and relates to the study of whole organisms or systems (Farmer, 1983). The terms 'holism' and 'holistic' were first used in 1926 by the South African Philosopher Jan Smuts, who expressed the tendency in nature to form wholes that are greater than the sum of their parts. The classical definition of holism is that people are multidimensional. Each dimension is considered to be inextricably linked to other dimensions, and change in one dimension, resulting from the internal or external environment, may result in change in the others. Therefore, in physical illness, a person may be affected spiritually, psychologically and socially. This explains the holistic view that assumes the person always responds as a unified whole, which is greater than the sum of its parts. The value of the concept of holism has been widely recognised by nurses, and the American Holistic Nurse Association provides a definition of holism as 'the concept of wellness: the state of harmony between mind, body, emotions and spirit in an ever changing environment' (1992: 278).

The main focus within the holistic perspective is on promotion of individual health and wellness and return to wellness, as opposed to illness. The heart of holism which is often overlooked is that the individual actively utilises their own inner resources to improve their quality of life and make healthy choices to support adaptation to their health challenge (Buckley, 2002).

The concept of holistic care is based on the holistic philosophy, and is an approach or value system held by the practitioner who provides care which recognises the patient as a whole person. Care delivered in this way is based upon aims, agreed between practitioner and patient, which will help facilitate the patient to achieve a degree of balance between some of the interacting and competing influences on the mind, body, spirit and environment in order that they move toward a condition of optimum health (Aggleton and Chalmers, 2000; Freeman, 2005). As holism implies a willingness to use a wide range of interventions and an emphasis on a participatory relationship between practitioner and patient (Pietroni, 1987), these would be essential elements within the approach to holistic care.

KEY POINTS

- The whole is greater than the sum of its parts.
- Holism refers to the concept of the whole person with physiological, psychological, sociological and spiritual dimensions which fully interact.
- Holism can be identified as a view of the person and an approach to care.
- Holistic care fully acknowledges the holistic needs of individuals and aims to provide mutually agreed care and self-care strategies which help facilitate the optimum of health.

DISCUSSION

The holistic approach acknowledges the contribution of conventional medicine but moves beyond the focus on the physical to include the contributions of emotions, mind, relationships with people and the environment and spirit as vital factors in health and illness (Benor, 1999). Medical and nurse education has been largely influenced by Engel's (1977) bio-psycho-social model, which has promoted a more balanced approach to the individual in health and illness. However, the holistic view can be considered more complete and encompasses the bio-psycho-social and spiritual dimension of the individual. The importance of the spiritual dimension lies in the recognition that people have spiritual needs and that these may be expressed in many and varied ways (Dossey et al. 2005).

Wholeness

Wholeness is an ideal all of us work to throughout our lives; it is not a description of us as we are, but is a value to which we aspire and is an important part of being a person. A person is a conscious human being who has purposes and intentions together with capacity to develop powers of reasoning, feeling, believing and acting (Griffin, 1993). Therefore, being a whole person is experiential and requires participation in roles and activities in life which demand a degree of balance in relation to self, family or significant others, community and the wider social context (Buckle, 1993). As inseparability is an essential characteristic of the holistic viewpoint, then although different dimensions of a person may be studied, these should not be considered as separate compartments of knowledge or understanding (Hopper, 2000).

Illness

When imbalance takes place within the person, they may demonstrate observable symptoms and a range of needs that require to be supported to help them return to health. Illness changes physical and social functioning and emotional well being and also affects the individual's health concept, which invariably leads to questions about the meaning of being ill (Strumberg, 2005). The spiritual dimension within each person that leads to a search for meaning and purpose in life is relevant to health and illness and the quest for wellness. Holism holds that treatment must involve all of these factors and therefore holism is a philosophy and a practice/treatment modality (McKenzie, 2002).

Holistic care

Consequently, the holistic view and approach to care provides nurses with an opportunity to assess the patient as a whole person rather than only their presenting problem, such as an illness or wound. McMahon and Pearson (1998) contend that if nurses are to practice holism and view the patient as a whole person, then they must have developed themselves and be in tune with their own values. Nursing care may be considered a therapeutic practice in itself (Freshwater, 2002; McMahon and Pearson, 1998). For this to be possible the nurse requires to be able to approach the individual as a whole person (McKenzie, 2002), exhibiting qualities that include self-awareness, mindfulness, compassion, empathy and respect for person, together with the motivation, commitment and value system to keep these qualities at the forefront of their practice (McMahon and Pearson, 1998). Holistic care actively encourages patients' involvement in their own care and the nurse is required to work in partnership with the patient, planning ways in which their needs will be met and engaging in holistic caring. Thus, the therapeutic relationship can be seen to be intrinsic to holistic care, and this demands a high level of ability on behalf of the nurse to communicate effectively and adapt to the requirements of different patients. Such an approach encompasses 'being with' the patient, demonstrating insight and empathy, providing information and patient-centred care.

Nurse education includes the concept of holism and holistic practice within curricula to support development of competencies necessary for holistic care. However, literature suggests that nurses do not always carry out the holistic care they have been taught in the classroom (McCaugherty, 1991). It is easily seen that it may be challenging to maintain a focus and commitment to holistic care within contemporary healthcare settings where the care is largely routinised, task orientated and physically focused. There is a struggle to deliver care of a holistic nature within a retracting workforce and a contemporary climate driven by agendas directed toward demonstration of cost-effectiveness and measurable targets for patient outcomes.

Pre-requisites for holistic care

The qualities and attributes necessary for holistic care require to be nurtured through education programmes which closely link education in theory and practice and where gaps are addressed (McKenzie, 2002). Education for holistic care must also support the maintenance of personal motivation through the skills of self-awareness, reflection on and in practice, ongoing personal and professional development. Nurses should be encouraged to participate in clinical supervision. This is centred on reflective practice, which promotes a re-emphasis on patient-centred care, provides a structure to challenge and apply research-based theories to practice and thus help empower the practitioner (Down, 2002).

An evidence base

There is a continued need for research which demonstrates that the response to disease is at the level of the whole person and that biological adjustment is a function of whole person adjustment. In addition, the state of disease cannot be known or understood without fully taking into account experiential reports or the impact of social influences on disease (Kolcaba, 1997).

CASE STUDY

Mrs Mary Walters, a fit 80-year-old widow who lives alone, was admitted to the orthopaedic ward having fallen and fractured the neck of her right femur. She was very distressed and unco-operative with nursing staff, insisting that she must go home and not stay in hospital. The registered nurse caring for her spends time with her to more fully assess her needs; through this she finds that Mrs Walters is very worried about her dog who is not being cared for in her absence; she is also concerned about whether she will still be able to look after him after her surgery. The nurse helps Mrs Walters contact her neighbour and sister in order to make immediate and longer-term arrangements for her pet. As her wider needs had been met, Mrs Walters was no longer distressed and unco-operative, and with support and ongoing reassurance from the nurse she was prepared for her surgery.

CONCLUSION

As the concept of holism illustrates, 'the whole is greater than the sum of the parts', and there is a need at all times to view people as whole beings with simple or complex needs that may not be purely physical in nature but spiritual, psychological or social. Holistic care requires our attention as it is at the heart of nursing and is a value and an approach essential to the provision of high-quality care for a wide range of individuals with needs which are unique to them. The contemporary constraints and changing contexts within healthcare pose challenges to nurses. This may in fact provide the impetus for them to re-focus on the value of holistic care, its contribution in nursing and to the patient. The humanistic imperative of care is the most important element in care itself, and holistic care may be seen as the aspiration and imperative by those who seek to enhance the humane and well-rounded approach to healthcare practice (Bloom, 2004).

FURTHER READING

Aggleton, P. and Chalmers, H. (2000) *Nursing Models and Nursing Practice*, 2nd edn. Basingstoke: Macmillan.

Freshwater, D. (ed.) (2002) *Therapeutic Nursing: Improving Patient Care through Self-Awareness and Reflection*. London: Sage.

McMahon, R. and Pearson, A. (1998) *Nursing as Therapy*, 2nd edn. Cheltenham: Nelson Thorns.

REFERENCES

Aggleton, P. and Chalmers, H. (2000) *Nursing Models and Nursing Practice*, 2nd edn. Basingstoke: Macmillan.

American Holistic Nurse Association (1992) 'Manifesto document'. *Journal of the American Holistic Nurses Association*, 10: 277–8.

Benor, D.J. (1999) *Wholistic Integrative Care*. Available online at www.wholistichealing research.com/wholisticintegrativecare.html (last accessed 25 Jan. 2007)

Bloom, W. (2004) *Solution: The Holistic Manifesto*. Carlsbad, CA: Hay House.

Buckle, J. (1993) 'When is holism not complementary?' *British Journal of Nursing*, 2(15): 744–5.

Buckley, J. (2002) 'Holism and a health-promoting approach to palliative care'. *International Journal of Palliative Nursing*, 8(10): 505–8.

Dossey, B.M., Keegan, L. and Guzzeta, C.E. (2005) *Holistic Nursing: A Handbook for Practice*, 4th edn. Sudbary, MA: Jones and Bartlett.

Down, J. (2002) 'Nursing and technology: clinical supervision and reflective practice in a critical care setting', in D. Freshwater (ed.), *Therapeutic Nursing Improving: Patient Care through Self-Awareness and Reflection*. London: Sage. pp. 39–57.

Engel, G. (1977) 'The need for a new medical mode – a challenge for biomedicine'. *Science*, 196: 129–36.

Farmer, B. (1983) 'Clinical ethics, the use and abuse of power in nursing'. *Nursing Standard*, 72(3): 33–36.

Freeman, J. (2005) 'Towards a definition of holism'. *British Journal of General Practice*, 55(511): 154–5.

Freshwater, D. (ed.) (2002) *Therapeutic Nursing: Improving Patient Care through Self-Awareness and Reflection*. London: Sage.

Griffin, A. (1993) 'Holism in nursing: its meaning and value'. *British Journal of Nursing*, 2(6): 310–12.

Hopper, A. (2000) 'Meeting the spiritual needs of patients through holistic practice'. *European Journal of Palliative Care*, 7(2): 60–2.

holistic care

Kolcaba, R. (1997) 'The primary holisms in nursing'. *Journal of Advanced Nursing*, 25: 290–6.

McCaugherty, D. (1991) 'The theory–practice gap in nurse education: its causes and possible solutions. Findings from an action research study'. *Journal of Advanced Nursing*, 17: 1055–61.

McKenzie, R. (2002) 'The importance of philosophical congruence for therapeutic use of self in practice', in D. Freshwater (ed.), *Therapeutic Nursing Improving: Patient Care through Self-Awareness and Reflection*. London: Sage. pp. 22–38.

McMahon, R. and Pearson, A. (1998) *Nursing as Therapy*, 2nd edn. Cheltenham: Nelson Thorns.

Pietroni, P.C. (1987) 'The meaning of illness-holism dissected: discussion paper'. *Journal of the Royal Society of Medicine*, 80: 357–60.

Strumberg, J. (2005) 'How to teach holistic care-meeting the challenge of complexity in clinical practice'. *Education for Health*, 18(2): 236–45.

Cross-References *Assessment, Communication, Compassion, Competence, Confidence, Empowerment, Environment, Professional development, Reflection, Value.*

28 Inequalities in health

Alison While

DEFINITION

Concern about health inequalities has its foundations in the social justice movement and has a long history in the United Kingdom with the recognition by Edwin Chadwick in the 1840s that mortality rates varied across social groups and living conditions (While, 1987). Health inequalities are different from health differences. While differences in health are naturally determined, inequalities in health are the consequence of influences in society, including social inequalities, which expose individuals to greater health risks and simultaneously reduce access to supportive services including healthcare.

KEY POINTS

- Health inequalities are socially determined.
- Health inequalities are important in terms of social justice.
- Evidence indicates that health inequalities have persisted despite various policy initiatives over the years.

DISCUSSION

The study of health inequalities began with a focus on mortality rates and attempts to explain the underlying causes of trends in the datasets (Beveridge, 1942; Chadwick, 1842; Farr, 1864; Rowntree, 1901). Evidence of social inequalities (see Table 2) provided the impetus for the foundation of the welfare state after World War II (Beveridge, 1942), and it was hoped that a comprehensive welfare state would reduce inequalities through publicly funded support at the time of need. However, first the Black Report (DHSS, 1980) and then an update of the Black Report (Townsend et al., 1992) confirmed persistent differences in the health experiences of different groups in the population expressed in terms of differential adult and child mortality and morbidity rates.

Table 2 *Health inequalities and their social gradient*

Social class	Health outcomes
I Professional	Lowest standardised mortality rates for men and women across all causes (coronary heart disease, cancer, accidents).
II Managerial and Technical III (N) Skilled (non-manual) III (M) Skilled (manual) IV Partly skilled	
V Unskilled	Highest standardised mortality rates for men and women across all causes. Highest prevalence of mental health problems, including alcohol and drug dependence.

A more recent independent inquiry (Acheson, 1998) noted that, while there have been health gains, not all sections of society have benefited equally, so that the differences in the health experience of different social groups have widened rather than narrowed. This analysis has been developed in terms of an explanatory model which argues the centrality of health determinants derived from the socio-economic circumstances of individuals and has resulted in a recognition that policies need to address a wide range of issues to reduce social inequalities and increase access to healthcare.

Socio-economic explanatory model

Dahlgren and Whitehead (1991) proposed a conceptual model (see Figure 12) comprising different layers of influence around an individual, with each layer building upon and interacting with each other. Thus an individual's biological make-up of genes, gender and age provide a fixed potential upon which influences act. Individuals live within a social context in which they interact with family members, friends and their immediate community, which influences the personal behaviour and may either damage or promote health. The support derived from the community can help mediate the effects of wider influences, such as living and working conditions (including the work environment, unemployment and housing) and access to services (including shops, leisure facilities, education and healthcare), over which the individual has limited control. These wider influences are shaped in turn by the socio-economic, cultural and environmental conditions within society.

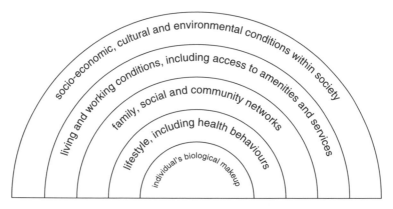

Figure 12   *Socio-economic explanatory model (adapted from Dahlgren and Whitehead, 1991)*

Importantly, this explanatory model emphasises the impact of the social structure upon health outcome, and highlights potential intervention points which may prevent avoidable morbidity and mortality. In other words, preventive action can reduce individual risk through attempting to change personal behaviour, interventions in the workplace or local environment may promote healthy behaviour, while interventions at the level of the social structure should reduce social and economic disadvantages.

The evidence supporting the socio-economic model is strong and clearly points to persistent inequalities in health across a number of dimensions, which include mortality, life expectancy and health status. The Acheson Report summarised its findings as 'Although in general disadvantage is associated with worse health, the patterns of inequalities vary by place, gender, age, year of birth and other factors, and differ according to which measure of health used' (1998: 10).

The Report (Acheson, 1998) argued strongly that the level of disposable income was a key determinant of health outcome. Poverty impacts upon standards of living and thus health choices as well as access to services, including access to education and other amenities. The Joseph Rowntree Foundation (www.jrf.org.uk) research provides a substantial body of evidence indicating the impact of poverty and resulting social exclusion upon children and their families and the long-term consequences in terms of inter-generational disadvantage which condemns some families to a life of disadvantage with few opportunities to improve their circumstances.

Access to healthcare

Access is concerned with whether those who need care can gain entry to healthcare. Healthcare provides services both at the beginning and at the end of life and in between those events through diagnosis and treatment services. A key issue is fairness related to access to those with equivalent health needs, with the evidence indicating that there are systematic variations in access to all components parts of the health services. Thus, those with the greatest health needs experience less access to preventive services, primary care and secondary care (Gulliford and Morgan, 2003). Indeed, little has changed since Tudor Hart (1971) argued that 'the availability of good medical care tends to vary inversely with the need for it in the population served' (1971: 405).

However, while the evidence suggests a variation in provision, there is also evidence that some social groups do not utilise services at levels which might be expected. Morgan (2003) has suggested that help-seeking behaviours play a major role in determining when and how health services are accessed, while others have argued that organisational and geographical barriers play their part in preventing access to preventive and curative services (Beech, 2003; Haynes, 2003). Additional access points have been introduced to primary care in the form of NHS walk-in centres and NHS Direct in an attempt to reduce organisational barriers, but their impact upon increased access is not yet evident. Geographical barriers range from regional variation in provision to more local service distribution between urban and rural areas. While there is improved regional equity as a result of a more fair distribution of health resources nationwide, the drive for increased efficiency and effectiveness has centralised services in urban areas with consequences for those living in rural areas who lack private transport and those with limited mobility such as older people and those with disabilities (Haynes, 2003).

CASE STUDY

Debbie is a single mother aged 20 who lives on benefits in a council flat in a run-down inner-city estate. She left school with no educational qualifications and has never worked. She has limited contact with her own family, having left home after an argument with her mother when she was 15 years old. Her father died at the age of 42 from a heart attack and her mother is in poor health having smoked up to forty cigarettes a day for many years. She has two children, Darren aged 3 years and Jaycee aged 9 months, who are slightly behind in their developmental milestones. Debbie is overweight and has been depressed and feels isolated. She has very low self-esteem and only ventures out of her flat to get essential shopping. Debbie's health visitor is her key health contact and visits her regularly. During her home visits she has immunised Darren and Jaycee with Debbie's consent and has introduced Debbie to the local toy library by accompanying her there. The health visitor is working with Debbie to develop her confidence so that she can attend the clinic's mother and toddler group and cookery and other classes which are held in the local community centre. Over the long term the health visitor hopes that Debbie will be able to join classes to develop her basic skills so that she may take up employment if she wishes.

CONCLUSION

Health inequalities are a key issue for all health professionals. Despite various policy initiatives, health experience continues to be determined in large part by socio-economic factors. Every encounter with a health professional has the potential to make a difference as to whether an individual gains maximum benefit from that health contact. An unsatisfactory interaction may dissuade an individual from seeking help on future occasions and may reinforce perceived access barriers. Health advice needs to be tailored and must recognise the individual's socio-economic circumstances so that suggested changes to health behaviour are realistic. Reduction in health inequalities requires action at not only governmental level but also at the level of health professional in their everyday practice.

FURTHER READING

Department of Health (2002) *Tackling Health Inequalities: Cross-cutting Review*. London: DoH. Available online at www.doh.gov.uk

Department of Health (2003) *Tackling Health Inequalities: A Programme for Action*. London: DoH. Available online at www.doh.gov.uk

Department of Health (2005) *Tackling Health Inequalities: Status Report on the Programme for Action*. London: DoH. Available online at www.doh. gov.uk

Gulliford, M. and Morgan, M. (eds) (2003) *Access to Health Care*. London: Routledge.

REFERENCES

Acheson, D. (1998) *Independent Inquiry into Inequalities in Health Report*. London: The Stationery Office.

Beech, R. (2003) 'Organisational barriers to access', in M. Gulliford and M. Morgan (eds), *Access to Health Care*. London: Routledge. pp. 84–103.

Beveridge, W. (1942) *Social Insurance and Allied Services*. London: HMSO.

Chadwick, E. (1842) *An Inquiry into the Sanitary Conditions of the Labouring Population of Great Britain*. London: HMSO.

Dahlgren, G. and Whitehead, M. (1991) *Policies and Strategies to Promote Social Equity in Health*. Stockholm: Institute of Futures Studies.

Department of Health and Social Security (1980) *Inequalities in Health: Report of a Research Working Group*. Chair: D. Black. London: DHSS.

Farr, W. (1864) *Letter to the Registrar General on the years 1851–1860; supplement to the 25th report of the Registrar General*. London: Registrar General's Office.

Gulliford, M. and Morgan, M. (eds) (2003) *Access to Health Care*. London: Routledge.

Haynes, R. (2003) 'Geographical access to health care', in M. Gulliford and M. Morgan (eds), *Access to Health Care*. London: Routledge. pp. 13–35.

Morgan, M. (2003) 'Patients' help-seeking and access to health care', in M. Gulliford and M. Morgan (eds), *Access to Health Care*. London: Routledge. pp. 61–83.

Rowntree, B.S. (1901) *Poverty: A Study of Town Life*. London: Macmillan.

Townsend, P., Whitehead, M. and Davidson, N. (1992) *Inequalities in Health: The Black Report and the Health Divide*. London: Penguin.

Tudor Hart, J. (1971) 'The inverse care law'. *The Lancet*, 1(7696): 405–12.

While, A. (1987) 'The early history of health visiting: a review of the role of central government (1830–1914)'. *Child: Care, Health and Development*, 13: 127–36.

Cross-References *Diversity, Empowerment, Environment, Equality.*

29 Leadership

Geoff Watts

DEFINITION

A particular feature of the development of organisational theory during the post-war period has been the emergence of leadership as a distinct entity from that of management. At the beginning of this period, Bennis (1959) was to define leadership as a process in which subordinates are influenced to behave in a desired manner; a definition of leadership indistinguishable from management. The notion of leadership as a medium for personal development emerged during the 1980s and is illustrated by Bass's (1985) view of leadership as a *transforming* process in which the leader creates visions of goals to be obtained and articulates ways to obtain those goals. By the 1990s, a definition of leadership was to emerge which completed the process of distinguishing between management activity and leadership activity. Rafferty proposed that 'Leaders are people who inspire ... and whom others will follow and trust in their integrity. Leaders care for people they are leading, and try to strengthen and promote them ... leaders facilitate, help, encourage and praise' (1993: 4).

KEY POINTS

- Leadership is complementary to, not a substitute for, effective clinical management.
- Leadership requires the exercise of power to effect change.
- Effective leaders within the NHS are required to challenge pre-existing guiding principles.

DISCUSSION

The emergence of leadership from out of the shadow of management raises the question of their relationship. Rather than seeing leadership as a replacement or substitute for the perceived failures of management, it is more pertinent to explore the manner in which leadership has come to be seen as complementary to the management process. McCormack and Hopkins (1995) illustrated this blend of skills by suggesting that clinical nursing leadership is about exerting (blending) influence, power and authority within a particular field.

The terms 'power' and 'authority' can sit uncomfortably within a modern-day discussion of leadership, as they seem to hark back to notions of managerial coercion, but the apparent dichotomy between the exercise of power and leadership had been addressed at an early stage in the post-war period. French and Raven (1959) identified bases of social power with which individuals potentially influence others. Although legitimate power, based on one's hierarchical position within an organisation, is recognised by French and Raven, so too is referent and expert power, which refer to a leader's potential to influence others by virtue of the leader's acknowledged experience and competence within their given field, as well as their capacity to act as a role model for other group members. The drawing of these distinctions between forms of power is a reflection of a key distinction between leadership and management. The manager's exercise of legitimate power is a permanent state, whereas the leader's exercise of referent/expert power is dependent upon a leader's capacity to bring knowledge and expertise to bear on the prevailing circumstances. Thus, it follows that in any given group of professional practitioners, although it is likely that there can be only one manager with legitimate power, there are potentially many leaders with expert power.

leadership

181

However effective the exercise of leadership, it cannot be an end in itself. Leadership is a means by which organisational development occurs. 'Development' implies advancement, movement or growth; ultimately change. Leadership is not about the preservation of the status quo, it is about the future. Leadership is change agency, and the power that the leader exerts is the power to influence others in the determination of future goals and directions (Bass, 1990).

Almost all discussions of the nature of change make reference to the work of Lewin (1951), who proposed a 'force field' model of change in which driving forces compete with restraining forces to move from a current to a future state. Effective change agency requires the leader to have an understanding of the restraining forces in operation. Nelson (2005) sees resistance as a major barrier to change which impedes progress within an organisation. This view suggests, however, that those who resist change are unhelpful and dysfunctional to an organisation. This idea was supported by Pratt (1980), who suggested that whenever change is proposed in an organisation, the people concerned will line up along the following continuum of response to change, ranging from enthusiasm to antagonism:

Enthusiasts – Supporters – Acquiescers – Laggards – Antagonists

According to Pratt's model, the *enthusiasts* are those with the initial ideas for change, *supporters* agree with and support change, *acquiescers* simply fall in line, and the *laggards* resist change and build obstacles to development. The *antagonists* actively reject the notion of change and become a focus of revolt.

It is possible, however, to superimpose on this horizontal continuum of response to change a vertical continuum of the legitimacy with which those positions are held, resulting in a four-dimensional model of response to change as shown in Figure 13. Within this model, four dimensions (A, B, C and D) of responsiveness to change are predicted. Position A denotes the legitimate enthusiast who supports change and appreciates the benefits. Position B denotes legitimate antagonists, who flag up problems out of genuine concern. Position C denotes the illegitimate enthusiast for change. They are often bored and wish change for the sake of change, but never take the lead or initiative. Position D denotes the classic illegitimate antagonist. They are the fearful, anxious, settled and complacent members of an organisation.

For the emergent leader the challenge would appear to be the development of strategies to cope with resistance to change. Thomas (1976) saw

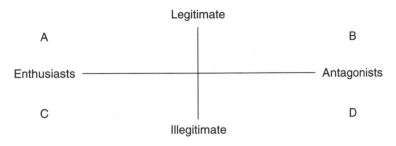

Figure 13   *A four-dimensional model of response to change*

such resistance to change as conflict arising from the differing perceptions or assumptions that people held about the value of the proposed change. Thomas suggested that leaders need to adopt a range of strategies to cope with such resistance, which he identified as:

- competing
- accommodating
- avoiding
- collaborating
- compromising

Effective leadership is about having access to all the strategies proposed by Thomas. It is not so much a question of which is the right or wrong conflict-coping strategy to adopt in any given situation so much as which is the most appropriate strategy. Clark (1997) has suggested that leaders need to encourage people to move from change avoidance to change acceptance, and cites Connor's (1993) view that the acceptance of change is a staged process involving denial of the need for change, anger at having to deal with change, bargaining to resolve conflict, depression due to doubt and lack of support, and finally acceptance of the reality of change. Connor acknowledged that this view of change acceptance is similar to, and indeed influenced by, the work of Kubler-Ross (1970) who discussed how the terminally ill are able to come to an acceptance of their impending death through support and open awareness. Since its inception, the National Health Service (NHS) in the United Kingdom has been subject to modification, re-organisation, re-direction, modernisation, reform and change. On the 50th anniversary of the NHS, Plamping suggested that 'despite considerable structural change and numerous attempts at reform, the underlying nature of the NHS has remained remarkably stable and many behaviours have not changed' (1998: 69). Plamping proposed that this situation may be as a result of uncertainty as to how the service should function, rather than what its function should be, and hypothesised that if there are guiding principles in operation within the NHS, then the service can only be reformed by challenging those principles. The NHS responded to the challenges for change presented to it at the beginning of the 21st century by establishing a leadership centre, under the auspices of The Institute for Innovation and Improvement, which was to publish *The NHS Leadership Qualities Framework* (NHS, 2002). This framework was designed to set the standards for outstanding leadership within the NHS, and to be applicable at all levels of function within the service, from senior managerial function to clinical leadership. The framework describes a set of fifteen key characteristics, attitudes and behaviours that leaders should aspire to in delivering the NHS plan (NHS, 2003). The key characteristics are organised into three clusters – personal qualities, setting direction and delivering the service – and each characteristic is presented within the framework in such a way as to allow service leaders to assess themselves against established criteria. The framework also allows for peer assessment of a leader's performance and thus affords those in leadership positions feedback from colleagues who work closely with them to deliver the service.

CASE STUDY

Charlotte, an experienced clinical nurse manager working in an acute hospital NHS Trust, was appointed to lead the nursing team in a newly established treatment centre. The centre was designed to function as a circuit, allowing patients to move smoothly through the various sections from reception, admission, assessment, treatment and discharge. This required staff to make significant changes to the way in which they were used to working. Within a few weeks of the centre opening, Charlotte became concerned that there were problems with the new system, with low staff morale and lack of commitment to the new procedures.

Charlotte concluded that as the operating protocols were clearly laid down, the issue may have been the manner in which she was leading the changes to staff working practices. Using the *NHS Leadership Framework*, Charlotte undertook a self-assessment of her leadership qualities, and invited a number of her colleagues to undertake a peer review using the same framework to allow a comparison of her findings.

This exercise revealed to Charlotte that although she had focussed on a drive for improvement and was deeply motivated to enhance the quality of service delivery, she needed to articulate for the staff a more compelling vision of the change and to communicate the rationale for change and modernisation to her staff to facilitate them working collaboratively to achieve the required change.

CONCLUSION

Whatever the quality of the leadership that is exercised, it can only be a means to an end: service improvement. Such improvement implies change. For change to be facilitated, those with leadership responsibility need to create new visions and goals, and to break down the adhesions of past practices. Leadership expertise must be developed at an operational level within the NHS as well as at a strategic level. It is a cliché that there is a Field Marshall's baton in the rucksack of every private soldier. There is leadership potential in every member of the health service workforce. It is less important for those delivering the service to learn about leadership than it is for them to learn about themselves as leaders.

FURTHER READING

Hughes, L., Ginnett, R. and Curphy, G. (2002) *Leadership: Enhancing the Lessons of Experience*, 4th edn. Boston, MD: McGraw-Hill Higher Education.

REFERENCES

Bass, B.M. (1985) *Leadership and Performance Beyond Expectations*. New York: Free Press.

Bass, B.M. (1990) *Bass and Stogdill's Handbook of Leadership*, 3rd edn. New York: Free Press.

Bennis, W.G. (1959) 'Leadership theory and administrative behaviour: the problem of authority'. *Administrative Science Quarterly*, 4: 259–60.

Clark, D. (1997) 'Leadership and Change'. Available online at www.nlink.com (accessed 31 Oct. 2006).

Connor, D. (1993) *Managing at the Speed of Change*. New York: Random House.

French, J. and Raven, B. (1959) 'The bases of social power', in D. Cartwright and A. Arbor (eds), *Studies of Social Power*. University of Michigan, MI: Institute for Social Research.

Kubler-Ross, E. (1970) *On Death and Dying*. Bedford: Tavistock Press.

Lewin, K. (1951) *Field Theory in Social Sciences*. New York: Harper Row.

McCormack, B. and Hopkins, E. (1995) 'The development of clinical leadership through supported reflective practice'. *Journal of Clinical Nursing*, 4(3): 161–8.

leadership

National Health Service (2002) *The NHS Leadership Qualities Framework*. Warwick: NHS Institute for Innovation and Improvement.

National Health Service (2003) *Introducing the NHS Leadership Qualities Framework. About the Framework'*. Warwick: NHS Institute for Innovation and Improvement. Available online at www.nhsleadershipqualities.nhs.uk (accessed 1 Dec. 2006).

Nelson, L. (2005) 'Managing the human resources in organisational change: A case study'. *Research and Practice in Human Resource Management*, 13(1): 55–70.

Plamping, D. (1998) 'Change and resistance to change in the NHS'. *BMJ*, 317: 69–71.

Pratt, D. (1980) *Curriculum Design and Development*. Oxford: Harcourt Brace.

Rafferty, A. (1993) *Leading Questions: A Discussion Paper on the Issues of Nurse Leadership*. London: King's Fund Centre.

Thomas, K. (1976) *Conflict and Conflict Management: Handbook of Industrial and Organisational Psychology*. Chicago, IL: Chicago Press.

Cross-References *Accountability, Coping, Empowerment, Managing change, Problem solving, Reflection, Teamwork.*

---

30 Manager

Jenni Templeman and Heather Cooper

DEFINITION

A manager is accountable for optimising human, material and financial contributions for the achievement of organisational goals (Manley, 1997). The primary remit of a manager is to implement the vision, policies, goals and objectives of the organisation. The concept of management is often used interchangeably with leadership and whilst discussion later draws a distinction between them, it is generally recognised by practising managers that they are often accepted as the same thing (Hannagan, 1998). Lucey (1996) stated that management is a practice not a science, yet the essence of management encompasses knowledge and performance and is viewed as getting things done through other people in order to achieve specific organisational objectives. Conversely, Dantley (2005) suggested that management is based on seven scientific principles which demonstrate the minutiae of the strategic agenda. Managerial tasks include planning, organising, co-ordinating and controlling the work of a group of employees.

KEY POINTS

- Role definition defines the necessary skills, knowledge and attributes required of a manager to enable achievement of organisational objectives.
- The management process is an organisational responsibility which utilises a multi-faceted, systematic approach.
- There are many management theories; however, these are broadly divided into the science and humanistic schools of thought.
- An eclectic array of management styles/behaviours are required to suit diverse situations in order to achieve organisational goals.

DISCUSSION

Management is a process which takes place at all levels in an organisation and is not only carried out by people with 'manager' in their job title. Many individuals carry out managerial functions, although perhaps not all of the same type or importance. It is the task a person performs that is important, not the job title. Current nursing curricula (NMC, 2004) provide learning opportunities for student exposure to management. However, anecdotal evidence suggests that new graduates in nursing need time to develop their clinical and leadership skills before attempting to take on management responsibilities. A recent initiative has identified this theory-practice gap and addressed areas for development, with competency-based criterion (Skills for Health, 2006). There are two schools of thought in relation to management theories:

- scientific management, which emphasises the task aspects of management; and
- human relations-based management, which emphasises the interpersonal aspects of managing people.

Scientific management

About 100 years ago it was believed that if a task was well designed and enough incentive was given to the task, then workers would be more productive. In healthcare this would equate to the number of clients

manager

187

bathed rather than the number of hours worked. This would necessitate an incentive to get the most work done in the least amount of time. Taylorism stresses that this is the best way to do a job and is usually the fastest way to do it (Dantley, 2005). The work itself is analysed to improve efficiency; for example, is it quicker to bring the phlebotomist to the client, or vice versa? Nurse managers who adopt the principles of scientific management pay particular attention to the type of assessments and procedures performed on a unit, the equipment that is needed to do this efficiently, and the strategies that facilitate efficient accomplishment of these tasks (Dantley, 2005). These nurse managers keep careful records of the amount of work accomplished and reward those who accomplish the most (Whitehead et al., 2007). It could be argued that by adopting a 'task orientation' method of management, clients may lose individualised healthcare delivery (Whitehead et al., 2007).

Human relations–based management

McGregor's (1960) theories (X and Y) are a good example of the difference between scientific management and human relations-based management. McGregor argued that theory X reflects a common attitude amongst managers; that most employees really do not want to work very hard and that it is the manager's job to make sure they do. To accomplish this, the theory suggests, a manager needs to employ strict rules, constant supervision and the threat of punishment (reprimands, threat of job loss) to create industrious, conscientious workers. The key elements of theory X can be summarised as:

- Work is something to be avoided.
- People want to do as little as possible.
- Use of control-supervision-punishment.

In an opposing viewpoint, theory Y managers believe that the work itself can be motivating and that people will work hard if their managers provide a supportive environment. A theory Y manager emphasises guidance rather than control, development rather than close supervision, and reward rather than punishment. This nurse manager is concerned with keeping employee morale as high as possible, and assumes that satisfied, motivated employees will do the best work. Employees' attitudes, opinions, hopes and fears are important to this type of nurse manager, and considerable time is spent on conflict management and promoting mutual understanding in order to create a conducive environment in which people can reach their optimal potential and ownership. Theory Y therefore supposes that:

- Work itself can be motivating.
- People really want to do their job well.
- The use of guidance-development-reward is beneficial. (Whitehead et al., 2007).

In current healthcare there can be seen to be a correlation between the quality of patient care, staff morale and effective nursing leadership. The degree of satisfaction staff achieve from their work is in part determined by the style of management they work under, and a proactive manager will impact on the team's performance and the quality of patient care (Clegg, 2000). The challenge facing the modern manager is maintaining control over the processes of an organisation, whilst simultaneously leading, inspiring, directing and making pertinent decisions to optimise present systems, structures and processes and remain open to future challenges.

Perceptions on leadership and management

Whitehead et al. (2007) drew the following distinctions between leadership and management:

- Leadership is based on influence and shared meaning, whereas management is based on authority.
- Leadership is informal, while management is a formally designated role.
- Leadership is an achieved position, compared to the assigned position of management.
- Leadership is part of every nurse's responsibilities, while managers are usually responsible for areas such as budgets, retention and recruitment of employees.
- Leadership requires initiative and independent thinking.
- Management is improved by the use of effective leadership skills.

Kotter (1990) stated that management was about coping with complexity, and good management further brought about a degree of order and consistency to core dimensions like the quality and profitability of

manager

products, whereas leadership, by contrast, is about coping with change, which is increasingly evident in our environmental, technological and political world. In practice, Kotter (1990) saw the activities of the manager encompassing planning, budgeting, organising and controlling, whereas the activities of leadership centred around giving direction, aligning the workforce and motivation.

The 'trait theory' (Stodgill, 1948) recognised that the qualities of leadership and management, as defined by Kotter, are considered combined prerequisites for the modern leader. The emphasis on leadership centres on interpersonal skills in a broader context, and is often associated with the willing and enthusiastic behaviour of staff members and is seen primarily as an inspirational process. In short, leadership is the process of motivating other people to act in a particular way to achieve specific goals. Leadership styles and organisational culture are associated with an increase in productivity and staff satisfaction (Almio-Metcalf, 1996; Bass, 1981). Goldsmith and Clutterbuck (1984) identified three key elements of leadership:

- Visibility of the leader.
- Clear statement of direction, with evidence of commitment from the team.
- Provision of clear objectives with financial balance.

Early theories did not explore the links between environment and leadership styles. Situational or contingency theories developed in the 1960s considered leaders in relation to their environment. Fiedlier (1967) developed his hypothesis around the premise that leaders' personal characteristics are stable and, therefore, so is the leadership style. Contrary to this theory, Vroom and Jago (1998) contend that leaders are perfectly capable of changing their behaviour from situation to situation, and argue that different environments necessitate different leadership styles.

Transactional leadership is seen to rely on the power of organisational position and formal authority to reward and punish performance (Clegg, 2000). Transformational leadership is held to be collaborative, consultative and consensus seeking, and ascribes power to interpersonal skills and personal contact (Markham, 1998). Transformational leaders concentrate on articulating a vision and mission, thus creating and maintaining a positive image in the minds of staff and superiors. This style of leadership is a pivotal factor in optimising team performance in the delivery of high-quality healthcare and best practice.

Managers hold multi-faceted, complex and responsible positions within healthcare organisations. Effective managers empower their staff to grow and develop as healthcare professionals while providing the highest quality care to their clients. Hannagan (1998) asserted that the best managers are probably flexible, applying the best style to cope with a particular situation. This suggests that the manager has to develop skills in more than one style.

An effective manager thus possesses a combination of qualities, for example, leadership, clinical expertise and business sense/knowledge. Historically, the nursing career structure was such that if an individual proved to have exemplified skills they were rewarded by promotion into management, but management expertise was often lacking. The current comparative lack of post-registration expertise necessitates competency skill development. This has recently been addressed by Skills for Health (2006) and forms an integral aspect of managers' lifelong learning facilitated through their personal development plan (PDP).

CASE STUDY

Sian was a senior sister of 18 months' standing. Her manager was on long-term sick leave and there was an expectation for Sian to 'act up' as the operational manager of the ward. Sian was considered a competent and confident clinical expert; however, her management skills were limited to managing the ward area. Staffing morale was considered at an all-time low and retention was poor. The primary objective for Sian was to gain the confidence of the staff to enable achievement of team cohesion and the delivery of quality care.

Sian soon realised that she needed to identify areas for development through her PDP. She identified that a short course on managerial training offered at the Trust would complement her new role and realise knowledge and skills fit for purpose. Sian then set out to identify the available resources and assistance from other managers to help achieve commitment, co-operation and cohesion from the team. This necessitated utilising a combination of different management theories and leadership skills in various situations and remaining open to change. With time, both Sian and the team grew personally and professionally and Sian's character, courage, knowledge and personality was infused not only within the climate and culture of the daily ward environment, but also the organisation as a whole.

CONCLUSION

The ethos of management occurs within the socialisation of each individual, and in nursing is developed and nurtured throughout the pre-registration pathway, creating a solid foundation for future post-registration career escalation. A value system that is shared and governed by the full spectrum of employees is crucial to achieving organisational and national agenda goals. Utilisation of these values will add impetus to the ever-changing climate of future healthcare delivery and avoid inertia. For a professional starting out in, or renewing, their career, the following advice is invaluable: 'Success is a journey not a destination' (Sweetland, 1960).

FURTHER READING

Lombardi, D.N. (2001) *Handbook for the New Health Care Manager*. San Francisco, CA: Jossey-Bass/AHA Press.

Whitehead, D.K., Weiss, S.A. and Tappen, R.M. (2007) *Essentials of Nursing Leadership and Management*, 4th edn. Philadelphia, PA: F.A. Davis.

REFERENCES

Almio-Metcalf, B. (1996) 'Leaders of managers'. *Nursing Management*, 3(1): 22–4.

Bass, B. (1981) *Bass and Stogdill's Handbook of Leadership*, 3rd edn. New York: Collier Macmillan.

Clegg, A. (2000) 'Leadership: improving the quality of patient care'. *Nursing Standard*, 14(30): 43–5.

Dantley, M.F. (2005) 'Moral leadership: shifting the management paradigm', in F.W. English (ed.), *The Sage Handbook of Educational Leadership*. Thousand Oaks, CA: Sage.

Fiedlier, F. (1967) *A Theory of Leadership Effectiveness*. New York: McGraw-Hill.

Goldsmith, W. and Clutterbuck, D. (1984) *The Winning Streak*. London: Penguin.

Hannagan, T. (1998) *Management Concepts and Practices*. London: Pearson Education.

Kotter, J.P. (1990) *Force for Change: How Leadership Differs from Management*. New York: Simon & Schuster.

Lucey, T. (1996) *Management Information Systems*, 7th edn. Guernsey: The Guernsey Press.

Manley, K. (1997) 'A conceptual framework for advanced practice: an action research project operationalizing and advanced practitioner/consultant nurse role'. *Journal of Clinical Nursing*, 6: 179–90.

Markham, G. (1998) 'Gender in leadership'. *Nursing Management*, 3(1): 18–9.

McGregor, D. (1960) *The Human Side of Enterprise*. New York: McGraw-Hill.

Nursing and Midwifery Council (2004) *Standards of Proficiency for Pre-Registration Nursing Education*. London: NMC.

Skills for Health (2006) *Career Framework for Health: Methodology Testing Report.* Bristol: Skills for Health.

Stodgill, R. (1948) 'Personal factors associated with leadership: a survey of the literature'. *Journal of Psychology,* 25: 35–71.

Sweetland, B. (1960) *I Will.* London: Wiltshire Book Company.

Vroom, V. and Jago, G. (1998) *The New Leadership.* Engelwood Cliffs, CA: Prentice Hall.

Whitehead, D.K., Weiss, S.A. and Tappen, R.M. (2007) *Essentials of Nursing Leadership and Management,* 4th edn. Philadelphia, PA: F.A. Davis.

Cross-References *Crisis management, Empowerment, Leadership, Managing change.*

31 Managing change

Linda Meredith

DEFINITION

Nurses function in an environment that is constantly being changed and reformed at both a national and local level. These reforms have modernised all aspects of their roles including the terms and conditions, their competencies within roles linked to the planning of personal and career development, and the requirement to update and change their practice (DoH, 2000, 2004). Effective strategies for managing change are dependent not only on the type of development involved, but also on the context in which it is implemented. Change can be viewed from several perspectives, including changes within an organisation that may be the result of restructuring in response to government initiatives, or a change in internal processes such as the implementation of a new sickness and absence policy. Change may be implemented by the individual responding to an organisational impetus, or implemented as an innovation in response to the production of new evidence from research, evaluation or audit. 'Change is what makes us know we are alive and conscious, and belief that we can bring about change is central to our understanding of ourselves as agents capable of change' (Hussey, 2002: 104). Change can be viewed as an inevitable progression for any individual, as this relates to the biological process arising from the notion that all life is in a state of flux. In human beings this relates to birth, development, ageing, illness and death. As nurses provide care within this context, change has to become an integral part of this care. This has led some authors to suggest that nurses should view change as an inevitable part of their role and as a normal life event that is linked to growth and development (Defeo, 1990).

KEY POINTS

- Change is an inevitable fact of life both at a personal and organisational level.
- An effective change strategy for transforming practice is one that involves those who will be implementing the change.
- Individuals need to be enabled to go through a period of transition in order to come to terms with major change.

DISCUSSION

Managing change in a healthcare context can be viewed from three perspectives: (a) strategies for implementing changes within an organisation; (b) implementing innovations in professional procedures that are linked to changing practice or individual behaviour; and (c) the individual's response to change. This chapter will briefly outline these three main perspectives and their application to managing change in healthcare.

Managing organisational change

The literature on managing change in organisations refers to strategies and theories that are generally not context specific, nor linked to any particular historical time and are applied indiscriminately to healthcare organisations. For example, Broome (1998) cited change theories and strategies that were written as a result of research on a wide range of organisations, yet it is suggested that they could be applied to multiple areas of nursing practice. Another classic model of change is Lewin's model of force field analysis that was devised in 1951 in the United States following research on housewives. This model is cited extensively in the literature as relating to the management of change in nursing and healthcare. More closely related to healthcare, one classic strategy regularly cited for the implementation of change is Bennis et al. (1993). This strategy identifies a series of approaches to managing change and gives an indication as to when they are applicable.

- *Power-coercive*: This is known as a top-down approach, where people in authority wield political, economic and sometimes moral power to instruct individuals to change. It is dependent on people who are basically compliant and who will generally do as instructed. Many national changes are implemented by adopting this strategy, for example, closing hospitals and changing service delivery as management directives.
- *Rational-empirical*: This is also a top-down strategy that is based on the assumption that people are rational and will be guided by reason. There is also the assumption that rational decisions will be made on a sound knowledge base. Changing professional practice following the results of audit, as evidence, is an example of when this strategy might be employed.
- *Normative-re-educative*: This strategy is a bottom-up approach and is based on the belief that people are social beings and need to be involved in all aspects of the changes to be made. Furthermore, it is expected that individuals prefer to adhere to their cultural norms and values. Therefore, change is based on trying to redefine and reinterpret existing norms and values, thus, developing commitments to new ones. (Bennis et al., 1993)

Implementing innovations

A large proportion of the literature on managing innovations in professional practice focuses on the challenges of implementing care that is evidence based. Bero et al. (1998) undertook a systematic review of the literature on the effectiveness of differing strategies for promoting behavioural change in the implementation of research findings in medical professional practice. Bero et al. (1998) found that the most effective strategies for promoting behavioural change were:

- The use of educational outreach visits to reinforce the use of evidence.
- Manual or computerised reminders.
- Multiple interventions such as audit and feedback in conjunction with local consensus agreement. These are discussions aimed at

gaining agreement from participating practitioners that the chosen clinical issue is important and the approach to managing the problem is appropriate.

- Educational meetings that involve discussion and practice.

The systematic review found that passive interventions had little or no effect, and these included distribution of educational materials such as clinical practice guidelines, audio-visual aids and electronic publications. Likewise, the use of educational meetings such as lectures which do not involve participants was seen as ineffective.

Individual responses to change

An individual's response to change has been identified as similar to a process of loss (Curtis and White, 2002; Knight, 1998). This may include one or several of the following: loss of power or influence (Ardern, 1999); loss of professional identity, expertise, competency, status, social relationships, control and familiarity (Salmond, 1998). Several authors have identified a process that an individual goes through as they come to terms with change (French and Delahaye, 1996; Knight, 1998; Perlman and Takacs, 1990). Perlman and Takacs have developed a comprehensive grief-change framework, which is made up of ten stages that the individual experiences as they come to terms with change. These stages include the grieving process as identified by Kubler-Ross (1978) and add on a further five steps. The individual begins in a state of equilibrium before the change commences, and then goes through the classic grief process of denial, anger and bargaining. These stages are the individual beginning to feel and their response to the reality of change. A new stage involves chaos, and includes the feelings of powerlessness, insecurity and the instability that ensue as it becomes apparent that change is inevitable. Depression and resignation are the stages where mourning for what was takes place. Openness and readiness are where the individual begins to identify with, and take on aspects of, the change. Finally, re-emergence is the evolvement of a new professional identity that is harmonious with their own values and assumptions (Schoolfield and Orduna, 1994).

CASE STUDY

One NHS Trust is planning to develop and implement a pain scale for use with patients following surgery. The intention is to evaluate the scale and implement it throughout the Directorate. The Directorate manager wants to involve as many staff as possible in the development and implementation. Therefore, a group is set up with representation from all nursing grades across all of the surgical wards as well as clinical specialists. The group is charged to develop a scale that reflects available evidence and good practice across the rest of the trust and other similar organisations. Following development, the scale is piloted on one ward. Training is organised to discuss the scale and give staff an opportunity to voice concerns. A coloured sticker is used on patient charts to remind staff to use the scale, and patient documentation is amended to require the score to be recorded. The use of the scale is audited for effectiveness and the results reported at the Trust clinical governance meeting. Similar initiatives for implementation across the directorate are set up with training provided, reminders sent out, and an identified nurse acting as a champion across the trust.

CONCLUSION

Change in the healthcare environment is occurring at a rapid pace at national, organisational and individual levels. Wright suggested that 'change itself is neither good nor bad, it is inevitable … Change will, must and should occur'(1998: 1). There are many facets to the management of change, and when exploring current literature it is clear that many assumptions are made. These include the fact that change is both desirable and inevitable, and that change needs to be a 'managed' process. Change is logical, rational and is more effective when it is a planned activity that follows a clear strategy identified before the change is implemented (Broome, 1998). The success of all change strategies is dependent upon support from people who will implement the change and the recognition that a period of psychological transition is essential in order to accept change.

FURTHER READING

Dalton, C. and Gottlieb, L.N. (2003) 'The concept of readiness to change'. *Journal of Advanced Nursing*, 42(2): 108–17.
McPhail, P. (1997) 'Management of change: an essential skill for nursing in the 1990s'. *Journal of Nursing Management*, 5: 199–205.

REFERENCES

Ardern, P. (1999) 'Safeguarding care gains: a grounded theory study of organizational change'. *Journal of Advanced Nursing*, 29(6): 7013–6.

managing change

Bennis, W.G., Benne, K.D., Chin, R. and Correy, K.E. (1993) *The Planning of Change.* London: Holt Rheinhart and Winston.

Bero, L., Grilli, R., Grimshaw, J.M., Harvey, E., Oxman, A.D. and Thompson, M.A. (1998) 'Closing the gap between research and practice; an overview of systematic reviews of interventions to promote the implementation of research findings'. *BMJ,* 317: 465–8.

Broome, A. (1998) *Managing Change.* London: Macmillan.

Curtis, E. and White, P. (2002) 'Resistance to change, causes and solutions'. *Nursing Management,* 18(10): 15–20.

Defeo, D.J. (1990) 'Change, a central concern of nursing'. *Nursing Science Quarterly,* 3: 88–94.

Department of Health (2000) *The NHS Plan: A Plan for Investment, A Plan for Reform.* London: HMSO.

Department of Health (2004) *The NHS Knowledge and Skills Framework and the Department Review Process.* London: HMSO.

French, E. and Delahaye, B. (1996) 'Individual change transition: moving in circles can be good for you'. *Leadership & Organization Development Journal,* 17(7): 22–8.

Hussey, T. (2002) 'Thinking about change'. *Nursing Philosophy,* 3: 104–13.

Knight, S. (1998) 'A study of the "lived" in experience of change during a period of curriculum and organizational reform in a department of nurse education'. *Journal of Advanced Nursing,* 27: 1287–95.

Kubler-Ross, E. (1978) *To Live Until We Say Goodbye.* Harlow: Prentice Hall.

Perlman, D. and Takacs, G.T. (1990) 'The 10 stages of change'. *Nursing Mangaement,* 16: 820–4.

Salmond, J. (1998) 'Managing the human side of change'. *Orthopaedic Nursing,* 13(5): 38–50.

Schoolfield, M. and Orduna, A. (1994) 'Understanding staff nurse responses to change; utilization of a grief change framework to facilitate innovation'. *Clinical Nurse Specialist,* 8(1): 57–64.

Wright, S.G. (1998) *Changing Nursing Practice,* 2nd edn. London: Arnold.

Cross-references *Accountability, Clinical governance, Communication, Crisis management, Data, information, knowledge, Educator, Empowerment, Evidence-based practice, Leadership, Realism, Reflection, Role model.*

key concepts in nursing

32 Managing technology

Neil Hosker and Peter Hinman

DEFINITION

Technological developments over the last half century have transformed the quality of patient care. In defining the meaning of technology in nursing, Barnard (2002) suggested it is associated with sophisticated machinery, objects, computers, scientific knowledge and technical skills that are designed to enhance healthcare through nursing and medical practice. Examples of technology include patient monitoring equipment, computers and information systems, development of drugs and new clinical and diagnostic procedures and equipment. All of these place an increasing requirement for nurses to be competent and skilful in their use.

Locsin (2005) defined nursing practice as the deliberate and continuous use of technologies for the purpose of knowing persons as a whole, with technological proficiency being described as an enhancement of caring. Barnard and Sandelowski (2001) believed that nurses have dehumanised, depersonalised and objectified patients by depriving them of their individuality, subjectivity and dignity as human beings by meeting the needs of the machinery and equipment rather than those of patients. For example, attending to a problem with an infusion pump rather than spending time with a patient or leaving a patient to answer a call bell. There seems to be a greater reliance on the finished product or task, such as readings of a blood pressure performed by an electronic sphygmomanometer, a peripheral reading of a patient's oxygen saturation by a pulse oxymeter and a cardiac rate visualised by a cardiotelemetry. These are obtained other than by personally performing the task, by employing the essential observational, auditory and tactile skills. Walters asserted that 'giving primacy to the technological culture of Western biomedicine has the potential to render invisible humanistic nursing practice' (1995: 338).

The burgeoning use of technology in nursing and healthcare has witnessed the development of curious terms such as telehealth (Audit Commission, 2004), telemedicine and telenurses (eHealth Insider,

2005). There is now the opportunity to use personal digital assistants (PDAs) in teleradiology, electrocardiogram monitoring and mobile documentation (Tachakra, 2006), particularly by mobile emergency response personnel. Concepts such as 'electronic care' (desktop computer management of care), more familiar in healthcare delivery, progressing to 'mobile care' with the use of wireless technology tools such as PDAs compatible with current nursing care applications, is a future and exciting development (Saba, 2001). On a less daunting note to technophobes, the use of technology in healthcare delivery is best evaluated by those who are exposed to it and appreciate its value, or directly using technology by complementing care delivery, much in the way that assistive technology is incorporated in rehabilitation and continuing care in the home. Examples in this context include text telephones for those with a hearing deficit, speech recognition software for the visually impaired, and unlit gas detectors for those with dementia and technically enhanced toys for children with specific learning needs (Bishop, 2003).

Technological developments are increasingly impacting on the work of the nurse whilst at the same time increasing the risk of errors being made and increasing the overall cost of healthcare. This brings with it a need for skilled and competent practitioners as greater demands are being placed on nurses to acquire relevant knowledge and skills.

KEY POINTS

- Patient safety.
- Competency.
- Organisation of nursing care.
- Technology and stress.
- Benefits.
- Attitude (or Perception) of healthcare staff and service users.

DISCUSSION

Davidson and Barber (2004) suggested that all patients on general wards are monitored with at least one piece of electronic patient monitoring equipment, either continuously or intermittently. There is a wide range of equipment available to nurses for use in their daily work, and depending on where a nurse works this equipment can be complex and have the potential to harm patients. Incorrect use of equipment is likely to be due to inadequate training and understanding of the equipment (Davidson and Barber, 2004). Quinn (2000) identified inadequate training as a particular issue with the increasing use of sophisticated equipment by nurses, especially with infusion devices, and links this to an increased risk to patients from adverse incidents.

Organisation of nursing care

Barnard (2000) states that technology in the form of equipment can be used to assess or monitor a patient while the nurse is not physically with the person and that this can influence how nursing care is organised. He argues that incorporating technology in nursing practice introduces patterns of activity focused on using the technology which changes how nurses work and introduces requirements for specific knowledge and skills. Technology can make nursing practice more time consuming and demanding, and the use of technology has been identified by nurses as one of the primary reasons they lacked time to be with people. It has also been described as a barrier, a distraction and reason for nurses not being able to attend to people on a personal level (Barnard, 2000). Again, Barnard boldly informs us that 'technology has the potential to destroy human dignity by reducing people to objects ... minimising the nurse's role as empathetic toucher' (1997: 127). A number of authors discussing the impact of technology on nursing point out that hands-on care still matters to patients, and technology cannot replace hand-holding and the human dimension of care giving (Gray and Martin, 2005).

Technology and stress

Coping with technology has been cited by nurses as a major source of stress (McGowan, 2001). The nature of the work of nurses means that they are more exposed to factors known to cause stress, and Harris (2001) suggested that stress in nurses can affect the efficiency of treatment. Harris cited the introduction of new technology as a significant cause of stress in nurses, with this in turn potentially leading to unsafe behaviour and increased incident rates. Coupled with this is the public's open access to healthcare knowledge; knowledge that was previously restricted to health professionals. Whether we view this as an intrusion or empowerment by the public as healthcare users, the availability of this knowledge means that they, as consumers, are a partner of the healthcare team (Saba, 2001). A patient armed with an abundance of material relating to their current health status, gleaned from the World Wide Web with which to convey to the healthcare professional, has its own stressors, a subject best afforded further independent research.

There are likely to be two dimensions associated with stress related to technology. The first is associated with using the technology itself, for example, whether a nurse feels comfortable or competent using the technology and being aware of the consequences to the patient and themselves if they use it incorrectly. The second is the impact technology has on the nurse's work patterns, for example, the setting up and checking of equipment, using computer systems, responding to alarms and potentially having less time to spend with patients. What remains a challenge is striving to uphold a caring concern for patients and their families amidst the 'technological fervour of today' (Ingadottir and Jonsdottir, 2006: 24).

Benefits

Dragon (2006) noted that more than one-third of the growth in health expenditure over the last decade could be attributed to technological change. With increasing costs there have been concerns about the benefits of some technologies, notably computer systems. Computer technology in the form of administrative and clinical record systems is increasingly being used by nurses. Started in 2003, Connecting for Health is the Government's ten-year project aimed at introducing standard computer systems across the NHS and eventually social care.

Computer systems can offer potential benefits around electronic health records, promoting multidisciplinary working, improving the efficiency of processes such as test ordering and results retrieval, and improved clinical communication both inside and across organisations. The use of any technological equipment, from the mobile telephone by an acute trust's bed manager to maintain constant contact with staff, to complex invasive monitoring devices by a critical care nurse, requires exploration of the use and comprehension of such equipment. The use of online packages together with software to provide instruction in their use extends to learning via computer technology and arguably saves time in getting to grips with these devices. Educating staff in the use of technical equipment along with mandatory and supplementary training is more accessible by the inclusion of e-learning or technically enhanced learning, in continuing professional development. A great benefit is the immediacy of this information providing 'on-tap learning,

learning available anytime, anywhere … a state of continuous learning' (Mackenzie-Robb, 2004: 2).

There are other benefits in the areas of information management and decision support. Parker (2004) highlights the ability to prevent medication errors by using bar-coded medications and 'rules' built into prescribing and administration systems to highlight medication inter-actions and contraindications. The management of non-patient informa-tion, such as policies, procedures and protocols in computer-based information management systems, allows nurses and other staff to be sure they are using the latest versions of documents which are based on recent evidence and best practice. This has obvious benefits over the still widespread use of paper-based documents which may or may not be the most recent versions and may or may not be complete. Nurses in relation to record keeping are notably more risk aware, and with the sphere of healthcare provision increasingly litigious, the implementation of computer-generated care directives has the potential to enhance the quality of medico-nursing documentation. Currell and Urquhart (2003), in a review of nursing record systems, found that although computerised care planning took longer to formulate, they did show improvements in meeting documentation standards. Though it is also important to acknowledge that where computer and information sys-tems are already in use, Ballard (2006) stated that there have been some difficulties adapting to the new technology, claiming that ward nurses continue to use established ways of working alongside, rather than fully adapting working practices to, computer systems in the workplace. This will have an inevitable negative impact on any benefits gained as nurses will be duplicating work and potentially fragmenting the clinical record and increasing the risk of adverse incidents.

CASE STUDY

Nurse Jones, a newly qualified registered nurse, was responsible for a patient who had recently been diagnosed as terminally ill. The patient, Mr Evans, was on a busy twenty-eight-bed medical admissions ward. Mr Evans was highly dependant and confined to bed on a pressure-relieving mattress, had an intravenous (IV) infusion in situ for hydration in his left forearm, as well as a drug infusion of broad-spectrum antibiotics via a central IV line. He was also prescribed subcutaneous morphine via a syringe driver. Nurse Jones had been shown how to use the syringe driver by a colleague and felt confident about setting it up and adjusting the dose rate. An hour or so after refilling the syringe driver, Mr Evans appeared to be moribund. The doctor was called and when he attended Mr Jones, noticed that almost all of the morphine in the syringe driver had been used. Shortly afterwards Mr Evans died. Nurse Jones was confident she had set up the syringe driver correctly and was devastated at the possibility she had made a mistake which she had perceived had resulted in the premature death of a patient. Nurse Jones later stated that she felt under pressure during the shift as she was one of only two trained staff on duty caring for many dependant patients with infusion pumps, monitoring equipment and the nurse call system all requiring attention.

CONCLUSION

Technology in its various forms is in widespread use by nurses in all branches of the profession, with its use increasing as more advances are made and applications are found. This places changing demands on those expected to use technology, particularly in relation to ensuring continuing competency and managing any stress associated with its use or the consequences to the nurse or patient of misuse or technology failure. Health professionals must ensure that the use of technology results in positive outcomes for those who must rely on them, while minimising the potential for unintended consequences (Marden, 2005). Organisations must have in place training and support programmes for staff to ensure that the risk of harm to patients and technology-related stress in nurses is minimised or eliminated.

FURTHER READING

Cook, A. and Hussey, S. (2002) *Assistive Technologies: Principles and Practice*, 2nd edn. London: Mosby.
Gillies, A.C. (2006) *The Clinicians Guide for Surviving IT*. Abingdon: Radcliffe.

REFERENCES

Audit Commission (2004) 'Press Release – Assistive technology: independence and well-being 4 – Evidence of how assistive technology can support independence'. Available online at www.audit-commission.gov.uk/olderpeople/olderpeoplereports.asp (accessed 4 Dec. 2006).
Ballard, E.C. (2006) 'Improving information management in ward nurses' practice'. *Nursing Standard*, 20(50): 43–8.
Barnard, A. (1997) 'A critical review of the belief that technology is a neutral object and nurses are its master'. *Journal of Advanced Nursing*, 26(1): 126–31.

key concepts
in nursing

Barnard, A. (2000) 'Alteration to will as an experience of technology and nursing'. *Journal of Advanced Nursing*, 31(5): 1136–44.

Barnard, A. (2002) 'Philosophy of technology in nursing'. *Nursing Philosophy*, 3: 15–26.

Barnard, A. and Sandelowski, M. (2001) 'Technology and humane nursing care: (ir) reconcilable or invented difference'. *Journal of Advanced Nursing*, 34(3): 367–75.

Bishop, J. (2003) 'The Internet for educating individuals with social impairments'. *Journal of Computer Assisted Learning*, 19(4): 546–56.

Currell, R. and Urquhart, C. (2003) 'Nursing record systems: effects on nursing practice and healthcare outcomes'. *Cochrane Database of Systemic Reviews 2003*, 3. Article No. CD 002099. DoI: 1002/14651858. CD002099.

Davidson, K. and Barber, V. (2004) 'Electronic monitoring of patients in general wards'. *Nursing Standard*, 18(49): 42–6.

Dragon, N. (2006) 'Patient care in a technological age'. *Australian Nursing Journal*, 14: 1.

eHealth Insider (2005) 'Nurses happier using telecare says international survey'.Available online at www.e-health-insider.com/news/item.cfm?ID=1263 (accessed 4 Dec. 2006).

Gray, L. and Martin, F. (2005) 'Electronic support for 21st century care'. *Age and Ageing*, 34: 421–2.

Harris, N. (2001) 'Management of work-related stress in nursing'. *Nursing Standard*, 16(10): 47–52.

Ingadottir, T.S. and Jonsdottir, H. (2006) 'Technological dependency: the experience of using home ventilators and long-term oxygen therapy: patients' and families' perspective'. *Scandinavian Journal of Caring Sciences*, 20: 18–25.

Locsin, R.C. (2005) *Technological Competency as Caring in Nursing: A Model for Practice*. Indianapolis, IN: Sigma Theta Tau International.

MacKenzie-Robb, L. (2004) 'E-learning and change management: the challenge'. Available online at www.vantaggio-learn.com/Vantaggio_CM.html (accessed 5 Dec. 2006).

Marden, S. (2005) 'Technology dependence and health-related quality of life: a model'. *Journal of Advanced Nursing*, 50(2): 187–95.

McGowan, B. (2001) 'Self-reported stress and its effects on nurses'. *Nursing Standard*, 15(8): 33–8.

Parker, P. (2004) 'Quantify technology's benefits'. *Nursing Management*, 35: 2.

Quinn, C. (2000) 'Infusion devices: risks, functions and management'. *Nursing Standard*, 14(26): 10.

Saba, V.K. (2001) 'Nursing informatics: yesterday, today and tomorrow'. *International Nursing Review*, 48: 177–87.

Tachakra, S. (2006) 'Using handheld pocket computers in a wireless telemedicine system'. *Emergency Nurse*, 14(5): 20–3.

Walters, A.J. (1995) 'Technology and the lifeworld of critical care nursing'. *Journal of Advanced Nursing*, 22: 338–46.

managing technology

Cross-references *Accountability, Communication, Confidence, Data, information, knowledge, Professional development, Record keeping, Risk management.*

33 Mentoring

Helen Carr and Janice Gidman

DEFINITION

The earliest act of mentoring is said to have originated from Greek mythology, in which Odysseus entrusted Mentor, an older wiser friend, to look after his son in his absence (Donovan, 1990). There is no single definition of mentorship, but there is a shared contemporary understanding that it is regarded as a process in which a person who is experienced, wise and trusted, guides an inexperienced individual to develop to their full potential (Short, 2002). Concepts of mentorship today have developed over the past twenty to thirty years from studies of disciplines that include academia, business and nursing. It is generally agreed that there are many benefits of mentorship for the organisation, mentee and mentor. Yoder (1990) suggested that early experience of mentoring is an important aspect for undergraduate and postgraduate nursing students, which positively influences their professional roles and perspectives and facilitates their transition to practice. Chow and Suen (2001) identified five key aspects of mentorship: assisting, befriending, guiding, advising and counselling. Within nursing, the term 'mentor' is used to denote the role of the nurse, midwife or health visitor who facilitates learning, but who also assesses students in the clinical setting (Nursing and Midwifery Council (NMC), 2006).

KEY POINTS

- Mentors enable learners to integrate theory and practice.
- Mentors are responsible for facilitating and assessing learning in practice and ensuring that students are fit for practice at the point of registration.
- Mentorship has its complexities, due to the demands of this dual role of mentor and practitioner that comes without any additional resources.
- Conflict can occur in balancing student learning needs against the demands of day-to-day workloads.

- To promote their development as autonomous practitioners, students need to take responsibility for their own learning needs.

DISCUSSION

Practice learning accounts for 50 per cent of pre-registration nursing education programmes. The clinical learning environment has been identified as central in integrating theory with practice for students in developing clinical skills. According to Carlisle et al. (1997), students cannot be expected to make this link for themselves and need mentor support to make effective links if they are to become highly competent practitioners and lifelong learners. Students value regular contact with their mentors, and the quality of mentorship they receive has a major impact on the quality of their learning during clinical placements. Neary (2000) conducted longitudinal studies in relation to mentorship from the perspective of both students and mentors which confirmed the conflict between the role of mentor and assessor, and also of other commitments including management, continued professional development and delivery of patient care within the dynamic context of the NHS. It is, therefore, essential that student learning in practice is a partnership approach between the student, mentor and lecturer, with all accepting responsibility for their role.

The role of the mentor

Nurses, midwives and health visitors wishing to become mentors must have current registration with the NMC, and professional qualifications equal to or at a higher level than the students they are supporting in the practice setting. All new mentors/practice teachers will be required to successfully complete an NMC-approved mentor preparation programme. Competencies and outcomes for mentors are discussed below and include:

- Establishing effective working relationships.
- Facilitation of learning.
- Assessment and accountability.
- Evaluation of learning.
- Creating an environment for learning.
- Contextualising practice.
- Evidence-based practice.
- Leadership.
  (NMC, 2006)

Establishing effective working relationships Promoting inter-professional working and learning involves mentors developing effective professional working relationships, within their own areas of practice and across other agencies and professions. Mentorship, however, can have its complexities, due to an already stretched caseload in which the practitioner has to balance student learning needs against the demands of day-to-day workloads. Ovretveit (1995) suggested that approaching problems as a team is more likely to produce creativity and a variety of potential solutions, which is important for the students to be involved in.

Facilitation of learning Mentors facilitate students to develop skills in problem solving, critical thinking, decision making and reflection, which are essential competencies for complex professional practice (NMC, 2004). Mentor preparation programmes also enable mentors to develop their skills to facilitate inter-professional learning with students. Recent developments in nurse education are leading to longer placements within programmes; for example, the 'hub and spoke' approach, which allocates students to a specific setting whilst encouraging them to access a wide range of alternative practice experience.

Assessment and accountability Assessment of proficiency is a vital part of the mentor's role to ensure safe and competent practitioners at the point of registration. This involves working in partnership with other team members to assess students, provide constructive feedback and identify future learning needs. In a national study, commissioned by the NMC, Duffy (2004) concluded that some mentors experienced difficulty in failing students. Consequently, the NMC have strengthened the accountability of mentors in assessing student competence and proficiency at the point of registration (NMC, 2006).

Evaluation of learning Mentors have a responsibility to evaluate the quality of the learning environment and to reflect critically on the teaching and learning strategies they have utilised with the student during his or her practice placement. Evaluation should not be seen as a process at the end of a placement as this does not provide mentors with the opportunity to clarify suggestions and comments. It should be an ongoing process, with designated time built into the placement to reflect on learning and to provide better understanding of the concerns of the student (Diamond, 2004).

Creating an environment for learning   For effective learning to take place the mentors must provide a safe learning environment for the students to feel integrated and involved within the team. Within practice areas, mentors promote the development of effective learning environments through inter-professional working and contributing to curriculum development, to maximise learning opportunities for students. Students reported that planned learning opportunities within practice had a positive influence on their perception of the placement (Metcalfe and Mathura, 1995). Within the classroom setting it is possible to control the learning environment; however, within practice there are more uncontrolled stimuli creating challenges for the mentor in facilitating student learning (Papp et al., 2003).

Contextualising practice   Mentors recognise the specific requirements of practice within their own context and also enable students to understand other professional roles and how these are being developed to meet the needs of service users. The learning environment for students in the community is very different from that in secondary care (hospital-based) in relation to addressing the students' needs against the clients' needs, particularly as the client becomes the host and the practitioner is a visiting guest.

Evidence-based practice   Mentors act as positive role models for students in promoting evidence-based practice. They support students to apply evidence in order to assist them in decision making to eliminate inappropriate and ineffective practices that could be potentially dangerous (Hamer and Collinson, 1999). Utilising evidence, however, does not guarantee that the treatment has been carried out effectively, and evaluation and monitoring are still essential.

Leadership   The mentor must also act as a role model by demonstrating effective leadership skills through personal qualities, setting direction and delivering the service. As nursing develops in line with the increasing complexities of patient care, leadership skills are an essential component of the role of a registered nurse. As a mentor there are many challenges to develop students' interpersonal and management skills, working in partnership with multi-professionals, multi-agencies and clients/patients (Carey and Whittaker, 2002).

mentoring

The role of the student

Higher education programmes in health and social care promote a student-centred andragogical approach to learning to meet the needs of the profession for lifelong learning, personal and professional development (NMC, 2004). Before commencing practice placements, students should be aware of their responsibilities for learning and for recording and reflecting on practice (Fell and Kuit, 2007). A phenomenological study which explored student learning in practice identified that students recognised their responsibilities for learning during clinical placements. Students reported that they learned more during placements if they were enthusiastic and motivated (Gidman, 2001). Peer support and mentoring, involving students learning with and from each other, have been identified as effective strategies to promote responsibility and independence, which increases students' self-confidence and learning (Lofmark and Wikblad, 2001).

CASE STUDY

Sue is a mature student nurse in the second year of her pre-registration nursing programme, and has been allocated to a community placement. Her mentor, Jane, is a district nurse team leader who manages a busy caseload within a challenging inner-city area. Prior to the placement, Sue undertakes a profile of the local area, identifying what services are available and any particular health needs. Sue accesses the local Primary Care Trust website for information and links to services. Sue has also researched Jane's role, so she is aware of the competing demands on her time.

At the initial meeting Jane is impressed, as Sue has already produced a list of what she considers are her strengths, learning needs and potential opportunities within the placement. Sue and Jane use a learning agreement to prioritise the outcomes for the placement and to agree dates for review and completion. One of Sue's particular interests is in addressing the health needs of ethnic minority groups and asylum seekers. Because Sue identified this at the beginning of the placement, Jane was able to accommodate her request by arranging for her to spend a day with a key worker for the local asylum communities.

Both Sue and Jane reflected that the placement was a positive experience as a result of having clear outcomes and action plans that were negotiated at the beginning and throughout the placement, and that it helped having time set aside to reflect. Due to Sue's enthusiastic approach, Jane was willing to give additional time and support.

CONCLUSION

Mentorship is a concept which remains difficult to define, but, increasingly within nurse education, is seen to be a short-term supportive relationship which both facilitates and assesses learning in the practice area. Mentors are experienced professionals who often experience conflict in their role due to the demands of patient care, management, student supervision and their own professional development. It is important that students accept responsibility for their own learning and it is evident that enthusiastic and motivated students learn more than those who are disinterested or passive. Several authors suggest alternative strategies to enhance mentorship, including peer mentorship, which provides additional support.

FURTHER READING

Canham, J. and Bennett, J. (2002) *Mentorship in Community Nursing: Challenges and Opportunities*. London: Blackwell Science.

Quinn, F. (2000) *Principles and Practice of Nurse Education*. Cheltenham: Stanley Thornes.

For effective leadership skills see www.nhsleadershipqualities.nhs.uk

For learning in practice see www.practicelearning.org.uk

REFERENCES

Carey, L. and Whittaker, K. (2002) 'Experiences of problem based learning: issues for community specialist practitioner students'. *Nurse Education Today*, 22(8): 661–8.

Carlise, C., Kirk, S. and Luker, K. (1997) 'The clinical role of nurse teachers within a Project 2000 course framework'. *Journal of Advanced Nursing*, 25(2): 386–95.

Chow, F. and Suen, P. (2001) 'Clinical staff as mentors in pre-registration undergraduate nursing education: students' perceptions of the mentors' roles and responsibilities'. *Nurse Education Today*, 21(2): 350–8.

Diamond, M. (2004) 'The usefulness of structured mid-term feedback as a catalyst for change in higher education classes'. *Active Learning in Higher Education*, 5(3): 217–31.

Donovan, J. (1990) 'The concept and role of mentor'. *Nurse Education Today*, 10(4): 294–8.

Duffy, K. (2004) *Failing Students*. London: NMC.

Fell, A. and Kuit, J.A. (2007) 'Placement learning and the Code of Practice'. *Active Learning in Higher Education*, 4(3): 214–25.

Gidman, J. (2001) *An Exploration of Students' Perceptions of Effective Clinical Learning*. Research report – Welsh National Board Development of Professional Practice, Occasional Paper 5, 15–18.

Hamer, S. and Collinson, G. (1999) *Evidence-Based Practice; A Handbook for Practitioners*. London: Bailliere Tindall & Royal College of Nursing.

Lofmark, A. and Wikblad, K. (2001) 'Facilitating and obstructing factors for the development of learning in clinical practice: a student perspective'. *Journal of Advanced Nursing*, 34: 472–7.

Metcalfe, D. and Mathura, M. (1995) 'Student's perceptions of good and bad teaching: report of a critical incident study'. *Medical Education*, 29: 193–7.

Neary, M. (2000) 'Supporting students' learning and professional development through the process of continuous assessment and mentorship'. *Nurse Education Today*, 20: 463–74.

Nursing and Midwifery Council (2004) *Standards of Proficiency for Pre-registration Nursing Education*. London: NMC.

Nursing and Midwifery Council (2006) *Standards to Support Learning and Assessment in Practice: NMC Standards for Mentors, Practice Teachers and Teachers*. London: NMC.

Ovretveit, J. (1995) 'Team decision making'. *Journal of Interprofessional Care*, 1: 41–51.

Papp, I., Markkanen, M. and von Bonsdorff, M. (2003) 'Clinical environment as a learning environment: student nurses' perceptions concerning clinical learning experiences'. *Nurse Education Today*, 23: 262–8.

Short, J.D. (2002) 'Mentoring: career enhancement for occupational and environmental health nurses'. *American Association of Occupational Health Nurses*, 50(3): 135–43.

Yoder, L.H. (1990) 'Mentoring: a concept analysis'. *Nursing Administration Quarterly*, 15: 9–19.

Cross-references *Educator, Leadership, Reflection, Role model.*

34 Nurturing

Frances Wilson and Jan Woodhouse

DEFINITION

The Cambridge Online Dictionary (2006) gives the following definitions for the word 'nurture': first as a verb – '1 to take care of, feed and protect someone or something, especially young children or plants, and help them to develop: 2 to help a plan or a person to develop and be successful: 3 to have a particular emotion, plan or idea for a long time': then as a noun – 'the way in which children are treated as they are growing, especially as compared with the characteristics they are born with'.

This latter definition, as a noun, links with the Wikipedia (2006) version, which places the concept of nurture squarely in the nature-versus-nurture debate, and comments that nurture is:

- Care given to children by their parents.
- Environmental factors that affect development.

These definitions help us to see that 'nurture' is instrumental in the development of an individual – be it child or adult – and we must remember that people, when they are ill, often psychologically regress to a childlike state (Bowman et al., 2006), that there is an emotional or personal quality attached to the concept and that nurture involves the act of caring.

KEY POINTS

- Nurturing is valued as a desirable skill in nursing.
- It is questioned whether it is an attribute that every nurse has.
- We can learn to nurture.
- There are definable aspects of the concept of nurturing.
- Nurturing is not confined to the patient–nurse relationship, therefore the concept has wider applications.

DISCUSSION

One could be forgiven for thinking that nurturing only takes place during our childhood years, an act between a child and their parent or carer. However, a more liberal interpretation would consider that nurturing occurs across the life stages. We may have particular people that have nurtured us through school, our current studies, or the ups and downs of life.

Hence nurturing may include all life experiences, and the degree to which we are nurtured will depend on environmental factors. These may include factors such as 'prenatal, parental, extended family and peer experiences plus ... influences such as the media, marketing and socio-economic status' (Wikipedia, 2006). At times, then, there might be an abundance of nurturing factors around, and at other times a dearth. An awareness of nurturing might help the nurse to increase the factors, so let us look as these facets individually.

Nature versus nurture

Nature might be regarded as the traits we are born with and may be demonstrated at an early stage of life. How parents react to their baby's needs, however, is a measure of a nurturing ability, and this is reflected in the definition of the noun version of nurture, cited above. The foundations of nurturing are set down in the early years. The effect of nurturing on nature has been recognised through history (Wikipedia, 2006). Philosophers have mused on problems such as how could two puppies from the same litter, when reared separately, become a fierce guard dog at one house and a loveable family pet at the house next door. The answer arrived at is the concept of nurture.

Consequently, how we are nurtured can have a lasting effect upon us. Environmental aspects affect nurture, and Raingruber (2003) cited upbringing and other human interactions and relationships as being instrumental in nurturing. So we learn about nurturing via our own experiences of being nurtured and by observing the nurturing of others. This can lead to the notion that how we were parented may well influence us as nurses and our interactions with clients/patients. For, as Raingruber points out, 'Nurture can influence nature, and nature can influence nurture'(2003: 111). If there is no nurturing within the environment around the individual, then this may give rise to the notion of deprivation. For example, two children raised in a poor district of the community may turn out very differently if one has been living in a warm and emotionally stable household, whereas the other has lived under angry and unpredictable conditions. The latter may say that they had an emotionally deprived childhood, the former may not. This aspect of emotional deprivation is important, as it can lead to distress and a variety of physical and mental health problems.

Nurture as a personal quality

We have discussed in the previous section the notion of nature and traits, so is being able to nurture a trait? If 'nurturing' is a trait, that is, the individual has it there from the beginning, this might lead to the idea that you can have a 'born nurse' or a 'born therapist' (Wheeler, 2002). However, we learn about nurturing experientially and we usually learn it from our early carers, our parents. So nurturing, as a personal quality, may be a subconscious trait that we pick up from our parents. As the chief nurturer in early life is often (but not exclusively) our mother, the concept of nurturing may often be seen as a 'feminine' quality (Evans, 1997).

As we grow and our social circle widens, then we may encounter others that nurture us, of either gender. Raingruber (2003) notes that humans have a need to connect with others, and so degrees of nurturing take place all the time. This connectedness with others means that nurturing receives mention in religious and spiritual education (Anthony, 2003), showing its value as a concept of compassion, that is, something that an individual can give to another. In giving, or nurturing, the focus of attention is on the other and their response (Raingruber, 2003). In order to maintain a focus on the other, Wheeler pointed out the importance of practitioners having 'insight and understanding of their own difficulties and motivation to deal with them ...' (2002: 435). In other words, it is difficult to nurture if you are centred on yourself rather than the other. Nurturing qualities include:

- Care for others.
- Compassion – something that an individual can give to another.
- Focus on other, and their responses.
- Personal insight and understanding.
- Respect for others.
- Positive approach and attitude.
- Value the other.
- Active listener.
- Encourage the other, including self-help.
- Teacher/role model.

This focusing on others is the essence of nursing and is important when considering the establishment of a therapeutic relationship, that is, the nurse acting as a caring person and teacher towards the patient (Pearson, 1991). However, a nurse may not have the capacity and the personal qualities that enable a focus on another, which may account for Moyle's comment that 'the therapeutic relationship does not come instinctively to a nurse' (2003: 104). If this is true, then maybe the nurturing we learned in our early years is an insufficient model for us to use in the process of learning to nurse. This would then lead us to consider further the act of nurturing, which may be dependent on nurses picking up on cues from 'nurturing nurses', that is, those who provide nurturing as part of their care.

The act of nurturing another

The concept of nurturing may have to be relearned, casting aside our childhood model and adopting that from others within the nursing profession. Raingruber (2003) commented that nurturing is focusing attention on the other and monitoring their responses. Moyle (2003) adds additional aspects to the act of nurturing, such as having a positive approach and attitude, respecting the values of others, being an active listener, encouraging expression of emotions and self-help in the other. Hence 'nurturing nurses' have these qualities and use them in their interactions with patients/clients, and act as role models for other nurses. Once these skills are acquired they usually do not remain exclusively with the patient–nurse relationship but may spread to other aspects, such as professional development, where the term of nurturing might be interchangeable with coaching.

Magneau and Vallerand (2003) undertook an extensive literature review of the relationship between the coach and athlete. A model emerged and it proves a useful model when thinking about the relationship between the nurturing nurse and their patient or client. The elements of the model, which Magneau and Vallerand call 'autonomy-supportive behaviours', are:

- Provide choice within specific rules and limits.
- Provide a rationale for tasks and limits.
- Acknowledge the other person's feelings and perspectives.
- Provide patients/clients with opportunities for initiative taking and independent work.
- Provide non-controlling competence feedback.
- Avoid controlling behaviours:

   – avoid overt control;
   – avoid criticisms and controlling statements; and
   – avoid tangible rewards for interesting tasks.

- Prevent ego-involvement in patients/clients.

This model is adaptable to any environment, be it athletics, healthcare or any situation where one person interacts with another. Where such behaviours occur it becomes a nurturing environment, and such an environment enables individuals to achieve their potential. Fasnacht (2003) noted that creativity flourishes in a nurturing environment. Similarly, Colwell and O'Connor (2003) point out that nurturing, if started early in the educational process, will enhance self-esteem. Student nurses, for example, need nurturing by their mentors, and the concept of clinical supervision enables both parties to explore issues encountered in practice in a supportive environment.

CASE STUDY

Helen, a student nurse, wishes to explore the following learning opportunities with her mentor through clinical supervision:

- Cultivate a therapeutic relationship with a patient that would, for example, allow them to regain confidence and independence in their own ability to return home.
- Embrace and promote the philosophy of care in the placement environment.

The student was caring for a patient who had sustained a fall at home. Although the patient had not sustained a fracture, she had been badly shaken, had loss of self-confidence and was expressing reluctance to return home. The philosophy-of-care aim of the unit was to provide therapeutic interventions and return patients to their own homes as quickly as possible. The learning relationship established between mentor and student can enhance and focus nurturing skills in the safety of exploring them through clinical supervision and then experientially. The nurse may develop a positive therapeutic relationship with a patient through experiential learning, reinforced through a patient's attitude, actions and feedback and reaffirmed with her mentor. The extent and effectiveness of the nurse–patient interactions will also be influenced by well-developed interpersonal skills.

The reaction of the student to the philosophy of care in the unit may be influenced by what is brought to the clinical area, such as expectations, knowledge, attitudes and emotions, that will influence their construction and interpretation of what they experience (Stuart, 2007). Helen's personal journey from child to adulthood within a nurturing environment may go a long way to developing the nurturing qualities used in giving care in personal or professional circumstances. This in turn will be maximised through a nurturing relationship between mentor and student. The opportunities afforded to the student to care for the same patient during their stay in the unit will allow a nurturing relationship to develop and reinforce the nursing philosophy.

Figure 14 may help to summarise the concept of nurturing applied to the development of a therapeutic relationship (see p. 218).

CONCLUSION

Nurturing is a desired attribute in nurses as our patients are often needy and vulnerable due to illness. We learn about nurturing at an early age and may often follow the nurturing pattern laid down by our parents or carers. However, in nursing, it has been suggested, the concept of nurturing may not come easily to an individual and therefore a student may seek out role models in order to acquire nurturing skills. Personal

nurturing

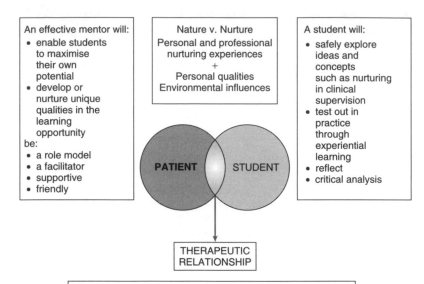

An effective mentor will:	Nature v. Nurture	A student will:
• enable students to maximise their own potential • develop or nurture unique qualities in the learning opportunity be: • a role model • a facilitator • supportive • friendly	Personal and professional nurturing experiences + Personal qualities Environmental influences	• safely explore ideas and concepts such as nurturing in clinical supervision • test out in practice through experiential learning • reflect • critical analysis

PATIENT   STUDENT

THERAPEUTIC RELATIONSHIP

The quality of the therapeutic relationship is determined by the attributes of the care giver (student supported by the mentor) and their ability to translate this into the interactions required with patients, clients, families and carers.

Figure 14   *Summary of the concept of nurturing*

attributes of nurturing have been identified which highlight that at the core is a focus on the concerns of the other rather than the self. The act of nurturing is not confined to the patient–nurse relationship but can be broadened to all those in the nurse's environment, hence it becomes a useful management skill too. Consequently, it has many different applications, but at the same time it is at the core of what is nursing.

FURTHER READING

Colwell, J. and O'Connor, T. (2003) 'Understanding nurturing practices – a comparison of the use of strategies likely to enhance self-esteem in nurture groups and normal classrooms'. *British Journal of Special Education*, 30(3): 119–24.

Stuart, C. (2007) *Assessment, Supervision and Support in Clinical Practice*, 2nd edn. London: Elsevier.

key concepts in nursing

REFERENCES

Anthony, F.V. (2003) 'Religion and culture in religiously affiliated schools: the role of teachers in nurturing inculturation'. *International Journal of Education and Religion*, 4(1): 17–40.

Bowman, G., Watson, R. and Trotman-Beasty, A. (2006) 'Primary emotions in patients after myocardial infarction'. *Journal of Advanced Nursing*, 53(6): 636–45.

Cambridge Online Dictionary (2006) *Cambridge Advanced Learners Dictionary.* Cambridge: Cambridge University Press. Available online at http://dictionary.cambridge.org (accessed 2 Feb. 2007).

Colwell, J. and O'Connor, T. (2003) 'Understanding nurturing practices – a comparison of the use of strategies likely to enhance self-esteem in nurture groups and normal classrooms'. *British Journal of Special Education*, 30(3): 119–24.

Evans, J. (1997) 'Men in nursing: issues of gender segregation and hidden advantage'. *Journal of Advanced Nursing*, 26: 226–31.

Fasnacht, P.H. (2003) 'Creativity: a refinement of the concept for nursing practice'. *Journal of Advanced Nursing*, 41(2): 195–202.

Magneau, G.A. and Vallerand, R.J. (2003) 'The coach–athlete relationship: a motivational model'. *Journal of Sport Sciences*, 21: 883–904.

Moyle, W. (2003) 'Nurse–patient relationship: a dichotomy of expectations'. *International Journal of Mental Health Nursing*, 12: 103–9.

Pearson, A. (1991) 'Taking up the challenge: the future for therapeutic nursing', in R. McMahon and A. Pearson (eds), *Nursing as Therapy.* London: Chapman Hall.

Raingruber, B. (2003) 'Nurture: the fundamental significance of relationship as a paradigm for mental health nursing'. *Perspectives in Psychiatric Care*, 39(3): 104–35.

Stuart, C. (2007) *Assessment, Supervision and Support in Clinical Practice*, 2nd edn. London: Elsevier.

Wheeler, S. (2002) 'Nature or nurture: are therapists born or trained?' *Psychodynamic Practice*, 8(4): 427–41.

Wikipedia (2006) Definitions of nature and nurture from www.wikipedia.com (accessed 14 Dec. 2006).

Cross-references *Caring, Compassion, Empowerment, Environment.*

nurturing

35 Pain

Paul Barber

DEFINITION

Prior to the 1960s, pain was seen as an expected symptom of disease rather than as a specific problem requiring appropriate treatment and care. However, since then a number of widely cited and accepted definitions of pain have been honed. McCaffrey stated that 'Pain is whatever the experiencing person says it is, existing whenever the person says it does' (1968: 95). According to the International Association for the Study of Pain, 'Pain is an unpleasant sensory and emotional experience associated with actual or potential tissue damage or described in terms of that damage' (1979: 249). The National Institute of Health defines pain as:

> a subjective experience that can only be perceived by the sufferer. It is a multidimensional phenomenon that can be described by the pain location, intensity, temporal aspects, quality, impact and meaning. Pain does not occur in isolation, but in a specific human being in psychological, economic, and cultural contexts that influence the meaning of the experience and verbal and non-verbal expression. (1986: 1)

The common denominator amongst these definitions is that tissue damage is not necessarily present, highlighting the importance of accepting an individual's report and the multidimensional experience of pain.

KEY POINTS

- Theories of pain help to contextualise current knowledge.
- Gate control theory helps explain modification of pain experience.
- Pain is multidimensional and requires equivalent assessment.
- Use of the analgesic ladder offers a step-by-step approach to the management of pain.
- There are many non-pharmacological approaches which can aid pain management.

DISCUSSION

Pain theories

There are a number of pain theories; however, the gate control theory is accepted as being the one that most successfully explains pain perception (Bond and Simpson, 2006).

Descartes (1644) proposed what is now known as the classical specificity theory. He theorised that a noxious stimuli would excite a point in the skin and, in turn, pull a delicate cord which rang a bell in the brain. This theory went relatively unchallenged until the 19th century (Melzack and Wall, 1996). Muller in 1842 and von Frey in 1894 built upon the classic specificity theory and made science aware of the location and distribution of sensory nerves. Another theory of the early 1900s discussed self-exciting loops of neurones lying in the dorsal horn of the spinal cord. This was known as the central summation theory, and although rudimentary by today's standards, did give us clues to a more complex and integrated pattern of pain perception, control and response.

Finally, peripheral pattern and the sensory interaction theory has provided valuable physiological concepts for the gate control theory (Melzack and Wall, 1996).

Physiology of pain

This section follows the gate control theory put forward by Melzack and Wall (1996). There are three basic structures involved in the transmission of pain impulses in this theory:

Peripheral nerves   Pain is detected by specialised receptors called nociceptors, which are high threshold and non-adapting in nature. There are millions of nociceptors in skin, bones, joints and muscles and in the protective membranes around internal organs. Nociceptors are more prevalent in the skin, muscles have fewer, and organs fewer still. The pain receptors respond to pressure, temperature and chemical changes. When the nociceptors detect a harmful stimulus they relay their pain messages by two distinct pathways: mylinated A delta fibres and non-mylinated C fibres (Tortora and Grabowski, 2003).

Spinal cord   When pain messages reach the spinal cord they compete with other neurones, such as touch, pressure or heat, for entry into the central nervous system. This is where Melzack and Wall (1996) refer to a gate being present. When the gate is open, pain impulses pass freely to the trigger cells and pain is perceived. However, if we apply massage or some form of thermal stimuli at the same time, pain perception is modified and therefore the gate is closed. Descending nerve pathways can also modify the degree of pain perceived by releasing neurotransmitters that amplify or diminish pain transmission (Besson and Chaouch, 1987).

Brain Pain impulses travel to the brain by two distinct pathways, the A delta fibres and the slower C fibres. These impulses arrive at the thalamus, which interprets the messages as pain and forwards them simultaneously to three specialised regions: the somatosensory cortex as a physical sensation, the limbic system for the emotional feeling component and to the frontal cortex which determines thought processes. The brain responds in a number of ways. One of the most important of these is to release our own analgesics. These are known as endorphins. Many methods of pain modification techniques are believed to act by stimulating these proteins therefore changing the nature of pain transmission (Wall and Melzack, 1999).

Pain assessment

Assessment of pain is a crucial part of the nursing role, and as such utilising a problem-solving process becomes a vital part of the equation. A pain assessment tool assists the nurse to be objective about an emotive and subjective experience. However, unless the patient is at the centre of pain assessment, the nurse is failing in their responsibility (Seers, 1988). Pain assessment tools nearly always rely on some form of scale. These introduce an element of objectivity to pain assessment. Three main approaches are used (McCaffrey and Pasero, 1999):

- *Numerical scales*: These scales range from a low number usually indicating a low level of pain to a high value number indicating worsening or more intense pain.
- *Visual scales*: These may be associated with numerical scales, but not always. The patient indicates the severity of their pain on a line that represents a continuum from worst ever pain to no pain at all. A pain thermometer or alternatively some form of likert scale would be examples of this approach.

- *Colour/faces scales*: Colour scales are especially useful for children and people who can associate their pain with a strong colour. The patient chooses which colour best represents their pain at its worst and at its least.

The McGill pain questionnaire is a tried-and-tested tool. This assessment tool suggests that the words people use provide an insight into pain quality, sensory, affective, evaluative and miscellaneous categories. The patient selects words to describe their pain and several scores can be calculated.

Pharmacology

The World Health Organisation (1996) offer what is commonly known as an analgesic ladder. This is a step-by-step escalation of a variety of analgesics depending upon the severity of pain experienced and is administered in standard doses at regular intervals:

- *Step 1:* The use of paracetamol and non-steroidal anti-inflammatory drugs (NSAIDS) such as Ibuprofen. These drugs work by inhibiting the production of prostaglandins in the body. Prostaglandins are local hormones which when released cause sensitisation of the nociceptors. One of the problems with this group of drugs is that by blocking prostaglandin synthesis they cause gastrointestinal problems such as peptic ulcer disease (Twycross and Lack, 1990).
- *Step 2:* If pain continues to be a problem the next step in the ladder is the use of a weak opioid. These are substances isolated from the opium poppy or synthetic relatives. This class of drugs works on a variety of receptors within the pain pathway. It is thought that they inhibit pain transmission by blocking opening of calcium channels in the neuronal membrane. They also act by making the membrane more porous so that the nerve loses potassium ions causing it to become hyperpolarised (Rang et al., 2003).
- *Step 3:* This involves the use of strong opioid drugs such as morphine. Opiates inhibit centres in the brain that control coughing, breathing and intestinal motility. Tolerance to opioid drugs also occurs, which means that taking a drug changes the body in such a way that you have to increase the dose to gain the same therapeutic effect. If the effect that is lost is a side effect like vomiting, or sleepiness, tolerance can be seen as a potentially good thing. However, if the effect is diminished pain relief, then it becomes problematic.

Adjuvants Portenoy (1998) describes these as a group of drugs and therapies that can be used alongside the drugs used in all three steps of the analgesic ladder. Adjuvants are used for their effects on the pain-relieving drugs that are being used in each step of the ladder. Drugs and therapies used as adjuvants enhance the pain-relieving properties of the analgesics that are primarily being employed in each step. Common categories of drugs that are prescribed include anti-depressants, anti-convulsants, local anaesthetics and steroids. Common therapies that can be employed as adjuvants include radio and chemotherapy.

Alternative approaches to pain control

Banks (2004) suggested that patients with chronic pain who do not respond to conservative therapies may require an interventional approach; the simpler of these are trigger-point injections, nerve blocks, spinal cord stimulation and intra-spinal drug administration. Mufano and Trim (2000) recognise that physiotherapy and occupational therapy can also be used to diminish pain and restore function. Heat, cold, vibration or ultrasound are all modalities that are used in order to modify pain perception. This is achieved by competing for entry into the central nervous system at the gateway in the dorsal horns of the spinal cord. A technique that is widely used and works in a similar way to that described above is transcutaneous electrical nerve stimulation (TENS) (O'Hara, 2004). Patients receiving TENS carry a small box-shaped device that transmits electrical impulses into the body through electrodes placed on the skin.

Dworking and Breitbart (2004) comment on how psychological approaches to pain relief have been found to be useful, and these include:

- *Cognitive re-focusing:* this approach enables the person to have a dialogue with themselves in order to prepare for a painful event.
- *Relaxation strategies:* these are useful for chronic pain and may include the use of music, massage or slow deep breathing.
- *Imagery techniques:* in which a person focuses mentally on a pleasant or peaceful experience or superficial body massage are also used alongside relaxation.
- *Complementary or alternative approaches:* are often used in combination with analgesics for pain relief.

CASE STUDY

Mabel, aged 76, presented at the Accident and Emergency department with a fractured neck of femur following a fall at home. A staff nurse was covering a colleague's break when Mabel's daughter approached him, upset, and asked when her mother could have some pain relief because she was 'obviously in agony'. To find out when she had last had analgesia, the nurse read Mabel's notes, which read: 'Patient comfortable, declined analgesia'. The nurse asked Mabel about her pain and she replied that she could 'cope with it if I don't have to move' and that she 'didn't like to make a fuss'. She said 'I can see how busy you all are. There are people who are really poorly here and they need you more.'

The nurse then explained to Mabel that she should not be 'coping' with pain, that it was important that her pain was managed effectively and there was no need for her to be in pain. He explained the importance of maintaining mobility while on bed rest as well as the physiological and psychological stress of persistent pain. The nurse reassured Mabel and her daughter that a range of analgesia was available and that dealing with her pain was as important as anything else he was doing. He stressed the importance of regular analgesia rather than waiting until she experienced pain to ask for help.

The nurse then requested a prescription for intravenous morphine and titrated it against Mabel's pain using an assessment tool until she was able to change position comfortably. She was also prescribed regular analgesia and encouraged to report any further pain. Her daughter reinforced this and Mabel stated 'that she understood', appearing relieved that she did not have to cope with the pain any longer.

CONCLUSION

Pain has a detrimental effect on people's physical, psychological and social wellbeing. The relationship between injury and pain response is not predictable. Many theories have tried to explain this relationship, the most current being the gate control theory. Effective pain management is a basic right which requires complex nursing skills. Regular pain assessment lies at the heart of this process. There are many tools to aid the nurse in quantifying the subjective experience of pain. However, the most fundamental tenet is that the person lies at the heart of the assessment process. An understanding of the pharmacological and alternative approaches to pain relief is paramount in nursing. This is in order for patients to be empowered when dealing with their own pain phenomena, for the nurse to act as an informed advocate, and finally for the nurse to become a knowlegable doer in the complex management of the pain experience.

FURTHER READING

Holdcroft, A. and Jagger, S. (eds) (2005) *Core Topics in Pain*. Cambridge: Cambridge University Press.

Linton, S.J. (2005). *Understanding Pain for Better Clinical Practice: A Psychological Perspective*. Edinburgh: Elsevier.

REFERENCES

Banks, C. (2004) *Chronic Pain Management*. London: Whurr.

Besson, J-M. and Chaouch, A. (1987) 'Peripheral and spinal mechanisms of nociception'. *Physiology Review*, 67: 67–86.

Bond, M.R. and Simpson, K.H. (2006) *Pain: Its Nature and Treatment*. Edinburgh: Elsevier Churchill Livingstone.

Descartes, R. (1664) 'L' Homme', trans M. Foster (1901) *Lectures on the History of Physiology During the 16th, 17th and 18th Centuries*. Cambridge: Cambridge Universty Press.

Dworking, R.H. and Breitbart, W.S. (eds) (2004) *Psychosocial Aspects of Pain: A Handbook for Health Care Providers*. Seattle, WA: IASP Press.

Frey, M. von (1894) *Bectra'g'e zur Sinnephysiologic der Haut. Ber. D. kgl. Sachs.Ges d. Wiss, Math-phys.K1 47*, 166–84.

International Association for the Study of Pain (1979) 'On a taxonomy of pain terms: a list with definitions and notes on usage'. *Pain*, 6: 249–52.

McCaffrey, M. (1968) *Nursing Practice Theories Related to Cognition, Bodily Pain, and Man–Environment Interactions*. Los Angeles, CA: University of California.

McCaffrey, M. and Pasero, C. (1999) *Pain: Clinical Manual*, 2nd edn. St Louis, MO: Mosby.

Melzack, R. and Wall, P.D. (1996) *The Challenge of Pain*, 2nd edn. London: Penguin.

Muller, J. (1842) *Elements of Physiology*. London: Taylor.

Munafo, M. and Trim, J. (2000) *Chronic Pain: A Handbook for Nurses*. Oxford: Butterworth Heinemann.

National Institute of Health (1986) 'The integrated approach to the management of pain'. *NIH Consensus Statement*, 6(3): 1–8.

O'Hara, P. (2004) *Pain Management for Health Professionals*. London: Chapman & Hall

Portenoy, R. (1998) 'Adjuvant analgesics in pain management', in D. Doyle, G. Hanks and N. Macdonald (1998) *Oxford Textbook of Palliative Medicine*, 2nd edn. Oxford: Oxford Medical Publications.

key concepts
in nursing

Rang, H.P., Dale, M.M., Ritter, J.M. and Moore, P.K. (2003). *Pharmacology*, 5th edn. London: Churchill Livingstone.

Seers, K. (1988) 'Factors affecting pain assessment'. *Professional Nurse*, 3(6): 201–205.

Tortora, G. and Grabowski, S.R. (2003) *Principles of Anatomy and Physiology*, 10th edn. New York: Wiley.

Twycross, R. and Lack, S. (1990) *Therapeutics in Terminal Cancer*, 2nd edn. Edinburgh: Churchill Livingstone.

Wall, P.D. and Melzack, R. (eds) (1999) *Textbook of Pain*, 4th edn. Edinburgh: Churchill Livingstone.

World Health Organization (1996) *Cancer Pain Relief.* Geneva: WHO.

Cross-References *Advocacy, Assessment, Caring, Communication, Empowerment, Holistic care.*

36 Problem solving

Jane Quigley

DEFINITION

Problems exist throughout daily life and sometimes help is needed in solving them. If an individual is in the midst of a problem situation it is often difficult for them to see a solution, and concentrating solely on the problem can sometimes make it seem even bigger, and a solution impossible. Sometimes too much energy is spent trying to change things that are beyond the individual's control instead of trying to find a solution to the problem, even if it is one they do not like. There are two main perspectives on which people can focus when problem solving: the *actual* problem and the *perceived* problem, where the person focuses on their internal feelings, values and beliefs rather than the actual problem. Within the *actual* problem-focused perspective there is problem solving, whilst in the *perceived* problem there may be an excess of feelings surrounding the problem, making it impossible to deal with. For many people reaching a solution to a problem can be difficult. Knippen and

Green defined problem solving by suggesting that 'problem solving is bringing a group of individuals together to analyse a situation, determine the real problem, look at every possible solution, evaluate each of the solutions, and choose the best one for their options' (1997: 98). Or as Nolan suggested, 'problem solving is the art of finding ways to get from where you are to where you want to be (assuming that you do not already know how). The problem therefore is the gap between the present situation and a more desirable one' (1989: 4).

KEY POINTS

- There are two main perspectives in problem solving – the actual and the perceived problem.
- Problem solving in healthcare has become a priority in the current climate of ongoing role and service redesign; individuals are forced to confront and cope with change in their professional and personal lives.
- Problem solving, decision making and seeking solutions are inexorably linked.
- Problem solving strategies generally entail a number of steps, including establishing the problem, identifying constraints or any alternatives, reaching a solution, and considering how the solution will be implemented.

DISCUSSION

Problems, whether actual or perceived, can occur at many levels and in many situations. On a professional level, individuals involved with healthcare deal with patients and clients who are ill, in pain, suffering either socially, physically or psychologically, and whose care requires problem identification and solving. Within the work environment, the health professional also has to deal with a multitude of factors, including such things as regulations, governance requirements, budget restrictions, staff cohesion and efficacy, local and national agendas resulting in role and service design, and changing patterns of healthcare. On a personal basis, modern-day life can also offer many challenges, sometimes compounded by the effect of an individual's professional responsibilities on such issues as childcare and maintaining a work–life balance. Consequently, they are required to seek solutions and coping strategies to overcome this. Individuals are thus constantly facing situations in and out of work that require them to make decisions, choosing between several courses of action, and they may well use a problem-solving approach to achieve a solution. Two main problem-solving approaches are action learning and mind/cognitive mapping.

Action learning

Action learning, whilst it is about the learning and development of people, takes place within the work setting and aims to address real problems by finding a solution. Garratt (1987) suggested that in order for problem solving to take place and be successful, it is essential to consider two major inputs. The first, the hard input, is the objective (or the problem) – for example, efficient use of resources, reduced costs – and the second, the soft input, such as personal feelings, experiences and relationships, both of which are inextricably linked.

Fry et al. (2000) noted that action learning is based on the relationship between reflection and action; the focus has to be on the problems that individuals bring and future planning action achieved within the structured support of the group. Fry et al. stated 'put simply, it is about solving problems and getting things done' (2000: 142).

McGill and Beaty (2001) also defined action learning as a continuous process of learning and reflection with the intention of getting things done. They considered that through action learning and with support from colleagues, individuals learn with and from each other by working on real problems and reflecting on their own experiences. McGill and Beaty (2001) also highlighted a positive aspect to action learning, that the process helps individuals take an active perspective towards life and problems and overcome the tendency to be passive towards the pressures of life. Ideally, in action learning participants are able to raise difficult questions, discuss sensitive issues, and share their learning in a supportive environment. An action learning set can be with peers from within an organisation or with professionals from different backgrounds. There are generally considered to be four steps for action learning (see also Figure 15):

- Describing the problem.
- Considering issues that you can control.
- Reflecting and deciding on action.
- Considering solutions.

Thus, action learning can be used as a tool for both personal and professional development and involves:

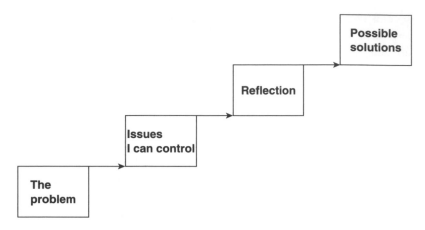

Figure 15   *Steps in the problem-solving process*

- Learning from others.
- The chance to ask questions, seek answers and gain support, as well as to expect challenge within a safe environment.
- The chance to learn from, and be supported by, a skilled facilitator of action learning.
- The opportunity to work on real problems and implement solutions in the workplace.
- Time for reflection on current practice – learning from action taken.

Mind or cognitive mapping

Another method of determining the problem and finding possible solutions is cognitive or mind mapping. In attempting to resolve a problem an individual's perceptions are shaped by values and beliefs, and a cognitive map enables concepts and their relationship to one another to be portrayed in a diagrammatical form.

A mind map is thus a diagram used to represent words, thoughts or other items linked to and arranged around a central key word or idea, in this case *the problem* (see Figure 16). It is used to generate, visualise, structure and classify ideas, and is an aid to problem solving and decision making. By using a diagram that represents connections and by presenting these connections it encourages a brainstorming approach to a problem. The mind map may involve images and/or words, with lines to link and connect them (Buzan, 2003).

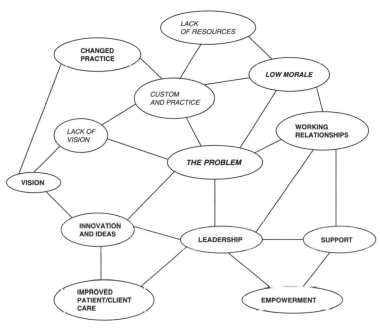

Figure 16   *An example of a mind map*

General aspects of problem solving

Problem solving requires skills such as open mindedness, positive attitudes, the ability to generate ideas, creative thinking, adaptability and the ability to manage change. It is often presumed that all individuals have the ability to 'problem solve' and use the aforementioned skills in their everyday work. However, the constant change within organisations can result in low morale, increased workloads, anxiety, stress and the inability to solve even the most simple of problems presented in everyday working life.

The ability to solve problems and find solutions is not always easy in bureaucratic organisations such as health, where even if a solution is found it may not be possible to influence and persuade others to accept the solution.

A simple technique to assist in problem solving is that of taking two pieces of paper and writing the headings 'Issues I can control' and 'Issues beyond my control'; the individual then writes down everything in relation to the problem on the appropriate page, reflects on the lists, and then tears up the 'Issues beyond my control' list. Energy should then be focussed on the things that can be controlled and influenced. Another way to look at problems suggested by Freeth (2003) is to ask questions such as: 'Think of someone you trust. What would they do?' and 'Who cares enough about you to help you?'

Active problem solving and seeking solutions involves such approaches as working through problems and coming to terms with change. Avoidance of problem solving can result in low morale, anger and reduced motivation. However, it must be stated that there are many reasons for such behaviours that could be outside the control of individuals, such as poor communication, lack of clarity, rules, regulations and local and national policies. There are a number of reasons why problem-solving strategies fail to achieve results, such as:

- Communication (or lack of it).
- Conflict and misunderstanding.
- The inability to listen.

Change is sometimes perceived as a threat, and lack of communication may result in the inability to consider a problem-solving solution, but individuals need to systematically evaluate problems to assist explanation and make plans for solutions. If an individual is in doubt about their own or their teams' ability to change and deal with current problems, it is worth considering how change has been implemented in the past using problem-solving skills to reach a solution to a problem or a change in practice.

CASE STUDY

A district nurse team was required to alter their shift pattern to longer days, starting earlier and finishing later. The team leader found that the staff were generally unwilling to consider changing their hours. As a team they seemed resistant to change and were always ready to put forward reasons to avoid changes, not looking for solutions to problems. The team leader found the increased pressure of the responsibility of trying to implement change stressful, and had difficulty solving the problem initially. She put this down to the general apathy towards the change, particularly in relation to two of the team members. The team leader approached these members of the team to seek and explore their views on the issues. One member of the team explained she was having trouble getting her children to school and her colleague had problems collecting her children from school. These they perceived as additional problems, but the solution was fairly simple as, in adopting the required change to shift patterns and starting earlier and finishing later, both could work shifts that solved both the perceived and the actual problems. In this instance the team leader used problem-solving skills such as effective communication and the ability and willingness to listen and negotiate to find a solution to a problem.

CONCLUSION

The number of ways in which individuals can respond to change is only limited by imagination, problem-solving skills and ability to seek a pathway to a solution. Problems and change are constants within healthcare and although individuals can change strategies for problem solving using different mechanisms, it must be remembered that not all problems can be addressed. However, with problem solving as a path to coping with and finding a solution to problems, healthcare professionals are able to go forward delivering care to patients and clients while developing on a professional and personal level. As G.K. Chesterton said: 'It isn't that they can't see the solution. It is that they can't see the problem' (1935: 686).

FURTHER READING

Improvement Leaders Guides, available online at www.modern.nhs.uk (follow links through 'improvement').
Pedler, M. and Boutall, J. (1992) *Action Learning For Change*. Bristol: National Health Service Training Directorate.
Wilson, G. (2000) *Problem Solving*. London: Kogan Page.

REFERENCES

Buzan, T. (2003) *Use Your Head*. London: BBC.
Chesterton, G.K. (1935) *Penguin Complete Father Brown*. London: Penguin.
Freeth, P. (2003) *6 Questions*. London: Communications in Action (CIAUK).
Fry, H., Ketteridge, S. and Marshall, S. (2000) *A Handbook for Teaching and Learning in Higher Education*. London: Kogan Page.
Garratt, B. (1987) *The Learning Organisation*. London: Fontana Collins.
Knippen, J.T. and Green, T.B. (1997) 'Problem solving'. *Journal of Workplace Learning*, 9(3): 98–9.
McGill, I. and Beaty, L. (2001) *Action Learning: A Guide for Professional, Management and Educational Development*, 2nd edn. London: Kogan Page.
Nolan, V. (1989) *The Innovators' Handbook: The Skills of Innovative Management – Problem Solving, Communication and Teamwork*. London: Sphere.

Cross-References *Coping, Guilt, Reflection, Sense of humour.*

37 Professional development

Maureen Wilkins and Annette McIntosh

DEFINITION

As nursing practice evolves and changes to reflect new patterns of healthcare delivery, growth in knowledge, technological advances and national agendas, professional development is essential for the maintenance and enhancement of care standards alongside the successful management of change. Any profession is characterised by a code of conduct, with members of the profession being required to take responsibility for their working practice, including a commitment to continuing professional development (CPD). The Nursing and Midwifery Council (NMC) address the requirements for CPD in their *Code of Professional Conduct*, stating that:

> As a registered nurse, midwife or specialist community public health nurse, you must maintain your professional knowledge and competence. You must keep your knowledge and skills up to date throughout your working life. In particular, you should take part regularly in learning activities that develop your competence and performance. (NMC, 2004: 9)

The terminology associated with CPD can be confusing, with various other terms addressing the concept, albeit with slightly different applications. These include continuing professional education (CPE), staff development (SD) and lifelong learning. CPE is generally applied to formal learning within a Higher Education Institute (HEI), while CPD, SD and lifelong learning are used to denote any learning that leads to personal and professional development, including that which occurs within the workplace. Specifically, CPD is considered by Madden and Mitchell to be:

> The maintenance and enhancement of knowledge, expertise and competence of professionals throughout their careers, according to a plan formulated with regard to the needs of the professional, the employer, the profession and society. (1993: 12)

KEY POINTS

- Professional development is essential for the enhancement of practice, the profession and the individual.
- To begin their CPD, newly registered nurses require a period of preceptorship.
- Registered nurses are required to engage in, and evidence, a minimum of 35 hours CPD activity over three years.
- CPD can be achieved through various means, from reflective work-based learning through to structured programmes of academic study.
- There are various influences and constraints on CPD; a key element is the support of clinical managers.

DISCUSSION

As stated previously, the concept of CPD in nursing is underpinned by the requirements for registered nurses to act in accordance with the NMC *Code of Professional Conduct*. The broader concepts in the code, such as protecting the public, upholding the reputation of the profession, accountability for practice and duty of care to patients and clients necessitate up-to-date knowledge, skills and abilities to ensure lawful, safe and effective practice without direct supervision (NMC, 2004). Specifically, CPD requires the practitioner to acknowledge their professional competence and boundaries, to facilitate others to develop their competence, and to deliver care based on current evidence, best practice and appropriate and validated research (NMC, 2004).

The context of CPD

The ongoing education of nurses has been subject to many developments over the years. The Briggs Report (Department of Health and Social Security (DHSS), 1972) recommended that post-registration education and specialist courses should be developed and organised as part of an ongoing educational process. The forerunner to the NMC, the United Kingdom Central Council (UKCC) recommended a comprehensive framework for post-registration education, providing opportunities for consolidation of learning for newly qualified nurses, for subsequent updating of knowledge and skills and for programmes leading to specialist practice qualifications (UKCC, 1986). A key focus at this time was for the education of student and registered nurses to foster flexible, critical, analytical and reflective practitioners. These qualities were seen as key in moving nursing from ritualistic care to practice based on evidence which was critically evaluated as opposed to unequivocally accepted (Ford and Walsh, 1994). Subsequent standards produced and implemented in 1995 by the UKCC addressed post-registration education and practice (PREP). CPD was seen as a process which would not only improve standards of care, but also enhance job satisfaction, career progression and retention (UKCC, 1994). These still current education standards require registered nurses to undertake a minimum of 35 hours learning activity during the three years prior to renewal of registration, to maintain a personal professional profile that records learning activity, and to comply with any request for the NMC to audit the meeting of the standards (NMC, 2006). The concept of CPD also underpins recent initiatives in designing frameworks for career progression, for knowledge and skill development and a move towards a competency-based workforce with an increasing emphasis on degree-level status for registered nurses. Key documents in this respect include *The NHS Knowledge and Skills Framework* (DoH, 2004).

Newly registered nurses

Various studies have highlighted the disparity and conflict between values espoused in the educational context and those in clinical practice (for example, Fealy, 1999; Melia, 1987). Preceptorship aims to reduce the impact of this phenomenon, referred to by Kramer (1974) as 'reality shock', often experienced by both student and newly registered nurses. The role of preceptor entails providing support and guidance through role modelling, reflective practice and reinforcing the concept of lifelong learning, thus enabling the newly qualified to make the transition to accountable practitioner (NMC, 2006).

PREP

PREP provides a framework for CPD, which, although not a guarantee of competence, is a key component of clinical governance (NMC, 2006). The NMC clearly indicates that in meeting the PREP (CPD) standard, the learning activity must be relevant to practice and assist the practitioner in providing the highest possible standard of healthcare. It also points out that there is currently no prescribed PREP learning activity so that any learning, whether formal or informal, that has influenced practice may constitute the evidence required to meet the standard.

While there is no approved format for recording the evidence of CPD, the NMC have produced a template for the organisation and recording of learning activity: a personal professional profile. Examples of the range of acceptable evidence include:

- Unstructured or informal activities/learning: for example, exploring elements of direct patient care; using informal teaching sessions within the workplace; and reviewing NHS documents.
- Structured or formal activities/learning: for example, in-service lectures; study days and courses.

As the NMC (2006) notes, key in the documentation of these activities is the reflection of how the learning has related to advancing practice. Professional learning in practice is seen by many authors to come from a systematic analysis and reflection upon experience (for example, Johns, 2000; Schon, 1987; Teekman, 2000). It is recognised that reflective thinking does not come automatically but requires active involvement and an environment conducive to, and supportive of, learning. Teekman (2000) noted from his research that reflection on practice is self-empowering for the individual as it adds to personal understanding and control, and that using a self-questioning strategy would lead to more proactive professional practice.

The structured or formal activities are often facilitated within HEIs in which nurse education has been situated since the mid-1990s. There are many educational opportunities available for registered nurses, including study days, stand-alone modules and undergraduate and postgraduate degrees. Some programmes of study, for example, those leading to specialist practitioner qualifications, are recordable with the NMC and the required element of supervised practice necessitates employer support. However, there is also a wide variety of part-time programmes available for registered nurses that, while not validated by the NMC, offer many opportunities for CPD. These frequently include flexible learning modes, including distance learning and work-based learning (WBL), which as the name implies concerns learning for, at or through work, normally with the formal involvement of the employer. Another mechanism for recognising learning occurring within the workplace is that of accreditation of prior experiential learning (APEL), in which evidence of learning can be used to gain either entry to a programme or general or specific exemption from module(s), where the prior learning is judged by an HEI to be of an equivalent level and credit value and which, for specific exemption, covers the subject matter that would be studied and assessed within a module.

In addition, and complementary to PREP activity, many clinical managers use an annual professional development plan (PDP) to provide a focus for identifying individual needs, implementing learning activities, and recording and reviewing progress. PDPs, therefore, take account of the individual's personal aspirations and professional development needs alongside the employer's requirements.

Influences and constraints

Ideally, it can be seen that nurses' CPD would be characterised by a strong commitment and a positive and proactive attitude to lifelong learning with practitioners acknowledging that their development and clinical competence are constantly evolving through structured processes, not just the ad hoc assimilation of skills and knowledge.

Indeed, research studies have shown that many individuals undertake CPD in line with the above premises (Dowsell et al., 1998; Murphy et al., 2006). Other factors have also been highlighted as being influential, including career progression, promotion, service requirements and work-related pressure (Dowsell et al., 1998; Murphy et al., 2006).

However, there are also well-recognised constraints that inhibit the CPD of nurses. These include a lack of employer support, poor funding, low staffing levels and difficulties in balancing home life with work and study responsibilities (Murphy et al., 2006). While it is recognised that professional development needs to be owned and managed by the individual, research shows that clinical managers and health services also have a clear role to play in supporting and guiding CPD to ensure that the ultimate goal of enhancement of clinical care is achieved (Murphy et al., 2006).

CASE STUDY

Rosemary, a theatre sister of twenty years' experience, is keen to ensure that staff are facilitated in their professional development, particularly as her own qualifications were gained in her own time, at her own expense. Rosemary's commitment to the CPD of her staff includes supporting attendance at in-house study days, conferences and modules in theatre-based practice. However, budgetary restrictions have meant that funding staff to undertake academic study is often not feasible. The CPD of two staff members has been prioritised by Rosemary following completion of the annual SD process, in line with the needs of the unit:

- Bob is a newly registered nurse with a Diploma in Higher Education. He needs sixty Level 3 credits to 'top up' to a degree and is keen to achieve this as soon as possible. His action plan for this year centres around completing his four-month period of preceptorship, whereupon he will be funded for two consecutive twenty credit modules that will be completed in his own time. One module will be a theatre-based theory module, the other addressing his development as a mentor to help support students' learning in practice within the theatre.
- Jane, Rosemary's deputy, completed her first degree five years ago and has since attended and presented at many study days and conferences, completed an in-house leadership programme and is now keen to embark on a postgraduate degree. Rosemary has agreed to support her studies on the basis that the programme addresses the advanced skills required within the department. Jane submitted a portfolio to her local HEI in support of an AP(E)L claim and achieved forty credits towards an MSc Advanced Practice.

CONCLUSION

CPD is an important concept within nursing and has the ultimate goal of enhancing an individual's knowledge and skills, which in turn aims to improve patient care. CPD can be achieved through various means, from work-based initiatives to structured programmes of study, and requires the commitment of service managers, educationalists, professional and government bodies and, not least, nurses themselves.

FURTHER READING

Nursing and Midwifery Council (NMC) web site: www.nmc-uk.org (accessed 25 Jan. 2007)

Quinn, F.M. (ed.) (1995) *Continuing Professional Development in Nursing; A Guide for Practitioners and Educators*. Cheltenham: Stanley Thornes.

REFERENCES

Department of Health and Social Security (1972) *Report of the Committee on Nursing.* Chair, Lord Briggs. London: DHSS.

Department of Health (2004) *The NHS Knowledge and Skills Framework (KSF) and the Development Review Process.* London: DoH.

Dowsell, T., Hewison, J. and Hinds, M. (1998) 'Motivational forces affecting participation in post-registration degree courses and effects on home and work life: a qualitative study'. *Journal of Advanced Nursing*, 28(6): 1326–33.

professional development

Fealy, G.M. (1999) 'The theory–practice relationship in nursing: the practitioner's perspective'. *Journal of Advanced Nursing*, 30(1): 74–85.

Ford, P. and Walsh, M. (1994) *New Rituals for Old: Nursing Through the Looking Glass.* Oxford: Butterworth-Heinemann.

Johns, C. (2000) *Becoming a Reflective Practitioner.* Oxford: Blackwell Science.

Kramer, M. (1974) *Reality Shock: Why Nurses Leave Nursing.* London: Mosby.

Madden, C. and Mitchell, V. (1993) *Professions, Standards and Competence: A Survey of Continuing Education for the Professions.* Bristol: University of Bristol Department for Continuing Education.

Melia, K. (1987) *Learning and Working: The Occupational Socialisation of Nurses.* London: Tavistock.

Murphy, C., Cross, C. and McGuire, D. (2006) 'The motivation of nurses to participate in continuing professional education in Ireland'. *Journal of European Industrial Training*, 30(5): 365–84.

Nursing and Midwifery Council (2004) *The NMC Code of Professional Conduct: Standards for Conduct, Performance and Ethics.* London: NMC.

Nursing and Midwifery Council (2006) *The PREP Handbook.* London: NMC.

Schon, D. (1987). *Educating the Reflective Practitioner: Towards a New Design for Teaching and Learning in the Professions.* San Francisco, CA: Jossey-Bass.

Teekman, B. (2000) 'Exploring reflective thinking in practice'. *Journal of Advanced Nursing*, 31: 1125–38.

United Kingdom Central Council (1986) *Project 2000: A New Preparation for Practice.* London: UKCC.

United Kingdom Central Council (1994) *The Future of Professional Practice: The Council's Standards for Education and Practice Following Registration.* London: UKCC.

Cross-references *Accountability, Educator, Mentoring, Reflection.*

---

38 Realism

Cathy Thompson

DEFINITION

Realism is the name given to a certain philosophical way of thought. Realism as a philosophy is the rational investigation of questions about existence, knowledge and ethics. For the purpose of this chapter, the definition of realism used will be the actual use of facts and their practical application rather than the theoretical possibilities.

KEY POINTS

- Realism is a state of being real as in 'the reality of the situation slowly dawned on me'.
- Nurses have to face the reality of the continuous state of change.
- Nurses are expected to have a high-level set of skills and understanding.
- Patients expect nurses to act in their best interests, and to make them feel safe, cared for, respected and involved.
- New skills have to be continuously acquired following registration as new roles emerge.
- Different career pathways are being developed and nurses need to be flexible where they will work as services are redesigned.

DISCUSSION

Bendall (1976; see Bendall, 2006) wrote about the gap between student nurses' theoretical knowledge of best practice and the way in which they actually delivered patient care in reality, and so the term 'theory-practice gap' emerged. This phenomenon has been explored in great detail and resulted in many changes to the nursing curricula. Some now say that the gap has moved and is now about the skills of nurses at the point of registration and beyond. There is a need to question what is happening in the healthcare setting which may be affecting student's, newly qualified and senior staff's view of reality. Nursing has changed radically in terms of the roles and responsibilities they now engage in and how care is delivered and organised.

Nurses of today have to work within a healthcare system which is subject to global and societal changes. The Department of Health (2006b) says that nursing is changing almost as fast as the setting in which it is practiced. Government policies (DOH, 2006b) set out clearly the reform programmes to which healthcare organisations have to respond. These policies are:

- Putting the needs and preferences of patients, users and the public first, and engaging people in service design.
- Moving more care out of hospital settings.
- Developing new ways of working.

realism

- New financial regimes.
- New working partnerships across health and social care, local and national economies.
- Staff need to be empowered to use their creativity to improve care.

The new realism is that nurses are now expected to help organisations achieve their performance targets and at the same time deliver patient-centred quality care. They have to ensure that the four-hour waiting time for patients attending Accident and Emergency is met so that the Trust does not breach their performance targets. Much debate has taken place about waiting times appearing more important than patients. Nurses need to understand the performance targets of the organisation and how this leads to a performance rating.

Performance rating is measured over several dimensions. The overarching dimension is quality (DOH, 2005), which is measured by compliance with:

- Standards for health.
- Existing targets.
- New targets.
- Children's services.
- Admissions.
- Diagnostics.
- Medicines management.

The dimensions do not remain static and the above were used for the ratings for the year 2005/6. In 2006/7 maternity care, accident and emergency and theatres will be used instead of children's services, admissions and diagnostics.

The *Standards for Better Health* (DOH, 2004) include core standards which must be assured, and progress must be demonstrated in meeting the developmental standards.

Trust ratings are available to the public, and the reality now facing health organisations and their staff is that patients have choices on where to be treated and this information will influence their choice of hospital, and with the new financial regime money follows the patient.

The effect of this is that nurses have to work with management to ensure organisational success or services will be lost, which will impact on the employment of professionals, and the care now delivered close to the patient's home may become unavailable. Nurses need to be delivered a curriculum that meets the care needs of their patients and families but incorporates the context in which care is delivered, and develops management, leadership, organisational knowledge and skills.

Care is delivered within a complex adaptive system, which means that health systems are complex and constantly adapting to their environments. Change is constant and is at individual, team, organisational, national and global levels. The reality of these changes are greeted with excitement by some, apprehension and stress by others.

Managers and academics can help nurses to practice effectively in these complex systems and adapt to rapid change and uncertain outcomes, by engaging in partnership work to ensure the curriculum constantly evolves to reflect the changing patterns of care and the new skills that nurses require.

Multidisciplinary teams are now emerging and skills are interchangeable, as is demonstrated by nurses undertaking roles previously the province of the medical staff, from inserting central venous pressure lines, bone marrow sampling, endoscopies and many more too numerous to list here. A new reality is occurring in nursing today, and the boundaries will continue to move.

The use of Wilber's (in Owen, 2004) model shown in Figure 17 may help nurses to gain an understanding of the reality of the situations and experiences they have. The nurse as an individual holds his or her own values and attitudes but at work as a professional has to demonstrate the qualities outlined in the upper right quadrant. The patient and their families also hold individual values and form their own team and are part of a social system. The upper left quadrant and the lower left quadrant of the diagram happen inside a person or a group and cannot be measured. The upper right quadrant and lower right quadrant can be observed and measured. Good nurse leaders will want to consider each of these boxes and how they relate to each other and to remember that the quadrants are not independent but interdependent.

Nurses of today will have to continue to lead ever-changing skill-mixed teams; they will need to know how to maximise the contribution of individuals and the team so that they are patient focused and quality oriented. Nurses are responsible for delivering the care patients want in areas where the 'flow rate' of patients is rapid, there are skills shortages, financial constraints and rising patient expectations. Nurses quickly learn that this is the reality of the workplace. Often learners and newly qualified nurses have learnt about an ideal state which allows them to achieve an award but does not prepare them for the reality they are

realism

	[INTERIOR]	[EXTERIOR]
[ME]	**Individual** Personal awareness Values Attitudes	**Professional** Personal capabilities Competencies Professional behaviour Measurable performance
[OTHERS]	**The team** Shared values Vision Language Culture	**Infrastructure** Social systems Organisational systems Technical environment

Figure 17   *Wilber's model of realism (adapted by Owen, 2004)*

experiencing and will continue to experience. The multidisciplinary team should have ownership and understanding of the lower left quadrant of the diagram to become a cohesive team. The lower right quadrant is the context in which nursing is practiced and impacts on the reality of nursing.

Social systems are changing, and patients when asked what a patient-led NHS feels like identified five dimensions (DOH, 2005):

- Access and waiting.
- Safe, high-quality, co-ordinated care.
- Better information, more choice.
- Building closer relationships.
- Clean, comfortable, friendly environment.

Nurses have to respond to these at individual, team and organisational levels. In today's world, patients are encouraged to tell their stories and are involved in programmes as patients/teachers. Nurses may initially find this challenging, but this approach brings realism about the patient's journey and can help nurses reflect on the care they give and the effect organisational processes may have on how the patient perceives their treatment.

To encourage realism in nursing, the use of stories needs to be explained as they offer a way to see and understand our world in a new light. They allow us to challenge ourselves and others and see our own areas of reality so that new insights become achievable (Owen, 2004) and then change can happen.

CASE STUDY

Mrs Briggs was invited along with other patients to a focus group which consisted of student nurses, qualified nurses, managers, medical staff, administrative staff and advanced nurse practitioners to tell her story about her experience as an inpatient in an acute hospital. The stories focused on how they felt their privacy and dignity had been protected.

Mrs Briggs said that most of her care was delivered by pleasant, respectful staff but pointed out that one incident can alter the whole experience. She recalled an incident where one member of the night staff insisted 'I could walk to the toilet on my own, despite the fact I have been unable to do so for 15 years. I requested I be taken on the commode; it was two hours later when a commode was pushed through the curtains.' This incident demonstrated that the individual nurse failed in her professional behaviour and sometimes when nurses reflect, they all see this incident as bad demonstration of practice, but may try to defend the act by blaming the system. Using Wilber's model of realism (Figure 17) to identify such issues may enable nurses to reach the conclusion that the individual as well as the system contributed to the neglecting of our duty of care.

In the real world nurses have to be proactive in challenging individuals, the organisation and the systems to ensure change takes place to eliminate similar incidents, and to ensure the patient's privacy and dignity is respected at all times.

CONCLUSION

The reality remains that patients need nurses to deliver the care they want, and the NHS reforms depend on the contribution of nurses. Nurses must remain true to the values of their profession in a rapidly changing environment. The reality is that the contribution nurses have made to delivering improvements in patient care has helped in reducing waiting times and has delivered high-quality care.

Change is constant, and realism is the act of accepting the reality, including facts. It does not matter whether a person likes or dislikes things as they are or appear to be: they are as they are. Emphasis needs to be placed on the importance of relationships. How people relate to each other affects what happens in the organisation, to the culture, the creativity and productivity. To have culture, people have to be real with one another and acknowledge work well done, and also trust each other. In this way working in partnership, patient-centred high-quality

realism

245

care can be delivered. Realism is the recognition of the true nature of a situation.

FURTHER READING

Department of Health (2004) *The NHS Improvement Plan*. London: Department of Health.

Hussey, T. (2000) 'Realism and nursing'. *Nursing Philosophy*, 1: 98–108.

Royal College of Nursing (2004) *The Future Nurse*. London: Royal College of Nursing.

REFERENCES

Bendall, E. (2006) '30th Anniversary commentary on Bendall, E. (1976) learning for reality'. *Journal of Advanced Nursing*, 1: 3–9.

Department of Health (2004) *Standards for Better Health*. London: Department of Health.

Department of Health (2005) '*Now I feel tall*', *what a patient-led NHS feels like*. London: Department of Health.

Department of Health (2006a) *Modernising Nursing Careers*. London: Department of Health.

Department of Health (2006b) *Our Health, Our Care, Our Say*. London: Department of Health.

Healthcare Commission (2006) *Developing the Annual Check in 2006/2007*. London: Commission for Healthcare Audit and Inspection.

Owen, N. (2004) *More Magic of Metaphor*. London: Crown House.

Cross-References *Assessment, Autonomy, Clinical governance, Confidence, Crisis management, Ethics, Problem solving.*

39 Record keeping

Anne Waugh

DEFINITION

The Nursing and Midwifery Council (NMC) (2004a) identifies accurate record keeping as a fundamental component of patient or client care and one which reflects the quality of a nurse's professional practice.

KEY POINTS

- The NMC (2005a) *Guidelines for Records and Record Keeping* sets out principles of good nursing practice.
- Patient safety and continuity of care is enhanced when records communicate relevant, concise information to other healthcare professionals and to patients and clients.
- Records can be used retrospectively by others:

  - locally for audit purposes, such as record keeping practice or standards of care, which forms part of the risk management process or to investigate complaints.

- The Audit Commission is a professional body such as the NMC or a court of law to establish circumstances surrounding a particular situation or event.

DISCUSSION

Registered nurses (RNs) are legally and professionally accountable for their records of care. The *NMC Annual Fitness to Practice Reports*. (NMC, 2004b, 2005b, 2006) provide information about professional misconduct cases, of which poor practice represents the greatest proportion; those due to poor record keeping were reported as 15 per cent in 2003–2004 and 6 per cent in 2004–2005. Although these figures suggest that record keeping may be improving, this vital aspect of practice benefits patient care and reflects the professionalism of nurses. This chapter considers the principles of effective record keeping and current influences on record keeping practice. The case study demonstrates how integration of these principles can maintain effective communication and prevent misunderstandings and complaints.

The *NMC Code of Professional Conduct: Standards for Conduct, Performance and Ethics* states 'You must ensure that the healthcare record for the patient or client is an accurate account of treatment, care planning and delivery' (NMC, 2004a: Clause 4.4).

Recognising the importance of the most fundamental aspects of care led the Department of Health to devise *The Essence of Care Benchmarks* in 2001. The best practice statements, or benchmarks, come with a resource pack to assist healthcare professionals rate their current practice against them. By changing aspects of current practice, progress towards meeting the benchmarks can be implemented and evaluated. The outcome for the record keeping benchmark is that 'patients benefit from

record keeping

Table 3 *Benchmarks for record keeping (NHS Modernization Agency, 2003)*

Factor	Benchmark of best practice
1. Access to current healthcare records	Patients are able to access all their current records if and when they choose to, in a format that meets their individual needs.
2. Integration – patient and professional partnership	Patients are actively involved in continuously negotiating and influencing their care.
3. Integration of records – across all professional and organisational boundaries	Patients have a single, structured, multiprofessional and agency record which supports integrated care.
4. Holding lifelong records	Patients hold a single, lifelong multiprofessional and agency record.
5. High-quality practice – evidence-based guidance	Evidence-based guidance detailing best practice is available and has an active and timely review process.
6. High-quality practice	Patients' records demonstrate that their care follows evidence-based guidance or supporting documents describing best practice, or that there is an explanation of any variance.
7. Security and confidentiality	Patients' records are safeguarded through explicit measures, with an active and timely review process.

records that demonstrate effective communications which support and inform high quality care' (NHS Modernization Agency, 2003: 2). The best practice statements that underpin this outcome are shown in Table 3. The NHS Clinical Governance Support Team (2004) provided an example of how engagement with this process led to a Standards Leaflet being devised to improve record keeping in an NHS Trust.

There is currently no national template for best record keeping practice, although this is likely to change in future with developments in information technology and projects such as the National Project for Information Technology (NPFIT) supported by the Department of Health. This will enable significant movement towards meeting several of the best practice statements in Table 3. At present documentation and recording practices are agreed locally, thus limiting the extent to which records may be shared between NHS Trusts.

Types of records

Health records may be either manual (paper) or electronic (computerised) and may be held by healthcare providers, patients themselves or children's parents. Patient-held records are often used in the community, and increasingly by people whose healthcare journeys take place across different settings and involve many healthcare professionals.

Records not only include assessment documentation, care plans and evaluations or summaries of progress, but also extend to charts such as those used to record vital signs, medication and fluid balance and incident forms. Increasingly interprofessional records are used, for example integrated care pathways. This single record is devised locally and used by all members of the multidisciplinary team (MDT). It has several advantages, including making the standards of care explicit and reducing the volume of individual documentation required, although their development is time-consuming (Wright and Tuffnell, 2002).

Principles of good record keeping

Bearing in mind people's right to see their records, even if they are not involved in writing them, and that they are likely to be scrutinised by others is a good starting point for accurate record keeping. Another is an often-quoted phrase 'if it is not recorded, it has not been done' (NMC, 2005a: 9). Records when read by others provide a measure of the author's professionalism.

Good practice involves the patient in all stages of their care, including what is recorded, and *The Data Protection Act* (The Stationery Office, 1998) provides people with the right of access to their records, both manual and electronic. Nurses are very often those who co-ordinate and maintain continuity of patients' care, and their records should provide clear evidence of care planned, decisions made and information shared. Patients' and relatives' requests or concerns should also be recorded, along with the actions taken to respond to them.

It is important to keep written information concise and relevant, a skill that must be learned and which involves professional judgment. A study by Martin et al. (1999) found that nursing records emphasised assessment at the expense of evaluation and patient outcomes. Furthermore, care was frequently recorded in different places by different nurses, resulting in records that did not fully reflect the care actually given.

Recording should be carried out as soon as possible after the event to maintain accuracy. This also prevents accumulation of information that requires to be documented, which may then become distorted or forgotten. An omission on a drug chart may result in a patient receiving their medication twice, which can have serious or even fatal consequences. All patient information must remain confidential and improper disclosure prevented (NMC, 2004a, 2005a). The principles explained below apply to both manual and electronic records.

All entries should be legible, factual, relevant and concise. Computerised records are easy to read; they overcome the problem of poor handwriting, are compact to store and can be easily accessed by members of the MDT. Recording of factual information maintains the accuracy of records; for example, '+ + +' does not accurately describe volumes and 'had a good day' does not state anything specific about a person or their progress. It also avoids value judgments and subjective statements which can be offensive. Abbreviations should only be used where agreed locally to prevent uncertainty. For example, between settings NAD may mean 'no abnormality detected' or 'not actually done', and CNS can stand for 'central nervous system' or 'clinical nurse specialist'. Jargon should be avoided so that others can easily understand the content and meaning of the record.

Manual records must be indelible, that is, made in ink, with any changes entered by neatly crossing through the error with a single line. This means that the original entry, the amendment and the reason for the change all remain legible. For this reason correction fluid must not be used. Written records include the date, time and signature. The signature is used, rather than initials, where possible and computerised records must be made using an individual user identity so that the author of each entry can be easily identified. Student nurses must have their entries countersigned by a RN who remains accountable for the care provided (NMC, 2005a).

Barriers

Nurses often work under pressure to complete their care. However, the busier one is, the more important it is to keep accurate, contemporaneous records. Being busy, heavy workloads and staff shortages are common reasons given for lack of time to keep records. Martin et al. (1999) found that many nurses would be unlikely to spend longer on record keeping even if more time was available, suggesting that record keeping was less important to them than hands-on care. Currell and Urquhart (2003) reported that nurses experienced difficulty in balancing the needs of clinical practice and administrative roles including record keeping.

The impact of poor record keeping

Being called to an NMC hearing can have a devastating effect on a nurse's personal and professional life. Hoban (2004) and Smith (2004) described situations where poor record keeping resulted in

NMC hearings, and the nurses' poignant reflections provide insight about how, with hindsight, this could have been avoided.

The Parliamentary and Health Service Ombudsman (2006) reported that during investigations into complaints or legal proceedings, recurring contributory factors included poor communication and poor record keeping. Increasing numbers of complaints and a culture of litigation have led to a huge and increasing financial burden on the NHS. The Audit Commission (National Audit Office, 2005) revealed that the cost of settling complaints and litigation has risen from £3.2 billion in 1999 to an estimated £7.8 billion in 2004. Imagine the impact of this resource if it could be diverted to patient care.

CASE STUDY

Imad was admitted to a care of the elderly assessment unit yesterday following a fall at home. He mentions to the night staff nurse that he has not received all his evening medication. She checks his nursing records, which confirm the information given during the ward handover that his medication regime had been simplified earlier in the day to improve his concordance after discharge. On checking his prescription chart she observes that the number of evening medicines have been reduced and that they have already been administered as the prescription chart is signed. The staff nurse returns to Imad and explains the situation. He now remembers that these changes had been discussed with him earlier. The staff nurse was able to resolve this query easily because the nursing documentation described the changes to the prescription chart and the reason why this was agreed. She was also able to provide reassurance that complex drug regimes can be hard to remember and are often not necessary. The staff nurse reflected that sometimes it is not easy to confirm all the necessary facts with patients as, being a busy ward, nurses can find it challenging to make time not only to provide good patient care but also to ensure that records are always accurate and up to date. Knowing that patients do not always remember health promotion messages and that new information needs to be reinforced, she drew a simple chart showing the revised medicine regime and went back and discussed this with Imad.

CONCLUSION

Good recording practice facilitates communication between healthcare professionals and between them and their patients/clients. It can promote high-quality care and provides an accurate factual record of care for audit and other purposes. As the impact of technology advances, old working practices will require review and new ones will emerge. Poor record keeping reflects a lack of professionalism and may have a devastating impact on nurses involved in investigations, complaints or litigation. It also leads to a huge drain on NHS resources.

FURTHER READING

Dimond, B. (2005) *Legal Aspects of Nursing*, 4th edn. Harlow: Pearson.

Hutchison, C. and Sharples, C. (2006) 'Information governance: practical implications for record keeping'. *Nursing Standard*, 17(20): 59–64.

Parliamentary and Health Service Ombudsman (2007) *Health – investigations completed*. Available online at www.ombudsman.org.uk/improving_services/selected_cases/HSC/index.html (accessed 13 Jan. 2007).

REFERENCES

Currell, R. and Urquhart, C. (2003) 'Nursing record systems: effects on nursing practice and healthcare outcomes'. *Cochrane Database of Systematic Reviews*, Issue 3.

Hoban, V. (2004) 'For the record'. *Nursing Times*, 101(27): 20–22.

Martin, A. Hinds, C. and Felix, M. (1999) 'Documentation practice of nurses in long-term care'. *Journal of Clinical Nursing*, 8(4): 345–52.

National Audit Office (2005) *Financial Management in the NHS – NHS Summarised Accounts 2003–2004*. London: Audit Commission. Available online at www.nao.org.uk/publications/nao_reports/05-06/050660_I.pdf (accessed 24 Nov. 2006).

NHS Clinical Governance Support Team (2004) *Essence of Care Eureka: Record Keeping Benchmark – Standards Leaflet for All Clinical Staff*. Available online at www.cgsupport.nhs.uk/downloads/Essence_of_Care/Eureka_Record_Barnsley.pdf, (accessed 24 Nov. 2006).

NHS Modernization Agency (2003) *The Essence of Care: Patient-focused Benchmarks for Clinical Governance*. London: The Stationery Office.

Nursing and Midwifery Council (2004a) *The NMC Code of Professional Conduct: Standards for Conduct, Performance and Ethics*. London: NMC.

Nursing and Midwifery Council (2004b) *Annual Fitness to Practice Report 2003–2004*. London: NMC. Available online at www.nmc-uk.org/aFrame Display.aspx?DocumentID=524 (accessed 24 Nov. 2006).

Nursing and Midwifery Council (2005a) *Guidelines for Records and Record Keeping*. London: NMC.

Nursing and Midwifery Council (2005b) *Annual Fitness to Practice Report 2004–2005*. London: NMC. Available online at www.nmc-uk.org/aFrameDisplay.aspx?DocumentID=1102 (accessed 24 Nov. 2006).

Nursing and Midwifery Council (2006) *Annual Fitness to Practice Report 2005–2006*. London: NMC. Available online at www.nmc-uk.org (accessed 25 Jan. 2008).

Parliamentary and Health Service Ombudsman (2006) *Annual Report 2005–2006: Making a Difference.* London: The Stationery Office.

Smith, S. (2004) 'Accurate record keeping must be a priority to ensure patient safety'. *Nursing Times,* 100(48): 18.

The Stationery Office (1998) *Data Protection Act.* London: The Stationery Office.

Wright, J. and Tuffnell, D.J. (2002) 'Implementing clinical guidelines', in J. Tingle and C. Foster (eds), *Clinical Guidelines: Law, Policy and Practice.* London: Cavendish.

Cross-References *Accountability, Assessment, Clinical governance, Data, information, knowledge.*

40 Reflection

Janice Gidman and Jean Mannix

DEFINITION

There is an extensive body of literature relating to reflection, originating from a range of sources including education, psychology and sociology. However, reflection is a difficult concept to define (Bulman and Schutz, 2004) and there appears to be a lack of clarity between different authors and disciplines in their use of terminology.

A commonly accepted definition of reflection is that it is:

> the process of creating and clarifying the meaning of experience (present or past) in terms of self (self in relation to self and self in relation to the world). The outcome is changed conceptual perspective. (Boyd and Fales, 1983: 101)

Johns presented a more holistic description (rather than definition) of reflection which incorporates both deliberate and intuitive learning and can take place either within or after practice:

> Reflection is being mindful of self, either within or after an experience, as if a window through which the practitioner can view and focus self within

reflection

the context of a particular experience, in order to confront, understand and move toward resolving contradiction between one's vision and actual practice. Through the conflict of contradiction, the commitment to realise one's vision and understanding why things are as they are, the practitioner can gain new insights into self and be empowered to respond more congruently in future situations within a reflexive spiral towards developing practical wisdom and realising one's vision as a lived reality. The practitioner may require guidance to overcome resistance or be empowered to act on understanding. (Johns, 2004: 3)

Johns thus views reflection as a process of learning through everyday experience, which facilitates the practitioner to move towards desirable practice. He contends that practitioners can use reflection to identify and explore contradictions between their vision of holistic practice and their actual practice. This may be particularly challenging within healthcare because of the deeply embedded social norms and traditions which often lead to resistance to change.

KEY POINTS

- Reflection is widely used as a teaching, learning and assessment strategy within professional education.
- Reflection is advocated to promote experiential learning during practice placements and the integration of theory and practice.
- Reflection is thought to promote problem-solving, critical thinking and decision-making skills.
- The key cognitive skills necessary to underpin reflection include self-awareness, description, critical analysis and synthesis.
- There is a range of approaches to reflection, and a number of models and frameworks are advocated to facilitate the process.

DISCUSSION

The concept of reflection within nursing has become an expectation in the development of competent reflective nurse practitioners. Reflection has been advocated as a means of integrating theory and practice, developing the ability to articulate and explore the knowledge embedded within practice and promoting change (Benner et al., 1996). Problem-solving, critical thinking and decision-making skills are essential competences for complex professional practice (Nursing and Midwifery Council (NMC), 2004).

Reflective practice is advocated as a teaching and learning strategy to facilitate the development of these cognitive skills (Burton, 2000).

Students need to develop a range of inter-related skills in order to engage in the complex cognitive process of reflection. These key skills include self-awareness, description, critical analysis and synthesis (Atkins, 2004). There is a wide range of approaches, models and frameworks available to facilitate reflection, which may involve verbal or written accounts, individual or group discussions, reflective journals and critical incident analysis. Facilitators of reflective practice need to be adequately prepared for their role, and this is now incorporated in the preparation of mentors and practice teachers who support both undergraduate and postgraduate nursing students. Mentors are required to spend time with students to facilitate reflection and experiential learning during practice placements and to enhance future learning.

Jasper (2003) advocated the use of journals to promote reflective practice, with these providing a record of experience and focus on the learning that occurred. She suggested that these accounts should include reflective commentaries and be written on an incremental basis over a period of time. The use of such journals contributes to continuing professional development for nurses, which is an ongoing requirement for registration (NMC, 2004).

Critical incident analysis is a widely used technique within professional education to explore and reflect on uncomfortable or puzzling situations (Rich and Parker, 1995). This is consistent with the educational theory proposed by the philosopher John Dewey, who is often described as the founder of reflection. Dewey's (1933) theory focused on the process of reflection as a means of making sense of the world, and emphasises perplexity as the stimulus for reflection. Schon is another influential theorist in relation to reflection; he proposed that reflection occurs when there are potential unexpected consequences to an action and suggested that healthcare involves '... a swampy lowland where situations are confusing "messes" incapable of technical solution ... in the swamp are the problems of greatest human concern' (1987: 42).

In contrast to the above perspectives, however, Francis (2004) contended that nurse education should promote reflection on everyday events, not just problematic ones, in order to challenge existing discourse and beliefs. Freshwater (2002) argued that practitioners need to be reflective in order to develop effective therapeutic relationships with their patients and to promote an equal power balance between professionals and patients. She also contended that student-centred approaches to

reflection

learning, including reflection on practice, promote the transformative learning which underpins therapeutic nursing. However, Freshwater cautioned that the appropriate assessment of reflection is a major issue for educationalists. Hargreaves (2004) argued that the imperative to achieve academically may discourage reflection that is open and honest. Indeed, she suggested that the formal assessment of reflective accounts may act as a barrier to the students' personal growth and integrity. The role of reflection in promoting empowerment is consistent with the description presented at the start of the chapter (Johns, 2004) and with the critical theory developed by the German sociologist and philosopher Jürgen Habermas. Habermas (1971) proposed that reflection has a role in the acquisition, development and consideration of knowledge as a means to promote the empowerment of the individual. A number of models and frameworks of reflection have been developed by educationalists to guide and structure the process of reflection, whether verbal or written. There is a debate in professional education about the value of reflective models and the formal assessment of reflection, which have the potential to either enhance or restrict the reflective process and the level of reflective thought (Gidman, 2006). It is outside of the remit of this chapter to discuss these; readers are directed to the further reading section to explore a range of reflective models and frameworks.

CASE STUDY

Suzy is a student nurse who has always been thoughtful regarding her practice and felt that this was her way of reflecting. She often wondered why a reflective model or framework was necessary. On her last placement, Suzy had a mentor who had excellent facilitation and communication skills and enabled Suzy to consider reflective practice in a different way.

During a shift with her mentor, Suzy began thinking about an issue in practice. However, rather than thinking only of how this made her feel and whether it was a good or bad experience, Suzy's mentor suggested that Suzy used a structured framework that encouraged further analysis including the political and professional issues related to the incident. When Suzy had reflected in the past she had always considered only the patient and her own role within the situation. By using a structured framework with her mentor, Suzy enhanced her reflective skills and also identified other areas to be taken into consideration.

Suzy had initially struggled with the complexity of this critical incident. However, the use of a structured framework became a catalyst for both Suzy and her mentor; as the complexity of the critical incident was deconstructed, the level of critical thinking required increased (this can be known as layers of reflection). Suzy had always found that a model of reflection had restricted her reflection; however, with the expertise of a mentor who guided, supported and facilitated reflection, Suzy was empowered to critically deconstruct her own practice and give consideration to the wider implications and drivers associated within nursing.

CONCLUSION

Reflection is a concept which remains difficult to define, but is widely advocated within professional education. Reflection is thought to promote experiential learning and to integrate theory and practice, and it is a requirement that mentors spend time with their students to facilitate this process. It is also a requirement that registered nurses demonstrate problem-solving, critical thinking and decision-making skills and continue their professional development throughout their careers. Reflection is a teaching and learning strategy which may facilitate this development. There are a number of approaches to reflection, which may involve verbal or written accounts and which may be structured and guided by models or frameworks.

FURTHER READING

Bulman, C. and Schutz, S. (2004) *Reflective Practice in Nursing*. Oxford: Blackwell.
Johns, C. and Freshwater, D. (eds) (2005) *Transforming Nursing Through Reflective Practice*, 2nd edn. Oxford: Blackwell.
Rolfe, G., Freshwater, D. and Jasper, M. (2001) *Critical Reflection for Nursing and the Helping Professions*. Basingstoke: Palgrave.

REFERENCES

Atkins, S. (2004) 'Developing underlying skills in the move towards reflective practice', in C. Bulman and S. Schutz (eds), *Reflective Practice in Nursing*. Oxford: Blackwell.
Benner, P., Tanner, C. and Chesla, C. (1996) *Expertise in Nursing Practice: Caring, Clinical Judgement and Ethics*. New York: Springer.
Boyd, E.M. and Fales, A.W. (1983) 'Reflective learning: key to learning from experience'. *Journal of Humanistic Psychology*, 23(2): 99–117.
Bulman, C. and Schutz, S. (2004) *Reflective Practice in Nursing*. Oxford: Blackwell.
Burton, A.J. (2000) 'Reflection: nursing's practice and education panacea?' *Journal of Advanced Nursing*, 31(5): 1009–17.

reflection

Dewey, J. (1933) *How We Think*. Boston, MD: Heath.

Francis, D.I. (2004) 'Reconstructing the meaning given to critical incidents in nurse education'. *Nurse Education in Practice*, 4: 244–9.

Freshwater, D. (2002) *Therapeutic Nursing: Improving Patient Care through Self-Awareness and Reflection*. London: Sage.

Gidman, J. (2006) 'Reflecting on reflection', in J. Woodhouse (ed.), *How to Teach in the 21st Century: Teaching Strategies in Healthcare Education*. Oxford: Radcliffe.

Habermas, J. (1971) *Knowledge and Human Interests*. London: Heinemann.

Hargreaves, J. (2004) 'So how do you feel about that? Assessing reflective Practice'. *Nurse Education Today*, 24: 196–201.

Jasper, M. (2003) *Beginning Reflective Practice*. Cheltenham: Nelson Thornes.

Johns, C. (2004) *Becoming a Reflective Practitioner*, 2nd edn. Oxford: Blackwell.

Nursing and Midwifery Council (2004) *Standards of Proficiency for Pre-registration Nursing Education*. London: NMC.

Rich, A. and Parker, D.L. (1995) 'Reflection and critical incident analysis: ethical and moral implications of their use within nursing and midwifery education'. *Journal of Advanced Nursing*, 22: 1050–7.

Schon, D. (1987) *Educating the Reflective Practitioner: Towards a New Design for Teaching and Learning in the Professions*. Aldershot: Avebury Academic.

Cross-References *Educator, Empowerment, Mentoring, Problem solving.*

41 Rehabilitation

Sandra Flynn

DEFINITION

Defining rehabilitation can be an extremely problematic task due to the variety of opinions that exist in the literature. The United Nations define rehabilitation as meaning:

> a goal-orientated and time-limited process aimed at an impaired person to reach an optimum mental, physical and/or social functional level, thus providing her or him with the tools to change her or his own life. It can involve measures intended to compensate for a loss of function or a functional

limitation (for example by technical aids) and other measures intended to facilitate social adjustment or readjustment' (2006: 1).

Rehabilitation is essentially a form of treatment or a series of interventions planned to facilitate a pathway of recovery from illness, injury, disease or addiction in order to promote an optimum level of function, independence and quality of life.

Rehabilitation may be required regardless of age, culture, social status or religion. It is important to consider the interpretation of human experience in relation to disability, disease or addiction as many individuals find themselves confronted by their sense of self, abruptly and significantly changed or challenged (Bishop, 2005). The focus of rehabilitation must centre upon the ability of the individual to navigate the psychosocial and physical roads of ill health to a desired destination of well-being. In order to assist this journey, a series of coping mechanisms and strategies must be employed to equip each individual to deal with what is effectively a unique personal and subjective life event.

KEY POINTS

- The primary goal of rehabilitation is functional or role restoration.
- The type, level and goals of rehabilitation are based upon and are responsive to individual needs.
- Rehabilitation programmes may be delivered within a variety of settings.
- Rehabilitation must be multi-professional and evidence based.

DISCUSSION

In daily life all individuals, regardless of health or illness, have differing life goals which exist as a motivational force. Life goals can inspire and contribute towards a sense of health and well-being (Emmons, 1986). During illness, disease, disability or addictions a person can be affected by negative physical or psychological feelings. This in turn can disrupt individual life goals, causing either a temporary or permanent interruption of these life pursuits (Hooker and Siegler, 1993; Wheeler et al., 1990). Coupled with this is the person's unique response to their illness or disability, which may be reflected in and influenced by such issues as interpersonal relationships, physical and mental functioning or interaction with the environment (Bishop, 2005). Rehabilitation includes a

rehabilitation

variety of activities aimed at enabling individuals with physical, psychological and social problems to reach and maintain optimal functional levels; for example, restoring skills, teaching new skills, provision of aids to assist activities of daily living and correcting or restoring speech.

Rehabilitation is both an art and science and aims to decrease impairments, prevent complications and improve, where possible, an individual's ability to perform significant activities. Historically, programmes of rehabilitation have been developed out of a need to respond to disabilities resulting from wars, natural disasters, occupational and road trauma (Disler et al., 2002). As a consequence, most programmes have centred upon a medical model of rehabilitation. However, in recent years the focus of rehabilitation has had a tendency to shift from a bio-medical to a bio-psychosocial model. This has subsequently provided a more person-centred approach where the emphasis is on empowerment, improving self-image and giving individuals values, choices, desired levels of independence and interdependence, self-esteem and above all control of their life (Scherer et al., 2006). This model has seen the emergence of a 'care partnership', whereby the main stakeholders work together to set realistic goals in order to achieve the best quality of life possible.

Rehabilitation goals are dependent upon the condition for which they are required, and because each person's circumstances are unique, each set of goals must be personalised and not standardised. Goals need to be set by the individual, family and rehabilitation team, ensuring that they are realistic, achievable and of interest to the person concerned. The United Nations report *Action Concerning Disabled Persons* advocates that the delivery of rehabilitation should take place as far as possible in the individual's 'natural environment' and provided within the 'existing health, social, educational and employment structures of society' (2006: 2).

Several models for rehabilitation exist in the literature, but generally these tend to be disease or condition specific. Examples are:

- Physical rehabilitation following stroke, cardiac events, brain injuries (Gillen and Burhardt, 2004; Matthews, 1999; Wilson, 1997).
- Psychological rehabilitation following mental ill health (Garske and McReynolds, 2005; Moxley and Finch, 2003).
- Drug rehabilitation following drug/alcohol dependency (Diclemente, 2006; Peele, 2004).
- Social/occupational rehabilitation which targets specific areas such as employment and social relationships (Matthews, 1999).

Rehabilitation services and programmes usually combine clinical, therapeutic and social interventions pertaining to the individual's needs and their environment and usually include:

- Diagnosis and treatment.
- Education in performing activities of daily living.
- Provision of technical and mobility aids.
- Counselling services.
- Social assessment.
- Specialised educational services.
- Vocational rehabilitation services, such as specialised employment schemes.
- Continuing care and assessment.

Rehabilitation programmes may take place in multiple settings, for example:

- In-patient; usually acute or community hospital settings.
- Outpatient; for individuals who can travel to hospitals, clinics, rehabilitation centres.
- Home or community, including schools, sports centres, places of employment.

In-patient rehabilitation tends to be primarily concerned with the treatment and care an individual receives whilst in hospital. However, continuing outpatient or community-based rehabilitation services are required in order to assist patients to maintain rehabilitation goals (Evans et al., 1998).

Any rehabilitation programme will consist of a number of professionals who form the rehabilitation team. Each team will differ according to the type of rehabilitation required. However, they may include medical staff, rehabilitation nurses, physiotherapists, occupational therapists, speech therapists, social workers, dieticians, rehabilitation psychologists, podiatrists, counsellors and audiologists. This is not an exhaustive list and the reader is directed to the further reading section of this chapter for more in-depth information.

The delivery of effective rehabilitation services is important from an economic viewpoint as finances affect improvements in healthcare technology. Within the last decade greater emphasis has been placed upon reducing lengths of hospital stay, resulting in an even greater need for the provision of community-based rehabilitation services.

Furthermore, the advances in healthcare technology have meant that life expectancy for patients suffering from specific types of injuries or illnesses, including lifestyle-related diseases, has now increased as, for example, with certain cancers or AIDS (Murphy et al., 2003).

Rehabilitation should not only provide for the training or re-training of individuals in order that they may make relevant life adjustments, but also above all to ensure the protection of human rights. According to Article 25 of the *Declaration of Human Rights*, these include the 'right to treatment, necessary social services, the right to security in the event of sickness and disability' (General Assembly of the UN, 1948: 76). The key to the success of rehabilitation programmes lies within the preparation of the services required and must include the expectations of the individual, their goals and desired outcomes, their customs and structures of the family and community in which they live.

CASE STUDY

John is a 62-year-old man who is employed full time as an electrician. He lives in a three-bedroom house with his 60-year-old wife Doreen, who is fit and well. Two weeks ago John fell off a ladder whilst working and sustained a fractured hip. He was admitted to hospital to internally fix the fracture.

Prior to his surgery, John's current level of function was assessed, following which a rehabilitation programme was developed by the multi-professional team. John decided, with support from the team, that his short-term goals would be to be pain free, return home to his wife and to regain full mobility and ultimately his long-term goals were to return to work on light duties, drive his car and finally be able to play football with his grandchildren again.

John's rehabilitation began with exercises designed to help improve the strength in his leg. The next step consisted of helping John to get in and out of bed, walking, turning and sitting in a chair. At first John was able to walk with the aid of a frame; this gradually progressed to walking sticks. As John was generally fit and well before his accident, his rehabilitation plan provided for an early discharge home. An occupational therapist undertook an assessment of John's home, providing equipment to assist with activities of daily living. Before his discharge from hospital he was provided with a programme of rehabilitation which would continue to help him cope whilst at home and prepare him for a possible return to work. Within a month John had met all of his short-term goals and was planning to return to work on light duties within the next two months.

CONCLUSION

Rehabilitation focuses upon a diverse and in-depth approach to a phenomenon where emphasis is placed firmly upon the relationship that exists between an individual, their family, society and the environment in which they live and work. Rehabilitation and medical care should complement each other, thereby enabling people with illnesses, disabilities, diseases and addictions reach their optimal levels of functioning. The focus of rehabilitation should not be one of cure but of preparation for adaptation and provision of new life skills. This adaptation may be temporary or permanent. Either way, each person brings into play a series of mechanisms for coping based upon their personal and subjective analysis of the problems faced.

Importantly, any rehabilitation programme or model needs to ensure that concordance exists between the individual, their family and the rehabilitation professionals. Rehabilitation must be tailored to the person's short- or long-term life goals, paying particular attention to all critical life domains, which are of considerable importance to each individual and to the success of each rehabilitation programme (Sivaraman-Nair and Wade 2003).

FURTHER READING

Matthews, D. (1999) *Rehabilitation Source Book (Health Reference)*. New York: Springer.

Moxley, D.P. and Finch, J.R. (2003) *Sourcebook of Rehabilitation and Mental Health Practice*. New York: Springer.

World Health Organisation (2001) *International Classification of Functioning, Disabilitiy and Health*. Geneva: WHO.

REFERENCES

Bishop, M. (2005) 'Quality of life and psychosocial adaptation to chronic illness and acquired disability: a conceptual and theoretical synthesis'. *Journal of Rehabilitation*, 71(2): 5–13.

Diclemente, C.C. (2006) *Addiction and Change*. New York: Guilford Press.

rehabilitation

Disler, P.B., Cameron, I.D. and Wilson, S.F. (2002) 'Rehabilitation medicine'. *The Medical Journal of Australia*, 177(7): 385–6.

Emmons, R.A. (1986) 'Personal strivings: an approach to personality and subjective well-being'. *Journal of Personality and Social Psychology*, 51: 1058–68.

Evans, R., Connis, R. and Haselkorn, J.K. (1998) 'Hospital-based care versus outpatient services: effects on functioning and health status'. *Disability and Rehabilitation*, 20(8): 298–307.

Garske, G.G. and McReynolds, C.J. (2005) 'Psychiatric rehabilitation: a means of de-stigmatizing severe mental illness'. *Journal of Applied Rehabilitation Counselling*, 36(4): 28–34.

General Assembly of the United Nations (1948) *Universal Declaration of Human Rights Act*. 217 A (III). United Nations Department of Public Information Reprint 2005.

Gillen, G. and Burkhardt, A. (2004) *Stroke Rehabilitation*, 2nd edn. London: Mosby.

Hooker, K. and Siegler, I.C. (1993) 'Life goals, satisfaction and self-rated health: preliminary findings'. *Experimental Ageing Research*, 19: 97–110.

Matthews, D. (1999) *Rehabilitation Source Book (Health Reference)*. New York: Springer.

Moxley, D.P. and Finch, J.R. (2003) *Sourcebook of Rehabilitation and Mental Health Practice*. New York: Springer.

Murphy, G.C., Young, A.E. and Reid, K. (2003) 'Contributions to rehabilitation from behavioural psychology: now and then'. *Behavioural Change*, 20(4): 218–22.

Peele, S. (2004) *7 Tools to Beat Addiction*. New York: Three Rivers Press.

Scherer, M., Blair, K., Banks, M.E., Brucker, B., Corrigan, J. and Wegener, S. *Rehabilitation Psychology*. Available online at www.apa.org/divisions/div22 (accessed Oct. 2006).

Sivaraman-Nair, K.P. and Wade, D.T. (2003) 'Life goals of people with disabilities due to neurological disorders'. *Clinical Rehabilitation*, 17: 521–7.

Wheeler, R.J., Munz, D.C. and Jain, A. (1990) 'Life goals and general well-being'. *Psychology Reports*, 66: 307–12.

Wilson, B.A. (1997) 'Cognitive rehabilitation: how it is and how it might be'. *Journal of the International Neuropsychological Society*, 3: 487–96.

United Nations *World Programme of Action Concerning Disabled Persons*. Available online at www.un.org/esa/socdev/enable/diswpa01.htm (accessed Dec. 2006).

Cross-References *Confidence, Coping, Dignity, Evidence-based practice, Holistic care, Realism.*

42 Relationship between the individual and society

Andy Lovell

DEFINITION

The relationship between the individual and society has always provoked intense debate, the parameters set by the notions of structure and agency, the extent to which one's actions are influenced or even determined by wider social forces. The question has been described as the most fundamental in sociological investigation, the fruitfulness of all enquiry being measured by the value of its contribution (MacIver and Page, 1950). A definition of this relationship requires consideration of three diverse, inter-related elements: social order, social change and socialisation. These elements vary according to theoretical persuasion, issues of consensus, conflict, control, negotiated order complicated further by factors of gender, 'race', sexuality, age, class and disability, and underpinned by change across time and space. The reader cannot ignore such factors, but they are clearly beyond the scope of this chapter.

KEY POINTS

- Society requires a balance between the influence of structure, such as family or education, and agency, whereby individuals are free to negotiate their own roles.
- Socialisation concerns the process by which individuals learn the culture of their society and internalise the key norms, values and beliefs.
- Each society has a number of culturally defined goals, which require a degree of conformity amongst its members and influence the maintenance of social order.

- Fundamental alteration to major societal dimensions such as culture, structure or the social behaviour of the population constitutes social change.
- The process of socialisation is mitigated by dimensions of social difference, which include social class, gender, age, ethnicity and sexuality.

DISCUSSION

Social Order

Maintenance of social order is an issue that challenges society as it adapts or tries to adapt to social change; it is a pervasive sociological concept and refers to the ways in which society retains its influence over recalcitrant members. Berger informs us that 'no society can exist without social control [and] the ultimate argument is violence' (1963: 84), the roles of the police, the criminal justice system and other state apparatus varying in their degree of complicity. Contemporary democracy requires sophisticated surveillance systems, tracking devices, multiple technologies, but even in such complex, developed societies, social order is never a given and the relationship with control is often ambiguous.

Foucault (1977) argues that modern disciplinary power increasingly reflects the particular mode of society, so that Western democracies come to rely less on direct force – what he refers to as failed forms of discipline – and more on the propensity of the individual to control the behaviour of him/herself and others. He argues that specific historical conditions enable society to employ particular mechanisms in the maintenance of social order. Surveillance technology, for example, requires the economic and political conditions prevalent within Western democracies, whilst a society embedded in different political, social, economic and cultural systems might rely on other approaches. Turner and Rojek (2001), in contrast, suggest that there has been a major social change away from the question of the maintenance of social order towards a preoccupation with the prevention of social disorder.

The maintenance of the health of the population would appear to be a central requirement of the maintenance of social order, but also forces us to address its complexity. Parsons (1951) formulation of the 'sick role' as a means of the way in which the medical profession monitors and regulates the amount of societal sickness through the sanctioning device of the medical certificate, demonstrates a classic account of the need for such mechanisms of social order. Medicine, however, has attracted criticism in relation to interpretation of its role as an instrument of social control (Zola, 1972), the medicalisation of life (Illich, 1975) and its relationship with capitalism (Navarro, 1976). Such powerful critiques reflected the particular social and cultural conditions of the period in which they were written, challenges to Western medicine necessitating specific societal circumstances.

Social Change

Social change refers to fundamental alterations in the patterns of culture, structure and social behaviour over time (Wander Zanden, 1993). The most prominent thinkers in society are primarily concerned with the 'salient characteristics of their time – and the problem of how history is being made within it' (Wright Mills, 1959: 183), though it is future generations who can accurately judge whether contemporary analysis was accurate. The Great Depression of the 1930s and World War II constitute two periods of marked social change during the last century. Giddens identifies the current era as being characterised by 'stunning social change, marked by transformations radically discrepant from those of previous periods' (1991: xv). He identifies the key features to be the collapse of Eastern Europe and the Cold War, the development of global systems of communication and the triumphalism of the capitalist system. Subsequent years, however, have witnessed an intensification of these same concerns, coupled with some others either escalating or emerging, such as climate change, mass extinction of species, the communications revolution and the 'war on terror'. Each era contains elements persisting over time, others declining or even disappearing, and some appearing unexpectedly on the political, economic and social landscape. It is the combination of different characteristics, such as economic collapse, mass unemployment and rural-urban migration, which produce an effect of social change.

A recent example of health-related social change concerns the advent of community care over the course of the last four decades. It began as an ideological movement in relation to the care of previously segregated groups, such as people with learning disabilities or mental health problems. Practical policy initiatives have been gradually implemented, which have transformed care practices, resulting in the demise of large institutions and affirming the family or other small-scale settings as most appropriate. The impact has been such that there has been a marked change in the ways in which we think about the delivery of care, not just to vulnerable individuals but also in relation to generic health services, many of which have been influenced by community care.

Socialisation

Socialisation refers to the process of social interaction by which we internalise the norms, values and beliefs essential for effective participation in society; the means by which a society's culture is transmitted across generations. Internalisation refers to 'the immediate apprehension or interpretation of an objective event as expressing meaning, that is, as a manifestation of another's subjective processes which thereby becomes subjectively meaningful to myself' (Berger and Luckmann, 1966: 149). In the absence of socialisation, society would be unable to perpetuate itself beyond a single generation. The individual and society are mutually dependent on socialisation; it blends the sentiments and ideas of culture to the capacities and needs of the organism (Davis, 1949). Culture comprises the mores, traditions and beliefs of how people function, and encompasses other products of human works and thoughts specific to members of an inter-generational group, community or population (Brookins, 1993). Socialisation is a lifelong process of inculcation, the key social systems being the family, education, religion, work, peer groups and the media. The relative influence of each agency varies across both time and space; the role of religion, for example, continues to play a powerful, life-defining role in the lives of many people, though declining church attendances and the increasingly secular nature of social life attests to the contrary. The role of the mass media and the role of interactive technology is consuming the current interests of many social commentators, but its overall impact on the socialisation process remains uncertain.

Socialisation is mitigated by many factors: the place in which one grows up, family structure, gender, financial security, ethnic background, experience of disability or mental illness. The development of the self in the social process, one's ability to 'take on the role of the other' (Mead, 1934), is complicated by these factors and the nature of the particular social system to which the individual belongs. Conformity to societal norms and values necessitates tolerance of difference, and society varies in the degree to which it regards those considered different according to prevailing circumstances. The attribution of deviance to people on the basis of their sexuality or intelligence, for example, may appear shocking at present, but was not always so, just as religious bigotry and racism appear susceptible to periodic reinvention.

CASE STUDY

Martin is 20 years old and lives at home with his parents; he has an older sister no longer living at home. He has cerebral palsy and a mild learning disability, which means that he has restricted but independent mobility, and communication problems to the extent that it takes some time before people understand what he is saying, less so for those close to him. Martin attended a mainstream school throughout his school years, though he fell short of gaining academic qualifications; he was provided with additional specialist support in the areas of speech and physiotherapy. Professional concern has always been on providing the family with the necessary help for their particular needs; despite considerable difficulties, there has never been concern about them being unable to cope.

Several decades earlier, the family's experience of specialist support and Martin's of social integration would very likely have been considerably different. The policy of community care demonstrates how social change has enabled people previously regarded on the margins of society to remain with their families. Furthermore, the relationship between Martin and society is now more reciprocal, with the anticipation that he might fulfil valued social roles within the family and the community; though he is not presently in employment, remaining dependent upon benefits, he is keen to acquire the skills to make him economically productive.

Martin's family background constituted the basis of his initial socialisation, the framework for learning about how things were rather than how things ought to be. His 'difference' from others was apparent very early, manifested through his appearance, mobility, speech and general physical awkwardness. Martin's parents were extremely aware of these differences and influenced the extent to which he became involved in playing with other children of his age and attended places where they would be present. They were a little concerned that he might be injured, had a desire to protect him from danger, ridicule or even being stared at because of his physical differences.

Martin's relationship with his cerebral palsy and learning disability has never been an easy one; he often becomes frustrated at his limitations, difficulties in being understood by others, and gaining acceptance and inclusion in the activities of his own age group. There have been serious challenges to barriers to social inclusion over recent years, but there are many unwritten rules that influence whether an individual becomes part of youth culture. Martin's anger tends to be concerned with issues of gaining fruitful employment, socialising in venues such as pubs and nightclubs, and gaining opportunities for developing relationships with women. This anger is sometimes manifested through a breakdown of communication between himself and those close to him, particularly his parents, and there have been occasions when he has displayed serious levels of aggression. He has, for example, become physically violent towards his mother and become almost uncontrollable in his rage, breaking furniture and striking out at others. This culminated in the use of emergency compulsory detention under mental health legislation. The resulting 48-hour period of detention was not renewed because the receiving consultant psychiatrist regarded Martin's behaviour not to be the result of mental illness or his learning disability. Further incidents of a similar nature have resulted in the involvement of the police, though charges have always been withdrawn.

CONCLUSION

Individuals living in society do so through the establishment of standards based on values. We become socialised into our societies by learning the behavioural requirements based on the traditions of our cultures, and these then govern how we overcome the conflicts and tensions that arise from human beings living together. Change in societies tends to occur slowly, as the new ways of behaving may not be readily accepted. This is also the case in healthcare settings, with new ways of delivering care looked upon with suspicion and old ways viewed as safe.

FURTHER READING

Scambler, G. (2002) *Health and Social Change: A Critical Theory*. Buckingham: Open University Press.

REFERENCES

Berger, P.L. (1963) *Invitation to Sociology: A Humanistic Perspective*. Harmondsworth: Penguin.
Berger, P.L. and Luckmann T. (1966) *The Social Construction of Reality*. Harmondsworth: Penguin.
Brookins, G.K. (1993) 'Culture, ethnicity, and bicultural competence: implications for children with chronic illness and disability'. *Pediatrics*, 91, 5(pt 2): 1056–62.
Davis, K. (1949) *Human Society*. New York: Macmillan.

Foucault, M. (1977) *Discipline and Punish: The Birth of the Prison*. London: Allen Lane.

Giddens, A. (1991) *Introduction to Sociology*. New York: Norton.

Illich, I. (1975) *Medical Nemesis: The Expropriation of Health*. London: Calder & Boyars.

MacIver, R.M. and Page, C.H. (1950) *Society: An Introductory Analysis*. London: Macmillan.

Mead, G.H. (1934) *Mind, Self and Society*. Chicago, IL: University of Chicago Press.

Navarro, V. (1976) *Medicine under Capitalism*. New York: Prodist.

Parsons, T. (1951) *The Social System*. London: Routledge & Kegan Paul.

Turner, B.S. and Rojek, C. (2001) *Society and Culture: Principles of Scarcity and Solidarity*. London: Sage.

Wander Zanden, J.W. (1993) *Sociology: The Core*, 3rd edn. London: McGraw-Hill.

Wright Mills, C. (1959) *The Sociological Imagination*. Harmondsworth: Penguin.

Zola, I.K. (1972) 'Medicine as an institution of social control: the medicalizing of society'. *Sociological Review*, 20: (4): 487–504.

Cross-References Communication, Environment, Reflection, Respect, Role model.

43 Researcher

Peter Bradshaw

DEFINITION

The word 'research' is derived from the French, and its translation into English means 'to investigate thoroughly'. Research is usually defined as a meticulous process of systematic inquiry aimed at establishing and discovering new knowledge and truths, or testing the explanatory power of existing understandings. The outcome of this intellectual endeavour is not only to extend knowledge, but also to contribute to the formulation of concepts and theories that make it applicable to practice. Research in nursing or midwifery is conducted within a number of frameworks associated with scientific or social scientific methods that are characterised by robust techniques for investigating phenomena encountered in practice. As an activity, therefore, research is based on gathering empirical, measurable evidence known as *data* that are then subject to the principles of reasoning and interpretation (Newton, 1687; Polit and Beck, 2006).

Research distils common sense. It broadens it and enhances its legitimacy by seeking logical relationships between everyday assumptions through its lucid, well-articulated system of explanation. It utilises abstract concepts in the course of its investigations, and aims consistently to relate and to apply its findings to the real world. Through its techniques, therefore, research into any discipline provides a systematically ordered, and evidence-informed, knowledge on which to base clinical decisions and to inform practice (Kuhn, 1962; Nagel, 1961; Polit and Beck, 2006).

KEY POINTS

In considering the nurse or midwife as a researcher, it is important to summarise the purpose of their activity before examining the rationale for what they do. Their research aims to:

- Better target services at those who need them by involving patients and their carers in deciding their preferences.
- Develop improved techniques for the assessment of patients and clients to enhance direct care.
- Construct and test tools used to collect data such as surveys and interview schedules to make research more effective.
- Construct and test theories that guide practice.
- Develop innovations in curriculum design and delivery to augment learning and teaching.
  (Hockey, 2000)

DISCUSSION

Research and epistemology

Any research activity is conducted within an epistemological framework. *Epistemology* defines a branch of Western philosophy that studies the nature and scope of the knowledge that explains scientific phenomena with a degree of certainty and exactness. In his treatise *The Structure of Scientific Revolutions* (1962), Kuhn traces the history and philosophical analysis of knowledge, the research that builds it and the way in which research is developed as an intellectual pursuit. This contends that a *scientific revolution* occurs when researchers produce new findings that cannot be reconciled with the general laws and previously accepted *truths* within a particular scientific discipline. To describe this occurrence, Kuhn coined the term *paradigm*. He thus postulated that a paradigm represents a generally accepted worldview about a particular theory. Kuhn emphasised the inconsistencies within all paradigms that have various levels of significance to the practitioners of any distinct branch of learning when something new is discovered. Consequently, paradigms are redefined over time, and this Kuhn calls *paradigm shift* as evidence that knowledge never stands still. The goal of research thereby is to produce new knowledge that takes three main forms:

- Exploratory research – this identifies problems.
- Experimental research – is intended to solve problems.
- Empirical research – that tests the feasibility of a solution using what has been observed and experienced from the data collected by the researcher.

Research and ontology

Fundamental to most research is the opportunity to contribute new understandings, ideally through findings that are applicable in as wide a context as possible (Polit and Beck, 2006). Yet, approaches to the conduct of research are ambiguous because the paradigms that guide them can be examined on a somewhat artificial continuum, each end of which has quite different ontological origins. *Ontology* concerns the perceptions and meanings of reality. How reality is interpreted, therefore, becomes as fundamental to the researcher as the epistemological dimensions of a study that concern the category of knowledge that it seeks to enhance.

Quantitative research paradigms

At one end of the continuum are classical definitions of research. These paradigms regard reality and knowledge as synonymous with the positivist view of science. They aspire to *objectivity*, and quantitative researchers are concerned with the hallmarks of a pure physical science because of its focus on conclusiveness and ability to predict cause and effect. From an ontological perspective, these researchers assume that reality consists of objective facts that can be analysed rigorously and expressed as numerical outcomes. Deductive reasoning guides the research and within this process, conclusions are reached that arise directly from the accumulated evidence.

Quantitative researchers know at the outset what they are going to measure and how they will achieve these precise measurements because the process of their study is structured in detail and in advance of it taking place. Large sample sizes are recruited that are representative of the population or phenomenon that is of interest and the data are gathered using structured research instruments. Tools such as question-naires or laboratory equipment are employed to collect statistical data by researchers who distance themselves from the subject matter of the study to create impartiality and minimise bias. The results confer *validity*, confirming that the researcher measured precisely what was intended, and also *reliability*, meaning that replication can occur. Common quantitative research techniques include randomised control trials, experiments, quasi-experiments and surveys.

It is argued that these paradigms analyse relationships between variables in a controlled, unprejudiced and value-free manner, producing theories that can be generalised to explain the same phenomena in similar populations elsewhere (Peat et al., 2002). For many decades, quantitative research enjoyed the position of being the prevailing paradigm associated with the generation and verification of theory (Peat et al., 2002). This has now been challenged through the belief that all synthesis, whether quantitative or qualitative, is a legitimate interpreta-tive endeavour (Bowling and Shah, 2005).

Qualitative research paradigms

These approaches contrast with quantitative research. In *qualitative* paradigms the ontological and epistemological origins stem from philos-ophy, anthropology and sociology, and their interpretations of the world and of truth challenge the classical definitions of positivist scientists. In these conventions, researchers contend that social reality cannot be captured solely by numerical means. Qualitative research thus places less importance on developing statistically valid samples, or on search-ing for statistical support for its findings. These researchers study phenomena in their natural setting, attempting to make sense of, or interpret them, in terms of the meanings people bring to them by using holistic perspectives to capture the complexities of human experiences (Parahoo, 2006). They argue that *subjectivity* is a key feature of reality that is to be discovered only through an open acknowledgement that the personal influences of the researcher and the researched cannot be ignored. Their interest thus lies in factors such as beliefs, values, attitudes and interactions, hence the qualitative paradigms seek a depth of understanding about human behaviour and the reasons that govern it. The researcher may, at the outset of a study, have only an approximate idea of what might be discovered, and the research design can emerge inductively as the work proceeds with an interest greater in process rather than outcomes (Miles and Huberman, 1994). This means that the researcher becomes personally immersed in the subject matter and builds abstractions, concepts and assumptions from details as these emerge from the data. The nature of qualitative research with its concern for how meaning is constructed from experience, frequently requires smaller but well-focused samples rather than large and random samples that are used in quantitative research. This typically involves fieldwork and the researcher physically goes to the people, setting, site or institution to participate in, observe or record behaviour in its natural setting. The qualitative researcher becomes the primary medium for data collection and analysis, and data are mediated through this human instrument, although the researchers will use inventories, questionnaires or technology to accumulate their findings. Researchers within these paradigms report their findings predominantly in words, and qualitative data is rich in meaning, time consuming to analyse, and is more reliant on the reader's interpretation for its generalisation. The notions of reliability and validity cannot be applied to evaluate the integrity of qualitative research. Rather, this is achieved through the following concepts (Lincoln and Guba, 1985):

- *Credibility*: establishes that the results are believable from the perspective of the research participants.
- *Transferability*: refers to the degree to which the results of qualitative research can be applied to other contexts or settings.
- *Dependability*: emphasises the need for the researcher to account for the ever-changing context within which research occurred.
- *Confirmability*: refers to the degree to which the results could be confirmed or corroborated by others.

It is undeniably the case that the polarisation between the quantitative and the qualitative research paradigms that have evolved are fundamentally ideological in nature (Hammersley, 1993). Researchers from each persuasion have contrasted their epistemological beliefs regarding scientific knowledge and ontological interpretations of reality, resulting in a sometimes false dichotomy that can be taken to extremes. Expressed simply, quantitative research investigates the *why* and *how*, whereas qualitative research focuses on the *what*, *where*, and *when*. The importance and strength of these debates however, is best seen in terms of their relevance to research into nursing or midwifery.

Research into nursing or midwifery

These emerging fields of study exist in a hinterland between medicine and the social sciences and concern complex human experiences that are shaped by physical, biological, social, psychological and spiritual influences. By necessity, therefore, not all research into nursing or midwifery can be conducted within a single paradigm. In developing knowledge and understandings about practice, paradigms and methods are employed that necessarily are eclectic in nature. What is more important than partisan perspectives is attention to how techniques can be integrated to yield more powerful results using mixed-methods research. Although inevitably there are nurse or midwife researchers who are wedded to a particular paradigm, qualitative research methods are frequently used together with quantitative methods to act synergistically to gain deeper insights into particular phenomena, or to help generate questions for further research.

CASE STUDY

A crucial task for the nurse and midwife is to be able to undertake a critical evaluation of existing research to inform clinical reasoning and decision making (Polit and Beck, 2006). The following brief analytical questions identify the principal features of research studies that are essential to their balanced analysis:

- *Title*: is it a clear, concise definition of what the study is about and what it might contain?
- *Authors*: do they give a guide to a known level of expertise indicating the likely quality of the report?
- *Abstract*: does it provide a succinct summary of aims and objectives, methods used, findings and how these relate to wider understandings of the topic?
- *Introduction*: does it provide a plain statement of the problem with its significance for practice, feasible research questions and transparent definitions of the key concepts under investigation?

- *Literature review*: does it locate the problem within related current research, and in doing so provide a rationale for the study?
- *Study design*: how is the study linked to broader theoretical understandings?
- *Methods*: do the methods address the problem comprehensively through full descriptions of the procedures of sampling, instruments, ethical considerations, data collection and analysis?
- *Results*: are the results adequately supported by the data, and is their presentation coherent?
- *Discussion*: is the researcher's interpretation of the results logical, and what were the limitations of the study?
- *Conclusions*: what claims are made for the study, are they justifiable, and what are the implications of the work for practice and for further research?

CONCLUSIONS

Nursing and midwifery are evolving fields of intellectual and clinical activity and this chapter has sought to demonstrate insights into how they might assume their rightful scholarly-oriented roles as they emerge and as they increase their research capability and capacity.

FURTHER READING

Bowling, A. and Shah, E. (2005) *Handbook for Health Research Methods: Investigation, Measurement and Analysis*. Maidenhead: Open University Press.

Lincoln, Y.S. and Guber, E.G. (1985) *Naturalistic Inquiry*. Beverly Hills, CA: Sage.

Parahoo, K. (2006) *Nursing Research: Principles, Processes and Issues*. Basingstoke: Palgrave Macmillan.

Polit, D. and Beck, C. (2006) *Essentials of Nursing Research: Methods Appraisal and Utilisation*. Philadelphia, PA: Lippincott, Williams and Wilkins.

REFERENCES

Bowling, A. and Shah, E. (2005) *Handbook for Health Research Methods: Investigation, Measurement and Analysis*. Maidenhead: Open University Press.

Denzin, N.K. and Lincoln, Y.S. (eds) (1994) *Handbook of Qualitative Research*. London: Sage.

Hammersley, M. (ed.) (1993) *Social Research Philosophy, Politics and Practice*. London: Sage.

Hockey, L. (2000) 'Introduction to the research process', in D. Cormack (ed.), *The Research Process in Nursing*. Oxford: Blackwell Science.

researcher

Kuhn, T.S. (1962) *The Structure of Scientific Revolutions*, 2nd edn. Chicago, IL: University of Chicago Press.

Lincoln, Y.S. and Guber, E.G. (1985) *Naturalistic Inquiry*. Beverly Hills, CA: Sage.

Miles, M.B. and Huberman, A.M. (1994) *Qualitative Data Analysis: An Expanded Sourcebook*. Thousand Oaks, CA: Sage.

Nagel, E. (1961) *The Structure of Science*. New York: Harcourt Brace.

Newton, I. (1687) 'Rules for the study of natural philosophy', *Philosophiae Naturalis Principia Mathematica*, Book 3, The System of the World, 3rd edn: the four rules as reprinted on pages 794–6 of I. Bernard Cohen and Anne Whitman's 1999 translation. Berkaley, CA: University of California Press.

Parahoo, K. (2006) *Nursing Research: Principles, Processes and Issues.* Basingstoke: Palgrave Macmillan.

Peat, J., Mellis, C., Williams, K. and Xuan, W. (2002) *Health Science Research: A Handbook of Quantitative Methods.* London: Sage.

Polit, D, and Beck, C. (2006) *Essentials of Nursing Research: Methods Appraisal and Utilisation.* Philadelphia, PA: Lippincott, Williams and Wilkins.

Cross-References *Data, information, knowledge, Evidence-based practice, Professional development.*

---

44 Respect

Moyra A. Baldwin

DEFINITION

Respect is often spoken about by healthcare professionals as being an important concept for client care. In defining respect, it is clear that there is a relationship between one person and another. It is politeness, honour and care shown towards someone or something that is considered important (http://dictionary.cambridge.org). Respect here includes an aspect of the behaviour of one person towards another. It also relates to attitude. It is an attitude of acknowledging the feelings and interests of another party in a relationship. In similar terms, ethics literature identifies respect as a principle by which people are valued.

Browne's concept clarification generated a definition of respect that encompasses the above notions of behaviour and attitude. Respect is '... a basic moral principle and human right that is accountable to the values of human dignity, worthiness, uniqueness of persons and self-determination ... respect is conveyed through the unconditional acceptance, recognition and acknowledgement of the above values in persons' (1993: 283). Browne continued by stating that respect, a 'primary ethic of nursing', is demonstrated by our attitudes, thinking and behaviour towards people.

KEY POINTS

- Respect involves behaving towards others in a way that values their uniqueness and individuality.
- Respect is an ethic of care and an attitude that recognises individuals' dignity.
- Respect requires nurses' knowledge, attitudes and behaviour to be consistent with valuing individuals.

DISCUSSION

Where respect is discussed in the literature it is often used in the context of respect for persons and reference to Downie and Telfer's (1971) classic text. Tadd (1998) claims that respect (for persons) is an ethical principle of paramount importance to healthcare professionals. To explain respect it is useful to see how the term is used in relation to persons. This chapter will explore the concept of respect in terms of (a) respect for the individual person, and (b) respect in practice.

Respect for the individual person

Henry and Tuxill (1987) state that in everyday use the terms 'person' and 'human' are often used interchangeably but there is a distinction between the two. It is in the distinction that perhaps we can see the meaning of respect and how respect is practised. The term 'person', according to Henry and Tuxill (1987), includes an aspect of judgement, like the word 'good'. The term 'human', on the other hand, does not. So when the term person is used it is key in applying value and respect to individuals, such as patients or co-workers. In valuing and respecting

respect

279

people, each person is considered as an individual. Respecting individuality avoids depersonalisation. If we take Browne's (1993) definition and the idea of person by Henry and Tuxill (1987), respect can be seen to denote accepting people as they are, themselves, treating them with dignity and valuing their individuality. Respect is therefore about a person's experience. Experience that has respect at its heart will be one in which the person experiences the right to exist just as much as another person who has individual strengths and needs.

Exploring the meaning and value of caring in the context of the nurse–client relationship, Thomas et al. (2004) elicited six themes. Caring involved love, respect, trust, mutuality, spiritual expression and enhanced personhood. Their research involved seven pairs of nurse practitioners and their clients. Respect as an aspect of caring was noted by six nurse practitioners and their clients. The last theme, enhanced personhood, involved clients feeling that they were being cared for holistically. Caring was shown by those practitioners whose interpersonal skills enabled clients' wellbeing and personhood. Thus, respect and personhood are encompassed in person-centred caring.

It is possible to be in a position of caring for a patient whom we may not like. The professional carer will put aside both bias and prejudice to be able to care for the patient, whether the patient is liked by the professional or not. Respecting the patient, the professional carer will be considerate and treat the patient as an individual. The professional will be able to care for the patient by engaging in a therapeutic client–professional relationship which affirms the individual as a person. The professional will convey an attitude that shows genuine positive concern for the patient. Professional practice such as this is what respect is about. This is the approach demanded by the Nursing and Midwifery Council (NMC) in its Code of Professional Conduct (2004: clause 2). The NMC requires its registrants to respect clients as individuals. Respect is to be demonstrated by preserving patients' dignity unrestricted by their individual differences such as gender, age, race, abilities, sexuality, economic status, lifestyle, culture, religious or political beliefs.

Respect in practice

It is a necessary condition of professional practice (NMC, 2004) that the registrant respects patients or clients as individuals. To do so, it is essential that the nurse has the necessary knowledge, attitude and skills that underpin respect.

Knowledge   The NMC (2004) claims that respect encompasses respecting the role patients play as partners in care and their preferences regarding their contribution and management to their care. To practice respect means that professionals need to work within professional boundaries and the law. In these terms the practitioners need to be knowledgeable about what constitutes a therapeutic relationship, and they need to make themselves aware of the law pertaining to the healthcare specialty or client group as well as the law pertaining to the country of practice. A therapeutic relationship for a terminally ill older person might be one that values and respects that individual's desire to stay in his own home despite the fact that professional carers believe that moving into a healthcare institution would be beneficial. One aspect of the law here would include consideration of the Mental Capacity Act (MCA) (DoH, 2005) so that professionals can be assured that the client has the capacity to make the necessary decision. Where capacity is impaired, respect can still be realised as knowledge of the MCA is applied. Because the patient lacks the capacity to make a complex decision it does not mean that the patient is unable to make less onerous, straightforward decisions.

Attitude   Respect is about affirmation, an ethic of care and attitude that recognises individuals' dignity. The professional can demonstrate these qualities by believing the client has the capacity to problem-solve and make decisions. Demonstrating respect for individuals relates to the ethics principle of autonomy (Downie and Calman, 1994). Conveying acceptance and a non-judgemental attitude will enable a patient to feel valued and respected, and will facilitate autonomy. Respect will be realised when professionals accept that people have the right to make decisions which may appear eccentric or even unwise (DoH, 2005). Demonstrating an attitude that respects the individual may involve the professional acting as the patient's advocate. This is especially important where the patient is capable of understanding and making a decision but unable to be understood because of communication difficulties. Respect demands that efforts are made to understand the patient by exploring issues that are relevant to the patient.

Walsh and Kowanko (2002), in studying the perceptions of dignity among nurses and patients, found that showing respect was one aspect. From the patients' perspective, dignity involved being 'seen as a person'. Similarly, dignity involved 'seeing the patient as a person' for nurses. As an aspect of and related to dignity, respect involves an attitude which preserves patients' individuality and personhood.

The healthcare professional who is sensitive and caring towards a person who undergoes a termination of pregnancy despite the professional's conscientious objection to abortion will be showing respect in practice. An attitude of understanding the patient being nursed in a prison setting, while challenging, will demonstrate respect when the carer can set aside prejudice and offer the incarcerated patient care, compassion and consideration. The patients being cared for in these circumstances will have respect shown to them by professionals whose attitude shows due regard to them as individuals and their feelings. To practise respect we have seen that knowledge and attitude are important. Additional requirements are the essential skills of communication.

Skills   In a healthcare professional's repertoire of skills there will be skills of verbal and non-verbal communication. Non-verbal communication can convey respect. The mere 'presence', 'being there' for the patient, and listening to the patient, shows respect. The Department of Health's survey of 'dignity in care' reports that for one respondent dignity 'is about respect ... It is about listening to patients and valuing them' (DoH, 2006: 5).

A client–professional relationship is a contract between the parties with the obligation of adhering to veracity. Beauchamp and Childress (2001) suggested that there are arguments for truth telling in the client–professional relationship. These are:

• In respecting others we express veracity by means of autonomy.
• Autonomy is based on disclosure and consent.
• Relationships depend on trust. Such trust is embedded in a reliance on and confidence in others to respect veracity.

The patient gains the right to truth telling with regard to diagnosis and procedures, while at the same time professionals gain the right to truthful disclosure from patients. When we communicate with others there is an implication that we will communicate truthfully. Respecting the patient means that we will not lie or misrepresent opinions, nor will we engage in deception. Veracity derives from respect for autonomy and fidelity. We communicate respect verbally by truth telling. In telling the truth, healthcare professionals demonstrate respect for others by means of respecting their autonomy. Autonomy is the basis of the rules of disclosure and consent. Patients cannot exercise autonomy unless the consent they give is informed. Such consent therefore depends on truthful communication. Indeed, according to Seedhouse (1988), knowing the truth enhances personal liberty because it involves autonomy. Respect for the person is implied in truth telling. Therefore, veracity is a principle to which professionals need to adhere if they are to show respect to and for people. A therapeutic caring relationship is one of partnership between health professionals and the patient. It is based on trust, and to facilitate respect communication needs to be open and honest. Respect for autonomy is advised by adhering to veracity; the sharing of truthful information about diagnosis and care with the patient will be enhanced by combining the verbal with the non-verbal skills of communication. The skilful use of verbal and non-verbal communication can convey respect.

CASE STUDY

Mrs Eleanor Norridge, a 68-year-old lady, was self-conscious of her visibly shaky hands and excessive saliva. These were symptoms of the Parkinson's disease that she had coped with for several years. She was admitted to a surgical ward to undergo surgery that was not related to her long-term illness. She confided in James, the ward nurse, that she was very embarrassed because of her 'dribbling' when she ate and that she wanted to sit on her bed, behind bed curtains, to eat her meals. James was concerned that Mrs Norridge might become isolated and worked with her to decide how best to accommodate her needs. Finding out how she usually coped at home, James and Mrs Norridge agreed that at mealtimes Mrs Norridge would have a napkin to protect her clothes, which would also reduce the amount of washing for her family. James ensured that the ward staff filled cups and glasses to only half full as Mrs Norridge usually used a heavy cup or glass for drinks, never filling these to the brim. As Mrs Norridge's bed was close to the ward's interview room, James negotiated that, when vacant, the room could be available for her to eat her meals. Staff were reminded to prepare the room for Mrs Norridge at mealtimes, when this was possible. James also gained permission to speak with his colleagues regarding reviewing Mrs Norridge's medication.

James's knowledge, attitudes and behaviour were consistent, respecting clients as individuals, by valuing Mrs Norridge as an individual. He showed respect in the way he preserved her dignity irrespective of her disability, valuing her individual needs. A therapeutic client–professional relationship of partnership existed between them.

CONCLUSION

Respect is a concept that we all wish to acquire from others and understand fully when we do not receive it. In this chapter, respect for the individual has been discussed in relation to caring for patients and respect for ourselves as professional nurses. Without respect for each other we are very much alone in a difficult sphere of both personal and professional operations.

FURTHER READING

Burnard, P. and Chapman, C. (2004) *Professional and Ethical Issues in Nursing*, 3rd edn. Edinburgh: Baillière Tindall.

Downie, R.S. and Calman, K.C. (1994) *Healthy Respect: Ethics in Healthcare*. Oxford: Oxford University Press.

Downie, R.S. and Telfer, E. (1971) *Respect for Persons: A Philosophical Analysis of the Moral, Political and Religious Idea of the Supreme Worth of the Individual Person*. London: Allen & Unwin.

REFERENCES

Beauchamp, T.L. and Childress, J.F. (2001) *Principles of Biomedical Ethics*, 5th edn. Oxford: Oxford University Press.

Browne, A. (1993) 'A conceptual clarification of respect'. *Journal of Advanced Nursing*, 18: 211–7.

Cambridge Dictionary (2006) Available online at http://dictionary.cambridge.org (accessed 27 Nov. 2006).

Department of Health (2005) *The Mental Capacity Act*. London: DoH.

Department of Health (2006) *Dignity in Care: Public Survey, October 2006. Report of the Survey*. London: DoH.

Downie, R.S. and Calman, K.C. (1994) *Healthy Respect: Ethics in Healthcare*. Oxford: Oxford University Press.

Downie, R.S. and Telfer, E. (1971) *Respect for Persons: A Philosophical Analysis of the Moral, Political and Religious Idea of the Supreme Worth of the Individual Person*. London: Allen & Unwin.

Henry, C. and Tuxill, A.C. (1987) 'Concept of the person: an introduction to the health professionals' curriculum'. *Journal of Advanced Nursing*, 12(2): 245–9.

Nursing and Midwifery Council (2004) *The NMC Code of Professional Conduct: Standards for Conduct, Performance and Ethics*. London: NMC.

Seedhouse, D. (1988) *Ethics: The Heart of Healthcare.* Chichester: John Wiley.

Tadd, G.V. (1998) *Ethics and Values for Care Workers.* Oxford: Blackwell Science.

Thomas, J.D., Finch, L.P., Schoenhofer, S.O. and Green, A. (2004) 'The caring relationships created by nurse practitioners and the ones nursed: implications for practice'. *Topics in Advanced Practice Nursing,* 4(4): 6–10.

Walsh, K. and Kowanko, I. (2002) 'Nurses' and patients' perceptions of dignity'. *International Journal of Nursing Practice,* 8: 143–51.

Cross-References *Advocacy, Autonomy, Caring, Compassion, Dignity, Problem solving.*

45 Risk management

Bob Heyman

DEFINITION

Risk assessment and management provide one means of attempting 'colonization of the future' (Giddens, 1991: 111) for individuals managing their own lives, and for professional carers. Defining risk management requires consideration of 'risk' and 'risk manager'.

Definitions of risk

The Royal Society depicts risk as 'the probability that a particular adverse event occurs during a stated time period, or results from a particular challenge' (1992: 1). This definition identifies four key risks elements: events, probabilities, adversity and a timeframe. It represents risks as naturally occurring phenomena, like heart attacks or epidemics, which exist independently of the observer. A contrasting perspective views risk propositions as statements of an observer's beliefs about and attitudes towards the future. Rosa defines risk as 'a situation or event where something of human value ... is at stake and where the outcome is uncertain' (2003: 57). This definition reframes adversity as value and probability as uncertainty. It does not cover timeframing, and takes for granted the existence of 'situations or events'. A formulation that covers all four of these elements defines risk as 'the projection onto the external world of uncertainty about the occurrence of a negatively valued event category within a selected time frame' (Heyman et al., in press). The definition of risks as 'projections' indicates that their origins in uncertainty can be lost sight of. In so far as they are accepted by the wider society as requiring management, risks become reified 'virtual objects' (Van Loon, 2002: 45). Although less pithy than the Royal Society definition, our alternative offers a more complex understanding of risk in which the observer plays a central role, as shown in Table 4 (Heyman, 2005).

Table 4   *Two views of risk elements (Heyman, 2005)*

Risk viewed as referencing natural phenomena	Risk viewed as referencing knowledge
Event	Category
Adversity	Values
Externally defined timescale	Timeframe
Probability	Expectation

This reframing does not matter much if stakeholders agree in their views about a risk, for example, that the overriding aim of care should be to minimise a child's risk of dying from cancer. However, service users may view their future differently, as, for instance, in the case of a frail elderly cancer patient who feels ready to die. Effective communication and willingness to try to appreciate the perspectives of others then become crucial to good risk management.

Definitions of risk manager

A useful distinction can be drawn between three categories of risk managers:

- A new occupational category of risk management specialists, including the UK National Patient Safety Agency and risk managers employed by NHS Trusts and other large organisations.
- Clinical professionals held accountable for risk management, particularly in retrospect when adverse events occur.
- Service users and carers concerned about the personal impact of specific risks on their own lives.

Constructive scepticism about the value of risk specialists (Power, 2005) should be maintained until their value is demonstrated. Reframing risk to include the active interpretive role of risk managers, broadly defined, brings service users and their carers to centre stage. Risk management theory in the field of business studies stresses the importance of clearly defining risk ownership (Chadbourne, 1999). However, in healthcare, risk ownership needs to be shared, and is frequently contested. For example, health professionals sometimes assume that they manage risks on behalf of their patients, whilst patients and carers may see themselves as the 'primary producers of their own health' (Stacey, 1976). Consensus about what risks should be prioritised – for example, litigation, mortality, quality of life – should not be assumed. Skilled risk management requires recognition of variability in risk perspective. Differences in social power, for instance between patients and service providers, will inevitably influence both the selection of risks as objects of concern and how they are managed, undermining official rhetoric about patient 'empowerment'.

The concept of health risk manager should encompass all three categories, namely risk specialists, clinical specialists and service users/carers, all of whom attempt to 'colonise the future'. These risk managers operate at the boundaries of current knowledge, between possessing the power to predict accurately, which removes uncertainty, and total ignorance. In these 'debatable lands', scientific claims to be able to predict and control the future, for example in relation to drug safety, are frequently contested, making risk management problematic.

KEY POINTS

- Health risk management can be directed towards the population, corporate, service and individual levels.
- Risk management requires trade-offs between safety and autonomy.
- Healthcare systems often develop a care ecology providing different balances of safety and autonomy.

DISCUSSION

Risk management contexts

Health risk management has received less research attention than has health risk assessment. The latter sometimes involves an organisational ritual rather than a process designed to benefit patients (Titterton, 2005: 88).

The diversity of contexts in which health risk management is attempted makes any kind of overview difficult. It may operate at four levels:

- Public health.
- Corporate sustainability, through clinical governance systems designed to detect and minimise clinical errors.
- The clinical environment.
- Clinical decision making involving individual patients.

Risk management issues associated with these four co-existing levels have distinctive characteristics, making generalised analysis of risk management problematic. For example, the operation of screening systems in health and social care can shift the focus of clinical attention from individuals to population risk indicators (Castel, 1991). Moreover, analysis at these levels will sometimes lead in contradictory directions. For instance, the inexorably rising rate of births by caesarean section above the rate recommended by the World Health Organization may result from consultants attempting to reduce the risk of litigation if a vaginal birth goes wrong (Habiba et al., 2006).

The safety v. autonomy dilemma

If safety and autonomy are defined broadly enough, tension between them can be seen to underlie any risk management problem which doesn't have a clear solution, such as a cure with minimal side effects. Pregnant women may, at one pole of the autonomy/safety dimension, give birth at home or, at the other, in a hospital environment catering for high-risk cases (Kirkham, 1989). Adults with learning disabilities living at home may be given a metaphorical passport allowing them to move freely about their locality, or may be supervised by carers on grounds of safety (Heyman and Davies, 2006). Frail older people may risk accidents and falls if they continue to live at home, or may be physically well looked after but lose control of their lives in an institution (Reed, 1998). Discharge of offenders with mental health problems from secure provision gives rise to the risk that they may reoffend, but ends their confinement (Heyman et al., 2004).

This initial analysis of the safety v. autonomy risk management dilemma needs to be qualified in two ways. First, the presumed safety of more controlling interventions such as caesarean sections, closely monitored hospital births and residential care for older people is and should be questioned. Risk managers balance safety with autonomy in relation to their beliefs about risks. Second, the more intense interference associated with interventions designed to maximise safety creates new iatrogenic risks. For example, institutionalised older people may lose the will to live (Reed, 1998). The birth process may be adversely affected by the stress associated with monitoring designed, ironically, to reduce risk (Lane, 1995; Mansfield, 1988).

Three implications of the safety v. autonomy dilemma for health risk management will be outlined. First, no single optimum solution to a dilemma is available. Decisions which enhance autonomy tend to limit safety and vice versa. A safety first attitude will not take account of the reasons why people want to take risks in the first place. This attitude needs to be replaced by a risk taking approach (Titterton, 2005: 15) which recognises that risks should sometimes be accepted. Such an approach can help service users to make informed choices based on systematic risk assessment and good communication. Moreover, skilled interventions, for example nurses imparting self-care skills to vulnerable patients before discharge, can to some degree change the terms of the dilemma, allowing a higher degree of autonomy to be achieved at the same level of safety.

Second, managing the safety v. autonomy dilemma can be facilitated by increasing the care options. For example, older people can be offered different levels of home support, or offenders with mental health problems can receive varying levels of supervision after discharge. Emergent care systems, often unplanned, can develop their own dynamics, some of which can be understood in terms of the metaphor of the health risk escalator (Heyman, 2005). For example, Lane (1995) discusses 'cascades of intervention' whereby a woman whose pregnancy is causing concern is monitored, responds with stress which gives rise to more intense monitoring and so on until a full-blown crisis triggers a caesarean section. Conversely, a downward risk escalator can carry the individual, not necessarily appropriately, towards autonomy as success in an environment involving higher degrees of monitoring is rewarded by progression to less and less constrained environments.

Third, adoption of a risk-taking approach requires a more reflective organisational and societal attitude towards the occurrence of adverse (negatively valued) events. In law, a professional risk manager cannot be held accountable if they can show that they accepted a 'reasonable' risk.

However, judgements about risk are heavily influenced by the 'hindsight effect'. Research (for example, Mitchell and Kalb, 1981) suggests that observers are swayed by knowledge of actual outcomes more than they realise. Powerful social forces work against adoption of a 'reasonable risk' approach to health risk management. Risk has become a 'forensic resource' (Douglas, 1990), a substitute for religious cosmology, which modern societies use to apportion blame and maintain a sense of control of the future. Fear of litigation gives organisations and professionals incentives to intervene, and lends itself to the emergence of blame cultures.

CASE STUDY

Jenny,[*] a single, self-employed mother in her forties bringing up a teenage son, has been diagnosed with early-stage anal cancer. Immediate surgery is indicated, and her consultant estimates that she has a 90 per cent chance of surviving the cancer for at least five years, but will need to rely on a colostomy bag for several months, with a 50 per cent probability that the bag will be required for the rest of her life. A colorectal nurse talks to Jenny a week after she has spoken to the consultant. Jenny accepts that she will need surgery. She shows little concern about her mortality risk, but discusses a number of issues which trouble her. She has always considered herself 'healthy', and is struggling to accept her changed health status. Jenny reports some guilt about past intolerance of an acquaintance who also relied on a colostomy bag. She is particularly worried about the implications of its use for her relationship with a new partner and wants to frankly discuss the implications for her sexual attractiveness. Jenny accepts having to rely on a colostomy bag for some months, but would hate to have to wear one permanently. However, she is confused about what the 50 per cent probability mentioned by the consultant actually refers to. She is concerned that her relationship with her adolescent son will be damaged, and that he will be unable to cope with the transition in his mother from provider to a person who needs support. Finally, she is worried about losing her customer base whilst unable to work as she is self-employed.

This example illustrates a number of the issues which come into health risk management. The clinical risks indicate that immediate

[*] I am indebted to Tony McGrath, Senior Lecturer in Colorectal Nursing at St Bartholomew School of Nursing and Midwifery, City University, for suppling the information on which this case study is based.

surgery is required. However, the decision to opt for safety raises a number of issues of importance to this patient which clinicians might not fully anticipate. She has not understood the quantitative risk information presented to her quickly in a distressing consultation. Skilled nursing communication based on good collaboration with the consultant could help this patient to fully understand the direct clinical risks which she faces, and also to work through the wider consequences for her self-concept and relationships with others.

CONCLUSION

Risk management is a specialist area of modern day healthcare in which professional clinicians are held accountable for their practice. This focuses on service users' needs and their own perceptions of what their healthcare needs are. Risk management can be aimed at individuals, services, organisations and populations. However, risk management often requires a trade-off between safety issues and a person's autonomy.

FURTHER READING

Berry, D.C. (2004) *Risk, Communication and Health Psychology*. Maidenhead: Open University Press.
Gigerenzer, G. (2003) *Reckoning with Risk: Learning to Live with Uncertainty*. London: Penguin.
Godin, P. (ed.) (2006) *Risk and Nursing Practice*. Basingstoke: Palgrave.
Titterton, M. (2005) *Risk and Risk Taking in Health and Social Welfare*. London: Jessica Kingsley.

REFERENCES

Castel, R. (1991) 'From dangerousness to risk', in G. Burchell, C. Gordon and P. Miller (eds), *The Foucault Effect*. London: Harvester Wheatsheaf.
Chadbourne, B.C. (1999) 'To the heart of risk management: teaching project teams to combat risk', Proceedings of the 30th Annual Project Management Institute 1999 Seminars & Symposium. Philadelphia, PA: Project Management Institute.
Douglas, M. (1990) 'Risk as a forensic resource'. *Daedalus*, 119: 1–16.
Giddens, A. (1991) *Modernity and Self-Identity: Self and Politics in the Late Modern Age*. Oxford: Polity Press.
Habiba, M., Kaminski, M., Da Fre, M., Marsal, K., Bleker, O., Librero, J., Grandjean, H., Gratia, P., Guaschino, S., Heyl, W., Taylor, D. and Cuttini, M. (2006) 'Caesarean section on request: a comparison of obstetricians' attitudes in eight European countries'. *BJOG: An International Journal of Obstetrics & Gynaecology*, 113: 647–56.

Heyman, B. (2005) 'Health risk escalators', in R. Bibace, J. Laird and J. Valsiner (eds), *Science and Medicine in Dialogue: Thinking Through Particulars and Universals*. Westport, CT: Greenwood.

Heyman, B. and Davies, J. (2006) 'The tension between autonomy and safety in nursing adults with learning disabilities', in P. Godin (ed.), *Risk and Nursing Practice*. Basingstoke: Palgrave.

Heyman, B., Alaszewski, A. and Shaw, M. (in press) *Risk, Safety and Clinical Practice*. Oxford: Oxford University Press.

Heyman, B., Shaw, M.P., Davies, J.P., Godin, P.M. and Reynolds, R. (2004) 'Forensic mental health services as a health risk escalator: a case study of ideals and practice', in B. Heyman (ed.), Special Edition on Risk and Mental Health, *Health, Risk & Society*, 6: 307–25.

Kirkham, M. (1989) 'Midwives and information-giving during labour', in S. Robinson and A.M. Thomson (eds), *Midwives Research and Childbirth*, vol. 1. London: Chapman & Hall.

Lane, K. (1995) 'The medical model of the body as a site of risk: a case study of childbirth', in G. Gabe (ed.), *Medicine, Health and Risk: Sociological Approaches*. Oxford: Blackwell.

Mansfield, P.K. (1988) 'Midlife childbearing: strategies for informed decision making'. *Psychology of Women Quarterly*, 12: 445–60.

Mitchell, T.R. and Kalb, L.S. (1981) 'Effects of outcome knowledge and outcome valence on supervisors' evaluations'. *Journal of Applied Psychology*, 66: 604–12.

Power, M. (2005) 'Organizational responses to risk: the rise of the chief risk officer', in B. Hutter and M. Power (eds), *Organisational Encounters with Risk*. Cambridge: Cambridge University Press.

Reed, J. (1998) 'Care and protection for older people', in B. Heyman (ed.), *Risk, Health and Health care: A Qualitative Approach*. London: Edward Arnold.

Rosa, E.A. (2003) 'The logical structure of the social amplification of risk framework (SARF): metatheoretical foundations and policy implications', in N. Pigeon, R.E. Kasperson and P. Slovik (eds), *The Social Amplification of Risk*. Cambridge: Cambridge University Press.

Royal Society, The (1992) *Risk: Analysis, Perception and Management: Report of a Royal Society Study Group*. London: The Royal Society.

Stacey, M. (1976) 'The health service consumer: a sociological misconception', in M. Stacey (ed.), *The Sociology of the National Health Service, Sociological Review Monographs*, 22. Staffordshire: University of Keele.

Titterton, M. (2005) *Risk and Risk Taking in Health and Social Welfare*. London: Jessica Kingsley.

Van Loon, J. (2002) *Risk and Technological Culture: Towards a Sociology of Virulence*. London: Routledge.

Cross-References Assessment, Caring, Clinical governance, Compassion, Competence, Holistic care, Nurturing, Problem solving, Teamwork, User involvement.

46 Role model

Dianne Phipps

DEFINITION

A simple definition from the *Oxford English Dictionary* suggests that a role model is 'a person looked to by others as an example to be imitated' (www.askoxford.com). However, this simple definition, when applied to nursing, does not do justice to the concept. Taken literally, this definition could mean that a nurse seen as a role model, and as such as someone that could be emulated by those aspiring to that position or profession, need only be copied in behaviour to achieve that title.

To be a role model as a nurse is to be much more than someone whose behaviour is copied. The Nursing and Midwifery Council (NMC) (2004) identify standards for conduct, performance and ethics for nursing including respect, obtaining consent before giving any care/treatment, confidentiality, co-operation with team members, maintenance of professional knowledge and competence, being trustworthy and minimising risks. This is the code that all nurses work to and some standards, such as being trustworthy, are less tangible, although just as important as others. It is all these skills, attributes, competencies and qualities that are considered by the observer when thinking of a nurse as a role model.

KEY POINTS

- Being a role model as a nurse brings its own responsibilities and rewards as well as stresses.
- Nurses as role models are more than people whose behaviour is copied.
- Expectations of skills possessed by nurses will differ between individuals, professionals, organisations and society.

DISCUSSION

Learning by watching and then modelling your own behaviour on that which is seen and respected (observational learning) has been well researched and reported (Bandura et al., 1961; Weiss et al., 1998). We do not necessarily have to experience the behaviour to know what the possible outcome or effect upon others may be if we have witnessed another performing the action. For example, if we see someone touch a hot surface, we don't necessarily have to touch the surface ourselves to know how it will feel (Bernstein et al., 2000). Both animals and humans learn in this way, as reports of young chimpanzees learning how to crack open nuts by watching their mothers doing the action proves (Bernstein et al., 2000).

Nurse education has embraced the concept of observational learning by enabling students to observe skills in the classroom from a lecturer demonstrating those skills before consolidating their learning and skills practice with people receiving healthcare (Wilford and Doyle, 2006). In this instance the nurse lecturer is a role model for the learners. When thinking of nurses being role models, we may consider others emulating their behaviour, those attributes which are seen as being desirable, skilful or caring. This may well be assisted by observing an 'expert' who is acting as our mentor (English, 1993). Student nurses are allocated a mentor to work alongside them in practice to act as a teacher and role model (Pellatt, 2006). As a nurse, the professional is guided by the NMC, which states that individuals who support learning and assessment in practice should 'act as a role model for safe and effective practice' (NMC, 2006). However, no guidance or definition of role model is given, so just what do people look for in a role model and how can the individual nurse live up to those expectations?

With regard to other professions, it is interesting to note that, in a study researching the characteristics that medical students think a role model, for them, should possess, the following were identified: 'excellent role models are mainly perceived to be those who exhibit personal characteristics such as dedication, honesty/integrity, respect and recognition of patients, their families and others, teaching ability and clinical skills' (Elzubeir and Rizk, 2001: 273).

As mentors, teachers and nurses, we need to be aware of what other people regard as beneficial characteristics. Studies of nursing attributes as described by the individual nurses themselves have delivered similar results, albeit that within differing specialisms, qualities and attributes of the 'good nurse' may differ somewhat. Zhang et al. (2001) studied competencies of fifty female nurses in China, who were asked to reflect on two critical incidents. From this, the researchers identified the most frequent competencies reported by the participants. These were:

- Interpersonal understanding
- Commitment
- Informational gathering
- Thoroughness
- Persuasiveness
- Compassion
- Comforting
- Critical thinking
- Self-control
- Responsiveness

These competencies or attributes that were self-reported by the nurses could be seen as indicators of a good role model.

Are these the same competencies that the recipients of our care want us to demonstrate? Again, this will depend upon the individual themselves, and the support they need to receive. For instance, the characteristics of a 'good nurse' may differ depending on whether the individual is having an acute episode of illness or needs to be supported to maintain their community residence. Attree (2001) interviewed forty-three acute medical patients and seven relatives about their experiences and perspectives of 'good' and 'not so good' care. The participants of the study highlighted the following issues that, for them, denoted 'good' care:

- Patient-focused
- Involves patients
- Acknowledges patients
- Individualised, holistic
- Related to need
- Needs anticipated
- Help offered willingly
- Close, sociable relationship
- Patients known as people
- Develops bond/rapport
- Open communication and information passage
- Demonstrates kindness, concern, compassion and sensitivity
- Available and accessible to patients
- Takes and spends time
- Feeling cared for and about

Other studies highlight similar findings, with communication and listening being seen as particularly important, and for some users of services (people with learning disabilities, children and disabled adults) respect was seen as a key competence (Rush and Cook, 2006).

Some nurses, whilst recognising and agreeing that they are perceived as a role model by and for others, also find it difficult to adapt certain behaviours, for example, smoking cessation (Strobl and Latter, 1998). This behaviour is not seen as being that of a good role model: '... the slightly ironic sight of a uniformed health professional with a cigarette in their hand' (Furniss, 2006: 510).

So, nurses are expected to be exemplary in thought and deed, to be a role model, both during work and in their leisure time. Nurses are in an excellent position to support students, educate users of services, the general public, other professionals and relatives simply by being themselves, doing their job and caring. However, it is true that a nurse is never 'off duty', and their actions and words are watched and listened to by all. This can be a possible source of stress for the individual, particularly if working in comparative isolation, with a new team, or when undergoing times of personal/professional difficulties.

CASE STUDY

Graham is a Home Leader for a new service, which offers 24-hour nursing care to people with complex learning disabilities. The house is registered as a nursing home and, as such, requires a qualified nurse to be on duty 24-hours a day, although at night this is achieved by means of a 'sleep over' system. Graham has been involved in recruiting staff to work in the service and feels that he has a good mix of experienced older and inexperienced younger staff. He is also a great believer in teamworking, and arranges teambuilding days supported by occasional social nights out. As a registered nurse, Graham always works alone as the only qualified nurse on duty, backed by a larger team of support staff.

Graham is aware that he is seen as a role model for these staff in what he does, how he does it, what he says and how he says it, for the duration of his shift, during teambuilding events and social activities. He is also aware of his position as a role model when supporting the people who live in the house to access community facilities, for members of the general public as well as to other professionals who visit the house or support individuals during interventions or activities.

Graham and the rest of the registered nurses working in the house have arranged to attend monthly clinical supervision sessions, supported by their employing organisation. They have found that these sessions have been most useful in discussing instances in a 'safe place' with their supervisor, and receiving feedback on their practice as a nurse, as a promoter of independence and inclusion for the people who live in the service.

CONCLUSION

To be a nurse is to be a role model who must be aware of his or her own expectations of what this means. The professional body to which the nurse belongs expects that person to be a role model and to mentor students. During clinical practice, the nurse will be demonstrating skills, attitudes and qualities to students and peers/team members. As always, the person in receipt of care is central to the nurse's purpose, and as such has his or her own expectations of 'good nursing'. Relatives too expect the nurse to display certain attributes of caring towards their loved one. As an inter-professional worker, the nurse may be a role model for other professionals and, in the public arena which he or she practices in, is looked to by society for guidance. Support systems may be sought and utilised by the nurse to enable them to embrace their status as a role model.

FURTHER READING

Pellatt, G.C. (2006) 'The role of mentors in supporting pre-registration nursing students'. *British Journal of Nursing*, 15(6): 336–40.
Rush, P. and Cook, J. (2006) 'What makes a good nurse? Views of patients and carers'. *British Journal of Nursing*, 15(7): 382–5.

REFERENCES

Attree, M. (2001) 'Patients' and relatives' experiences and perspectives of 'Good' and 'Not so Good' quality of care'. *Journal of Advanced Nursing*, 33(4), 456–466.
Bandura, A., Ross, D. and Ross, S.A. (1961) 'Transmission of aggression through imitation of aggressive models'. *Journal of Abnormal Social Psychology*, 63: 525–82.
Bernstein, D.A., Clarke-Stewart, A., Penner, L.A., Roy, E.J. and Wickens, C.D. (2000) *Psychology*, 5th edn. Boston, MD: Houghton Mifflin.
Elzubeir, M.A. and Rizk, D.E.E. (2001) 'Identifying characteristics that students, interns and residents look for in their role models'. *Medical Education*, 35(3): 272–7.
English, I. (1993) 'Intuition as a function of the expert nurse: a critique of Benner's novice to expert model'. *Journal of Advanced Nursing*, 18: 387–93.
Furniss, L. (2006) 'Just nipping outside for a quick smoke'. *British Journal of Cardiac Nursing*, 1(11): 508–9.
Nursing and Midwifery Council (2004) *The NMC Code of Professional Conduct: Standards for Conduct, Performance and Ethics*. London: NMC.

Nursing and Midwifery Council (2006) *Standards to Support Learning and Assessment in Practice: NMC standards for mentors, practice teachers and teachers*. London: NMC.

Oxford English Dictionary, available online at www.askoxford.edu (accessed 15 Nov. 2006).

Pellatt, G.C. (2006) 'The role of mentors in supporting pre-registration nursing students'. *British Journal of Nursing*, 15(6): 336–40.

Rush, P. and Cook, J. (2006) 'What makes a good nurse? Views of patients and carers'. *British Journal of Nursing*, 15(7): 382–5.

Strobl, J. and Latter, S. (1998) 'Qualified nurse smokers' attitudes towards a hospital smoking ban and its influence on their smoking behaviour'. *Journal of Advanced Nursing*, 27(1): 179–88.

Weiss, M.R., McCullagh, P., Smith, A.L. and Berlant, A.R. (1998) 'Observational learning and the fearful child: influence of peer models on swimming skill performance and psychological responses'. *Research Quarterly for Exercise and Sport*, 69(4): 380–94.

Wilford, A. and Doyle, T.J. (2006) 'Integrating simulation training into the nursing curriculum'. *British Journal of Nursing*, 6(15): 604–7.

Zhang, Z., Luk, W., Arthur, D. and Wong, T. (2001) 'Nursing competencies: personal characteristics contributing to effective nursing performance'. *Journal of Advanced Nursing*, 33(4): 457–74.

Cross-References *Accountability, Caring, Compassion, Dignity, Educator, Leadership, Manager, Respect, Sense of humour, Teamwork, Value.*

47 Sense of humour

John Struthers

DEFINITION

Hyrkas's concept analysis on humour includes a succinct definition of a sense of humour:

A sense of humour consists of: humour production, comprehension, humour appreciation and humour attitude. In other words, a sense of humour includes recognition of oneself as humorous, recognition of others' humour, a propensity to laugh and a perspective that allows an appreciation of life's absurdities. It incorporates a general attitude of playfulness and a coinciding ability to play on ideas. (2005: 216).

The ability to perceive humour is dependant on a person's cognitive ability. A person's sense of humour is an accumulation of many interrelated factors. These factors include their gender, geographical location, personality disposition, upbringing, culture, education, life experiences and maturity. The amalgam of all these variables creates a person's view of the world, through which they create a frame of reference for interpreting events. As each person's world view is unique to them, no humour can have a guarantee that it will be received in the same vein it was sent.

KEY POINTS

- A sense of humour is unique to each person.
- The use of humour can be both beneficial and harmful depending on how it is sent and received.
- A sense of humour is a valuable acquisition in delivering healthcare.

DISCUSSION

A person's sense of humour relies on their personality traits and cognitive schema to utilise their executive functions of the brain to problem solve the sending and receiving of humour. Humour requires the 'ability to detect the incongruity between the joke stem and punch line followed by resolution of the incongruity by establishing coherence of the punch line with the joke' (Ward, 2006: 305). Apologies for the amount of concentration required to understand the preceding quote, but it illustrates the complexity of investigating humour. Humour disappears when placed under the microscope of investigation, as spontaneity is lost. Such difficulties underpin exploration of this key concept. Humour's abstract nature makes it difficult to capture its essence. Although key ingredients of a good sense of humour may be identified, the question as to whether they can be taught so they become integrated into a healthcare worker's rapport is not without difficulty. Struthers (1999), when researching community mental health nurses' use of humour with clients, identified the problem of too much analysis leading to paralysis. The precise moment for the injection of humour can be lost if too much time is spent on deciding if the humour is appropriate.

Winbolt (2002) cautions against using contrived humour, as the results may be disastrous.

Various explanations of humour have been written as far back as 340 BC by Plato and Aristotle (Ferguson and Campinha-Bacote, 1989). A good 'sense of humour' was thought to be derived from the four body fluids of choler, melancholy, blood and phlegm being in balance. Although investigations into use of humour has developed from the aquatic nature of body fluids, the notion that your sense of humour impacts on your communication style from which others form an opinion of you has not changed. This factor is of concern when communication forms the basis of so much healthcare.

Dobson (2006) provides a useful description of four categories of how a person may demonstrate their sense of humour. The labels given to these types of humour are reasonably self-explanatory and are used here only as convenient headings to shape the discussion.

Put-down humour

This type of humour is usually aggressive and can be used to criticise and manipulate others. The put downs are usually done through the use of sarcasm, ridicule or teasing. Such use of humour in this form can be described as a socially acceptable form of aggression. Research into teasing (Tragesser and Lippman, 2005) in psychology students in America indicates that its use may not be all negative. Subjects valued a 'solidarity' function of teasing humour within groups. However, the findings of the research concluded that the use of teasing as a means of expressing 'superiority' was more common.

Bonding humour

People whose sense of humour enables them to use bonding humour can create happiness and fun within a group. Their use of jokes, witticisms and ability to create humorous quips can break the ice and lighten the mood. Such people also feel comfortable about being humorous about their own shortcomings. Where 'mistakes' happen in performance, such as the nurse accidentally spilling the client's blackcurrant drink on the ward floor then perhaps commenting, 'Thank goodness it wasn't on my carpet'. In this situation 'We see beyond the mask of cool professionalism to the ordinary individual behind' (Giddens, 2001: 91). Taylor (1994) detailed the value of being 'ordinary' within practice nursing, providing patient accounts of the value of a sense of humour in interactions. Similarly, the use of humour has been considered within education.

'Hate me' humour

Overuse of 'hate me' humour should carry a health warning. The person using such an approach centres themselves as the butt of the joke. A sprinkling of this sense of humour can assist in integration. However, 'hate me' humour, if used excessively, can reflect and create low self-esteem, low mood and reduced feelings of self-worth. The use of humour to create continual self-put-downs may be representative of insecurities in a person's 'life script' stemming from earlier experiences (Joines and Stewart, 2002). However, isolation rather than integration may result due to the unease felt by others.

Laughing at life

Dobson describes this sense of humour as someone who doesn't take him/herself too seriously. 'Someone with this outlook deploys humour to cope with challenges, taking a step back and laughing at the absurdities of everyday life' (2006: 76).

Healthcare workers by the nature of their work come into contact with life-changing and life-threatening conditions. The breaking of 'bad news' to a person about their condition will have significant impact on their mood and sense of humour. However, through time their sense of humour may evolve to encompass the beneficial aspect of humour in association with their current health state. A sense of distance between oneself and the issue is reinforced when it can be considered in a humorous manner (Hargie, 2000). Effective listening is a key skill when responding to another's humour. Observation of the non-verbal expressions of humour and the way in which laughter is produced can all give clues as to the appropriateness of timing of a humorous response. Laughter alone is not evidence of humour (Hargie, 2000).

CASE STUDY

A case study is deliberately not given in relation to the concept 'sense of humour'. No matter how elaborate and detailed the description of the case study may be, each use of humour is singularly unique. The relationship between those involved, the context, language and perceptions are bound within the unfolding of the event. No given phrases or humorous remarks are represented within a case study as a caution to healthcare workers thinking that such statements with practice may be evidence of a sense of humour. Instead, read the following and reflect on shaping your own style.

Wise words about the use of humour in healthcare

These points are from my own experience:

- Consider ethical implications of the content of jokes and humour.
- Do not risk offending, especially with regards to ethnicity, religion, sexuality.
- Be cautious about practical jokes in relation to health and safety.
- Using humour in caring relationships is not about being a comedian.
- Laugh with people, not at them.
- Have the courage to apologise if you have been misguided with your use of humour.
- Be sensitive to other's sense of humour.
- Be open to appropriate humour directed at you.
- Don't over play the use of humour; its spontaneity and timing are part of its magic.

CONCLUSION

The value of reflecting and considering how your sense of humour is perceived by others can lead to developmental insights. Or you may underestimate the value others put on your humorous contribution when, for example, you take the heat out of a situation or keep things in perspective. Using humour remains a serious business.

FURTHER READING

Hyrkas, K. (2005) 'Taking "humour" seriously: an analysis of the concept "humour"', in J.R. Cutcliffe and H.P. McKenna (eds), *The Essential Concepts of Nursing*. Edinburgh: Elsevier.

REFERENCES

Dobson, L. (2006) 'What's your humor style'. *Psychology Today*, 39: 74–8.
Ferguson, S. and Campinha-Bacote, J. (1989) 'Humour in nursing: did you hear the one about?' *Journal of Psychosocial Nursing and Mental Health Services*, 27(4): 29–34.
Giddens, A. (2001) *Sociology*, 4th edn. Oxford: Polity Press.

Hargie, D.W. (2000) The *Handbook of Communication Skills*, 2nd edn. London: Routledge.

Hyrkas, K. (2005) 'Taking "humour" seriously: an analysis of the concept "humour"', in J.R. Cutcliffe and H.P. McKenna (eds), *The Essential Concepts of Nursing*. Edinburgh: Elsevier.

Joines, V. and Stewart, I. (2002) *Personality Adaptations*. Nottingham: Lifespace.

Struthers, J. (1999) 'An investigation into community psychiatric nurses' use of humour during client interactions'. *Journal of Advanced Nursing*, 29(5): 1197–204.

Taylor, B.J. (1994) *Being Human: Ordinariness in Nursing*. Melbourne: Churchill Livingston.

Tragesser, S.L. and Lippman, L.G. (2005) 'Teasing: for superiority or solidarity?' *The Journal of General Psychology*, 132(3): 255–66.

Ward J. (2006) *The Student's Guide to Cognitive Neuroscience*. Hove: Psychology Press.

Winbolt, B. (2002) *Difficult People: A Guide to Handling Difficult Behaviour*. London: Seaford Institute for Social Relations.

Cross-References *Communication, Coping, Ethics, Guilt, Realism.*

48 Teamwork

Alan Gee

DEFINITION

The definition of what constitutes a 'team' or team approach in the nursing arena is often the subjective perception of those who constitute the dynamics of that particular team's membership. In other words, it is dependent on those who make up the team and the roles that they are expected to carry out in order to achieve the best possible outcome for the patient or client within the available resources.

Irrespective of the individual's perceptions of what constitutes their team structure (which is based on their background and unique clinical experience), this key concept is based on common expectations of the whole team membership, including a common understanding of goals, educational requirements, role expectancies and leadership (Tomey, 2004). These common expectancies need to be present in order that a team can function effectively and may, of course, be provided by a varied array of health-related personnel brought together to meet the individual needs of a client or client group. This is a view encapsulated in what is one of the most appropriate definitions of a nursing team by Marquise and Huston: 'the collaboration of ancillary personnel in providing care to a group of patients under the direction of a professional nurse' (2006: 333).

Despite the many known means for organising nursing provision, including total patient care, primary nursing, case management and functional nursing, it is evident that the common ethos in approaches in recent years is that of team care. This development highlights the need for increased knowledge, interpersonal and practical skills. It also suggests that if this approach is to be effective there needs to be greater understanding of teamworking strategies, potential benefits to the client, and the development opportunities for the practitioner.

KEY POINTS

- There are benefits to nurses (particularly newly qualified nurses) from being part of a team in the form of access to an extended experience and knowledge base.
- The effects of the team on the patient–nurse relationship may or may not be conducive to patient care.
- Leadership, structure and communication are key elements in the application of team nursing interventions.
- There are significant resource implications in regard to the development of team nursing strategies.
- Changes in team dynamics can have significant effects, both positive and negative, on care provision.
- Team care includes individuals from other care professions.

DISCUSSION

Starting from the premise that the team is 'the collaboration of ancillary personnel in providing care to a group of patients under the direction of a professional nurse' (Marquise and Huston, 2006: 333), it can be seen that nursing care is often provided by all grades of clinical staff and from varying professional doctrines.

The basis of team care, however, has its origins in past healthcare services. Following the end of World War II, there was a shortage of nursing staff in public services due to continued high demand following the advent of the new National Health Service and the effects of five years at war, including dietary and other health needs. Whilst the numbers of voluntary and auxiliary staff had increased during the war years, there was a need to improve services using a finite budget and largely unqualified auxiliary staff. Many people believed that a system had to be developed that accompanied the then dominant nursing approach of functional nursing and reduced fragmented care. The result was the development of a team nursing strategy whereby ancillary staff provide care to meet client needs under the direction of professionally trained staff, and in turn an apparent increase in patient satisfaction (Tomey, 2004), which suggests that team nursing is not a new concept.

In this system of provision, the team leader is responsible for knowing all relevant information about the clients that his or her team are caring for, and the duties of the team leader will vary accordingly. This will be based on the needs of the client and the team, though primarily dictated by a qualified practitioner. Whilst we will highlight potential problems with this approach later, it is evident that there are significant benefits to the development of advanced nursing interventions and in particular to the newly qualified nurse.

The role of the team in healthcare provision often appears varied and complex, but generally has common aims and objectives in providing quality care, staff support and continuity in provision of a twenty-four-hour service. This is particularly important in the training of first-level nurses following their post-qualifying period. They are often still consolidating their practice experience and knowledge base and may refer to more experienced and senior colleagues in the transfer of information and standards of practice (Sheaffer and Mano-Negrin, 2003). The team approach helps provide a support network for their continued education and sound decision-making skills for the benefit of the client and promote 'best practice'. It is also important to note that teamwork builds a strong continuity of care ethos that supports the patient through extended healthcare provision and ensures that individual care plans are followed accurately to ensure a fast and speedy recovery.

However, there are also some potential disadvantages of being in a strong team network. The training of students in the pre-registration programme can be viewed as being geared towards promoting autonomous practice and one-to-one decision-making partnerships between the patient and nurse, in the search for best quality care that is needed and wanted by the patient concerned. Furthermore, the negotiation of these partnerships constitutes what could be deemed a 'contract' aimed at working towards the client's recovery and getting them back to their normal living environment as soon as possible.

Being part of a team has the potential to affect the dynamics of this one-to-one relationship, and may often mean that a nurse's decision is 'swayed' by the views of more experienced colleagues. This is common practice within the ward environment, and may mean that a nurse becomes entrenched in the traditional care provided by a team rather than question the validity of the care provided on an individual basis. This prevents innovation in advancing services, best practice and is in general against the clinical governance directives, code of conduct, re-negotiated care and government National Service Framework (NSF) guidelines. It may be suggested that from some perspectives, teamwork is not conducive to healthcare. The key components of effective teams are given in Figure 18.

- Clear sense of direction
- Talented members
- Clear and enticing responsibilities
- Efficient operating procedures
- Constructive interpersonal relationships
- Active reinforcement system
- Constructive external relationships

Figure 18   *Key components of effective teams*

CASE STUDY

Having qualified eight months ago, David was pleased to have gained his first nursing position on a general surgical ward where, like many clinical areas, there is a fast turnaround of patients, never enough staff and constant pressure to discharge patients as soon as possible. He had completed his preceptorship some two months earlier and whilst he knew the staff team were under constant pressure to meet targets, he had appreciated the support and guidance the team had provided in ensuring he had a chance to consolidate his practice and evidence base. He now viewed the team not only as his colleagues but also as his friends.

Following a weekend off, David was looking after Charlie, who at the age of 82 had been to surgery for clinical debridement of a laceration following a fall one week earlier which was failing to heal. Twenty-four hours after surgery, the wound was healing fairly well. Charlie was due to be discharged. However, because of Charlie's age and skin condition he was still at risk of infection and a slow healing process. The care plan David put together for Charlie involved the use of a dressing, usually used for this type of wound and in common use throughout his clinical area. However, following discussion with a colleague on another ward who was 'testing' a new dressing, David had been reading a research article sponsored by the dressing manufacturers which guaranteed a 30 per cent reduction in healing time and potentially an earlier discharge for Charlie. On approaching colleagues with his suggestion of using the new dressing on Charlie, David was met with reasons not to use the dressing, including not being established as best practice, cost effectiveness and availability, and also that as discharge was imminent he could leave the district nursing team to change the dressing regimen following discharge.

David decided to go with the traditional dressing used in the clinical area even though inside he felt that the new dressing, whilst an unknown quantity, would be more beneficial to Charlie to promote his healing.

CONCLUSION

The advancement of nursing structured approaches is paramount in the current healthcare environment in developing a service that can meet the demands of a growing and increasingly varied client base. In meeting this challenge, a greater understanding of the role individuals play within teams is essential if we are to meet the directives set by government in expanding access and providing quality services within restrictive budgets.

In a climate where there are reported cut-backs in provision, development of expensive new medications, technologies and general pressure on resources, we must consider the approach taken to nursing care. At present, team nursing appears to be the dominant philosophy of NHS provision, but it has not always been seen as the best way of managing services for the population it serves, and this philosophy may already be changing.

Considering the constant change in public demand from National Health Services and resources available to meet that demand, it is inevitable that future provision will have to adapt and thus change the dynamics of team structures in order to meet this need. Developments in the political climate at the time of writing are advocating the development of a practitioner with a wider care provision remit that incorporates the roles of physiotherapists, nutritionists, social workers and occupational therapists, for example, and where traditional nursing roles are just a small element of this provision.

It can be seen that practitioners will have to become more knowledgeable outside of their professional evidence base and take on a role that implements more than what is considered to be conventional nursing care. Whatever happens in future, however, it is important to remember that care must remain on a professional basis, have a sound knowledge base and be delivered on a one-to-one negotiated basis between the patient and the care provider. It is imperative that support continues to be provided for newly qualified staff in order to achieve optimal care, and whilst a team approach is one way of achieving this, it is now necessary to look further to other professional, voluntary, business and private sector practices to develop new approaches to care provision.

FURTHER READING

Huszczo, G.E. (1996) *Tools for Team Excellence: Getting Your Team into High Gear and Keeping it There.* Mountain View, CA: Davies-Black.

Marquis, B.L. and Huston, C. (2006) *Leadership Roles and Management Functions in Nursing,* Philadelphia, PA: Lippincott, Williams and Wilkins.

REFERENCES

Marquis, B.L. and Huston, C. (2006) *Leadership Roles and Management Functions in Nursing,* Philadelphia, PA: Lippincott, Williams and Wilkins.

Sheaffer, Z. and Mano-Negrin, R. (2003) 'Executives' orientations as indicators of crisis management policies and practices'. *Journal of Management Studies,* 40(2): 573–606.

Tomey, A.M. (2004) *Nursing Management and Leadership.* St Louis, MO: Mosby.

Cross References *Communication, Crisis management, Leadership, Managing change, Professional development.*

Julie Dulson

DEFINITION

User involvement refers to the process of involving users of a service, in this case healthcare, in the decision-making processes related to that service (Hickley and Kipping, 1998). This can be at the most basic level of a user being involved in decisions regarding their own care, from timing and frequency of appointments to choice of interventions, to a more complex level of involvement where users are making decisions regarding service delivery and the training of healthcare professionals.

KEY POINTS

- The policy context regarding user involvement highlights the fact that this concept has become a central focus of healthcare provision.
- The continuum of user involvement which is dependant upon the power that they have to influence decisions.
- Whist there are barriers to (and potential solutions for) effective involvement there are equally solutions to them.

DISCUSSION

The policy context

User involvement has become a central focus of healthcare provision over the last decade (Anthony and Crawford, 2000). This is evidenced by the discussion of user involvement in Department of Health publications and policy, such as *The National Plan* (DoH, 2000) and *Involving Patients and the Public* (DoH, 2001). Furthermore, there has been a shift of focus from consultation to partnership and collaboration; that is, it is no longer acceptable to merely ask users for their views but rather the users should be partners in their care. This is evidenced by the promotion of recovery and social inclusion (Repper and Perkins, 2003) within health services and has led to a change in focus in healthcare delivery, which Barker and Whitehill (1997) classify as caring *with* people as opposed to caring *for* people.

There has also been a large increase in the user movement (Felton and Stickley, 2004). Everett (1994) suggests that in recent years, users have developed themselves into a forceful social movement. However, despite this movement and increasing policy rhetoric, it has been suggested that true involvement of users in their care is still unusual (Simpson, 1999).

User involvement continuum

Hickley and Kipping suggest that the amount of involvement a user of services can have in those services will be dependent upon the 'power they have to influence decisions' (1998: 84). They suggest that this power can be highlighted by considering user involvement in practice on a continuum. They describe four stages from information/explanation at one end to user control at the other. Underpinning the four stages are the philosophical beliefs regarding the rationale for user involvement:

- *User control*: Here the power is fully redistributed to the users. The user or group of users will make the decision whether or not to involve others in the decision-making process.
- *Partnership*: Here users and service providers have an equal standing (and equal power), and decisions are made jointly. To ensure that this approach is effective it is necessary that all parties have access to the same information and have the same abilities for interpreting that information.
- *Consultation*: Providers ask for users' views, but do not necessarily act upon those views.
- *Information/explanation*: Here the users are provided with information, but are not included in any processes regarding their treatment.

Barriers to user involvement and their solutions

A study by Evans et al. (2003) regarding oncology service users' perceptions of their involvement in decisions regarding their care found that professional attitudes were a considerable barrier to effective involvement. Many users in the study reported that they felt that by asking questions and asking for information they were challenging the authority of the professionals involved, and some felt that their attempts to be involved were not wanted.

To address this, Forrest et al. (2000) suggest that it is very important to identify exactly what you want the user to do and clarify the purpose of their involvement. Masters et al. (2002) also agree that role definition is essential to effective user involvement. It should be clearly defined exactly what the purpose of the user's involvement is to be, and the limitations of their role. Langton et al. (2003) emphasise the importance of agreeing the outcome of the service user involvement in advance. They suggest that this will help to ensure that all those involved are clear regarding their role and their expectations.

It is necessary to have a clear organisational philosophy highlighting why user involvement is so important to the organisation (Morgan and Sanggaran, 1997). This philosophy should be evidenced at every level of the organisation, which means that users should be present at every strategic meeting that occurs within the organisation. However, user involvement at committee level can be criticised as a way for organisations to give status and credence to their plans but can have limited value. To ensure that this does not happen, it is of paramount importance to support and train users appropriately.

The need for training and support has the potential to create many organisational issues. For example, who will manage the service user (Masters et al., 2002)? Will there be one person who is responsible for the management of all involved, or will individual staff members be responsible for supporting the users that they involve in their own area of work? Placing that responsibility upon individual staff members may in turn create a reluctance to involve users due to the extra work that will be involved. This could also create training considerations for the staff members themselves. For example, how will the individual staff members be trained to identify the training and support needs of the users? Further, how will it be identified that the individual staff member is capable of offering the necessary support and supervision? In a study by Masters et al., lecturers who were asked to be involved in a project aiming to involve users in curriculum design stated that they needed 'training and support in involvement' (2002: 317).

Representation of users is often discussed as a potential barrier to user involvement (Hopton, 1997). The discussions centre upon the concern that no one service user can truly ever represent the views of anyone but their own. Felton and Stickley (2004) discuss the concerns of mental health lecturers regarding this issue. For example, when, if ever, does a user become an ex-user? Is an experience fifteen years ago the same as an experience last week? Is an admission to hospital in London the same as an admission to hospital in rural Cheshire? Can a user who has experience of care and services for people with one diagnosis truly comment on the care and services available to individuals with another completely different diagnosis? It could be argued not, although there are certainly common themes. For example, a person admitted taken to Accident and Emergency following a minor car accident may be able to make comment upon the impact of admission to hospital, but they would have little to offer when discussing services for terminal illness. To help address the problem of representation, service providers could target user groups and so recruit users who are able to represent a range of users' perspectives. However, McAndrew and Samociuk (2003) suggest that the debate regarding representativeness of users is often overplayed.

A study by Crawford et al. (2003) identified the importance of adequate financial provision for effective user involvement. However, when discussing payment it is important to consider the rate at which users are paid. It can be suggested that users should be paid the same rates as the other professionals they are working alongside. However, McAndrew and Samocuik (2003) argue that paying users comparable rates has many difficulties, not least in that it may seriously limit the amount of involvement each organisation can afford, particularly in today's current economic climate. They argue that it may be more appropriate to devise a sliding scale of payment and fit the payment for the task. This would then mean that users who are delivering training, for example, are paid a higher rate, and those who are contributing to service planning or interviewing potential staff are paid a lesser rate. There are also difficulties in paying users who are in receipt of benefits. The majority of benefits have a set maximum weekly amount a person can earn in excess of their benefits; earning in excess of this in any one week will cause that person's benefits to cease. They will then have to reapply for them, which can result in that person being without finances for up to three weeks.

Finally, it is important to consider access. Users may have physical problems or disabilities which present difficulties accessing buildings, for example. It may also be necessary to consider the timing of meetings, particularly for mental health service users. A group of core symptoms of schizophrenia, for example, are negative symptoms which include lack of motivation and lethargy. This can make it increasingly difficult for such users to be able to attend at nine o'clock in the morning. It may also be important to consider the availability and accessibility of transport. Users may have to rely on public transport, which can be costly. In such circumstances users should be reimbursed for travel expenses on the day, or preferably before they travel.

CASE STUDY

The following is an example from the writer's own experience of involving users in the education of pre-registration nursing students. The students involved in this particular example were first-year adult-branch students, and the aim of the teaching session was to introduce the students to key concepts associated with mental health nursing. The students had been informed that two visiting lecturers from practice would be leading the session. At the beginning of the session the students were asked to write down three words that came into their minds when they heard the term 'psychosis'. The words they suggested included terms such as violent, unpredictable, aggressive, manic and frightening.

The rest of the session was led by the visiting lecturers. Towards the end, the lecturers revealed that they both had a history of serious mental health problems; one had experienced psychotic episodes and the other had a diagnosis of bipolar affective disorder. The shock around the room at that time was clearly visible. After the lecturers had left, I asked the students to reflect upon the experience and there were a number of themes to their discussion. First, all expressed regret that the visiting lecturers had heard the way that they had described psychosis, such as frightening and violent. By involving users in that session, the students were able to learn a great deal regarding the personal experience of mental health problems, but also – and perhaps more importantly – they were able to challenge their own perceptions regarding what it means to have mental health problems.

Furthermore, education and training of health professionals is frequently viewed as the most appropriate place to develop change and to promote appropriate values and attitudes. This was certainly the case here; those nurses will take their revised beliefs about mental health nursing with them throughout their careers. User involvement can, therefore, be far more than improving services for a group of users, it can change the face of nursing – how fantastic is that?

CONCLUSION

Whilst there are many barriers to user involvement, they can all be addressed with effective strategic planning. Whilst it is vastly important to avoid user involvement becoming tokenistic, it is equally important not to let fear of tokenism prevent user involvement from happening. If you view user involvement on a continuum, then you can see that each act of involvement is at least a step in the right direction.

FURTHER READING

Anthony, P. and Crawford, P. (2000) 'Service user involvement in care planning: the mental health nurses' perspective'. *Journal of Psychiatric and Mental Health Nursing*, 7: 425–34.

REFERENCES

Anthony, P. and Crawford, P. (2000) 'Service user involvement in care planning: the mental health nurses' perspective'. *Journal of Psychiatric and Mental Health Nursing*, 7: 425–34.

Barker, P. and Whitehill, I. (1997) 'The craft of care: towards collaborative caring in mental health nursing', in S. Tilley (ed.), *Views of Practice and Education*. Oxford: Blackwell Science.

Crawford, M.J., Aldridge, T., Bhui, K., Rutter, C., Manley, C., Weaver, T., Tyrer, P. and Fulup, N. (2003) 'User involvement in the planning and delivery of mental health services: a cross-sectional survey of service users and providers'. *Acta Psychiatrica Scandinavica*, 107: 410–4.

Department of Health (1999) *The National Service Framework for Mental Health*. London: DoH.

Department of Health (2000) *The National Plan*. London: DoH.

Department of Health (2001) *Involving Patients and the Public*. London: HMSO.

Evans, S., Tritter, J., Barley, V., Daykin, N., McNeil, J., Palmer, N., Rimmer, J., Sanidas, M. and Turton, P. (2003) 'User involvement in UK cancer services: bridging the policy gap'. *European Journal of Cancer Care*, 12: 331–8.

Everett, B. (1994) 'Something is happening: the contemporary consumer and psychiatric survivor movement in historical context'. *Journal of Mind and Behaviour*, 15: 55–70.

Felton, A. and Stickley, T. (2004) 'Pedagogy, power and service user involvement'. *Journal of Psychiatric and Mental Health Nursing*, 11: 89–98.

Forrest, S., Risk, I., Masters, H. and Brown, D. (2000) 'Mental health service user involvement in nurse education; exploring the issues'. *Journal of Psychiatric and Mental Health Nursing*, 7(1): 51–60.

Hickley, G. and Kipping, C. (1998) 'Exploring the concept of user involvement in mental health through a participation continuum'. *Journal of Clinical Nursing*, 7: 83–8.

Hopton, J. (1997) 'Who are we listening to?' *Nursing Times*, 93(41): 44–5.

Langton, H., Barnes, M., Haslehurst, S., Rimmer, J. and Turton, P. (2003) 'Collaboration, user involvement and education: a systematic review of the literature and report of an educational initiative'. *European Journal of Oncology Nursing*, 7(4): 242–52.

key concepts in nursing

Masters, H., Forrest, S., Harley, A., Hunter, M., Brown, N. and Risk, I. (2002) 'Involving mental health service users and carers in curriculum development: moving beyond classroom involvement'. *Journal of Psychiatric and Mental Health Nursing*, 9(3): 309–19.

McAndrew, S. and Samociuk, G.A. (2003) 'Reflecting together: developing a new strategy for continuous user involvement in mental health nurse education'. *Journal of Psychiatric and Mental Health Nursing*, 10: 616–21.

Morgan, S. and Sanggaran, R. (1997) 'Client-centred approach to student nurse education in mental health practicum: an inquiry'. *Journal of Psychiatric and Mental Health Nursing*, 4: 423–34.

Repper, J. and Perkins, R. (2003) *Social Inclusion and Recovery: A Model for Mental Health Practice*. London: Balliere Tindall.

Simpson, A. (1999) 'Creating alliances: the views of users and carers on the education and training needs of community mental health nurses'. *Journal of Psychiatric and Mental Health Nursing*, 6: 347–56.

Cross-References *Accountability, Communication, Dignity, Ethics, Managing change, Problem solving, Respect, Teamwork.*

50 Value

Tony Warne and Sue McAndrew

DEFINITION

Values are a fundamental part of the human condition. A value is a belief, principle, standard, quality or a philosophy that is meaningful. Whether we are consciously aware of them or not, every individual has a core set of personal values. Personal values might include the commonplace, such as the belief in hard work and honesty, to the more psychological, such as self-reliance, concern for others and loyalty. All our behaviours, judgements and actions are based upon values. Value judgements, for example, are dependent upon beliefs and experiences of everyday life. They are also concerned with what we would like our experience to be.

value

Values have three important characteristics:

- Values are developed early in life and are very resistant to change. Values develop out of our direct experiences with people who are important to us, particularly our parents. Importantly, values result from how people behave towards us, and not from what it is the tell us.
- Values enable us to define what is right and what is wrong. Importantly, values do not involve external standards in setting out what is right or wrong; rather, our understanding of what is wrong, good or bad is intrinsic. However, we might internalise other values, such as social values, into our own value system; for example, society makes a value judgement on the unmarried mother. Being a doctor or solicitor is valued highly as a professional career.
- Values themselves cannot be proved correct or incorrect, valid or invalid, right or wrong. If a statement can be proven true or false, then it cannot be a value. Values tell what we should believe, regardless of any evidence or lack of evidence.

Values are not simply cognitive beliefs but include an emotional element. As values are enacted, they also come to constitute an individual's identity. Values can also be shared by groups of different individuals, groups made up of similar individuals (professions and so on) and collectively by the wider society (see Table 5).

Table 5   *Common personal, organisational and societal values*

Personal values	Organisational values	Societal values
Respect for others	Safety	Authority
Self-reliance	Co-operation (teamwork)	Education
Honesty	Standardisation	Democracy
Integrity	Discipline	Celebrity
Concern for others	Continuous improvement	Protection (of law)
Accuracy	Loyalty	Equality
Justice	Competency	Personal freedom
Creativity	Innovation	Tradition
Family	Systemisation	Wealth
Decisiveness	Co-ordination	Service (to others)
Chastity	Flexibility	Patriotism
Privacy	Skill	Equal opportunity

For nurses, professional identity refers to the nurse's understanding of what it means to be a nurse and to do nursing (Warne and Stark, 2004). The individual nurse's identity is defined as the values and beliefs held by the nurse that guide their thinking, actions and interaction with the patient and others (Fagermoen, 1997). It represents the individual nurse's philosophy of nursing, serving as a basic frame of reference for practice.

KEY POINTS

- Values are beliefs, principles or a quality that is meaningful.
- Values are resistant to change.
- Values are individual but can be shared.
- Values provide a philosophy for practice.

DISCUSSION

As nurses we are involved in our patients' suffering, and it has been argued that how we manage these interpersonal aspects of nursing is dependent upon the autonomy and courage of the individual nurse (Begat et al., 2005). To be able to meet these challenges we need to be clear about why we think and act as we do, a process that is about better understanding of self (McMurray, 1995). The identification of individual values and beliefs is crucial in the development of the 'authentic self' (Fawcett et al., 2001). We need to be authentic in our relationships with patients, and in so doing better understand how we might express our concern and caring for other people. In this sense, personal knowing is not 'knowing one's self' but rather knowing how to be authentic with others, knowing one's 'personal style' and of 'being with' another person. This is a crucial step in developing an effective nurse–patient relationship, and one that recognises the importance of such relationships to successful nursing care (Andrews, 2003; McCormack, 2004; Peplau, 1952).

Gaining an understanding of self arises from the individual being clear about the values that are important to them. Just as with personal values, which are acquired in early life, professional values will start to be formed during the nurse education programme and educational processes. For example, nurses learn the importance of ethical practice, being the patient's advocate and caring (Tovey, 1999). Whilst gaining an understanding of self is important, in the context of nursing practice, the

value

wider respect for values is central to delivering patient-centred practice (Warne and McAndrew, 2005; Williams and Tappen, 1999). It is important that we learn to develop a clear picture of what our patients value about their lives, and how the individual patient is making sense of what is happening to them. This will require the nurse to be genuinely interested in the welfare of each patient, to be able to be tolerant, able to listen attentively to them and be non-judgemental and open to their opinions and point of view. Helping an individual to find meaning in their care may help them to tolerate the incongruity of their existing situation and help them plan for the future (Repper, 2000). In this way we can help provide practical help to maintain or promote those desired relationships, roles and activities that are valued by the patient. In situations where the patient cannot exert any control over their illness, environment and care, for example when admitted to hospital in pain and distress, then we can, through learning to listen to what the patient values, help reduce the sometimes dehumanising processes of hospitalisation (Armstrong, 2006).

One of the problems in consistently working in this way concerns the level of congruence between values that are espoused and those values used in practice. For example, the Royal College of Nursing (RCN) defined the value base of nursing as being based upon ethical values which respect the dignity, autonomy and uniqueness of human beings, the privileged nurse–patient relationship, and the acceptance of personal accountability for decisions and actions (RCN, 2003). These are espoused values. Such values in nursing are universal; for example, the American Nurses Association (ANA) *Code for Nurses* describes nursing values such as respect for persons, beneficence and justice as being crucial to modern nursing practice (ANA, 1998). However, these espoused values might not be the ones that are used in practice. So nurses need to consciously and periodically set out to uncover the values and beliefs which influence their relational being/knowing/doing; and as a consequence, actively consider how these values might be expanded or transformed (Hartrick, 1997). This is also an important activity, as often nursing values can be overshadowed by the values of the organisation, which may well cause conflict and tensions. Begat et al. (2005) found in their study that where nurses' personal values are at odds with the organisational values reflected in policies and rules, nurses are often forced to compromise their moral integrity for the sake of the organisation they work for. Watson (2002) noted that it is the nurses' values that give them the courage to contemplate other possibilities for action rather than simply conforming to the prevailing point of view and practice. Unless we can become more aware of the values we hold which influence us, we are unlikely to become effective nurses, competent and skilled in providing patient-centred care.

CASE STUDY

A student nurse working in an infertility clinic was asked to complete an assessment on a young lady who appeared to be a similar age to the student and was attending for the first time to pursue the possibility of having artificial insemination. The young lady explains to the nurse that unfortunately her partner had to go abroad on business at very short notice and she did not want to miss the appointment to attend the clinic. The nurse was reassuring and continued with the assessment, discussing various aspects of the procedure and gaining insight into the young lady's general health status, her psychological well-being and her social circumstances. The nurse is attentive in listening to the lady's desire for a baby and asks pertinent questions relating to the lady's partner and if he had been upset by not being able to attend for the appointment. At this point the lady becomes agitated, flushed and stops having eye contact with the nurse. The nurse inquires if she is all right, to which the lady responds by saying that there has been some confusion and that her partner is in fact a woman. The women had been in a relationship for ten years and had now made the decision to have children. From the nurse's perspective she had assumed, being brought up in a heterosexual culture, that anyone wanting children and attending an infertility clinic would, like her, be heterosexual. Her value system was one whereby children should only be brought up in a heterosexual relationship. The relationship she had developed with the lady during the assessment process came to an abrupt end.

CONCLUSION

Everybody has a core set of personal values. These are acquired and developed early on in our lives. These values shape and influence our thinking and behaviour. Understanding this process is crucial in developing a sense of self. As nurses we need to have this sense of self in order to better help the patients and their carers we come into contact with. Our personal values might not be shared by others. We need to find out from our patients and carers what they value and what is meaningful to them. If we fail to do this, we might be behaving in a way that is offensive and unhelpful to our patients. This can make what might already be a distressing and difficult experience into one that is more so. It is clear that the organisations we work in may also have differing values than those we hold. At times this can cause tension and conflict. Being more aware of our own core values and being committed to and applying those values can help to better consider and offer alternative ways of doing something.

FURTHER READING

Basord, L. and Slevin, O. (2003) *Theory and Practice of Nursing*, 2nd edn. Cheltenham: Nelson Thornes.

Cronin, P. and Rawlings-Anderson, K. (2004) *Knowledge for Contemporary Nursing Practice*. London: Mosby, Elsevier.

Pattison, S. and Pill, R. (2004) *Values in Professional Practice: Lessons for Health, Social Care and Other Professions*. Oxford: Radcliffe.

REFERENCES

American Nurses Association (1998) *Code for Nurses with Interpretive Statements*. Kansas City, KS: ANA.

Andrews, G. (2003) 'Locating a geography of nursing: space, place and the progress of geographical thought'. *Nursing Philosophy*, 4: 231–48.

Armstrong, A. (2006) 'Towards a strong virtue ethics for nursing practice'. *Nursing Philosophy*, 7: 110–24.

Begat, I., Ellefsen, B. and Severinsson, E. (2005) 'Nurses' satisfaction with their work environment and the outcomes of clinical nursing supervision on nurses' experiences of well-being – a Norwegian study'. *Journal of Nursing Management*, 13: 221–30.

Fagermoen, M. (1997) 'Professional identity: values embedded in meaningful nursing practice'. *Journal of Advanced Nursing Practice*, 25: 434–41.

Fawcett, J., Watson, J., Neuman, B., Hinton-Walker, P. and Fitzpatrick, J. (2001) 'On nursing theories and evidence'. *Journal of Nursing Scholarship*, 33(2): 115–19.

Hartrick, G. (1997) 'Relational capacity: the foundation for interpersonal nursing practice'. *Journal of Advanced Nursing*, 26: 523–8.

McCormack, B. (2004) 'Person-centeredness in gerontological nursing: an overview of the literature'. *International Journal of Older People Nursing*, 13(3): 31–8.

McMurray, J. (1995) *The Self as Agent: The Form of the Personal*. London: Faber and Faber.

Peplau, H. (1952) *Interpersonal Relations in Nursing*. Philadelphia, PA: Putnam's Sons.

Repper, J. (2000) 'Adjusting the focus of mental health nursing: incorporating services users' experiences of recovery'. *Journal of Mental Health*, 9(6): 575–87.

Royal College of Nursing (2003) *Defining Nursing*. London: RCN.

Tovey, E. (1999) 'The changing nature of nurses' job satisfaction: an exploration of sources of satisfaction in the 1990s'. *Journal of Advanced Nursing*, 30(11): 150–8.

Warne, T. and McAndrew, S. (2005) 'The shackles of abuse: unprepared to work at the edges of reason?' *Journal of Psychiatric and Mental Health Nursing*, 12: 679–85.

Warne, T. and Stark, S. (2004) 'Service users, metaphors and team working in mental health'. *Journal of Psychiatric and Mental Health Nursing*, 11: 654–61.

Watson, J. (2002) *Postmodern Nursing and Beyond*. London: Churchill Livingstone.

Williams, C. and Tappen, R. (1999) 'Can we create a therapeutic relationship with nursing home residents in the later stages of Alzheimer's disease?' *Journal of Psychosocial Nursing*, 37: 28–35.

Cross-References *Advocacy, Caring, Communication, Ethics, Evidence-based practice.*

value

Index

Figures and diagrams are shown in *italics*. In addition to cross-references in this index please also refer to the list of cross-references at the end of each chapter.